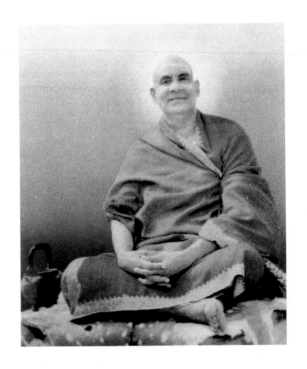

Dedication

*In humility we offer this dedication to
Swami Sivananda Saraswati, who initiated
Swami Satyananda Saraswati into the secrets of yoga.*

Asana Pranayama Mudra Bandha

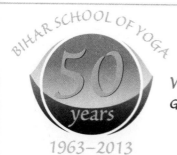

BIHAR SCHOOL OF YOGA
50 years
1963–2013
GOLDEN JUBILEE

WORLD YOGA CONVENTION 2013
GANGA DARSHAN, MUNGER, BIHAR, INDIA
23rd-27th October 2013

Asana Pranayama
Mudra Bandha

Swami Satyananda Saraswati

Yoga Publications Trust, Munger, Bihar, India

Published by Bihar School of Yoga
    First edition 1969
    Reprinted 1971
    Second edition 1973
    Reprinted 1977, 1980, 1983, 1989, 1993, 1995, 1996
    Third (revised) edition 1996 (by Bihar Yoga Bharati with
        permission of Bihar School of Yoga)
    Reprinted 1997, 1999

Published by Yoga Publications Trust
    Reprinted 2002, 2004 (twice), 2005, 2006
    Fourth (revised) edition 2008
    Reprinted 2008, 2009, 2012

ISBN: 978-81-86336-14-4

Publisher and distributor: Yoga Publications Trust, Ganga Darshan, Munger, Bihar, India.

Website: www.biharyoga.net
        www.rikhiapeeth.net

Printed at Thomson Press (India) Limited, New Delhi, 110001

Contents

Preface

The first edition of *Asana Pranayama Mudra Bandha*, published in 1969, was derived from the direct teaching of Swami Satyananda Saraswati during the nine month Teachers Training Course conducted at Bihar School of Yoga, Munger, in 1969. The second edition was published in 1973 to commemorate his Golden Jubilee Birthday. At this time, the text was completely revised and new material was added from class notes taken during the 1970–71 Sannyasa Training Course, which was the last course that he personally conducted.

In response to popular demand and to meet the requirements of a university text, APMB was revised and updated under the direction and inspiration of Swami Niranjanananda Saraswati, the successor of Swami Satyananda Saraswati. This text is currently being used as the main practical text for the teaching of asana, pranayama, mudra, bandha and shatkarma around the world by yoga teachers from every tradition and path.

Since publication of the first edition, interest in yoga has spread widely. Now APMB is used in ashrams, centres and yoga schools in every country as the standard textbook for teachers and students alike. The techniques presented have been assimilated by fields as diverse as medicine, education, entertainment, business, sports and the training of spiritual aspirants.

The science of yoga applies itself to all aspects of life. This revised edition presents basic yogic practices including *asanas*, postures; *pranayamas*, breathing techniques; *mudras*, positions or gestures which represent the psyche; *bandhas*, locks for channelling energy; and *shatkarmas*, cleansing practices. All of these techniques purify the body, mind and energy systems to prepare the ground for higher practices of meditation and for the ultimate experience of cosmic consciousness. Also included is a section introducing the *chakras*, psychic centres, and other aspects of the subtle body.

The effects of yogic practices during and after performance are currently being researched by scientists and doctors around the world. Their results show that asanas, pranayamas, mudras and bandhas are a potent means to restore and maintain physical and mental health.

Asana Pranayama Mudra Bandha is designed for yoga students, spiritual seekers and for those studying yoga in depth. Although many health professionals consult this text as a guide when constructing programs to provide clients with physical, mental and emotional balance, these techniques are not primarily for the sick but for the healthy.

When learning the practices of yoga, the guidance of a competent teacher is recommended. People with specific health problems or who are undergoing a period when extra care is needed, such as pregnancy, need individual guidance, not techniques learned from a book, not even this book. This text provides yogic practices and information for personal evolution. When practised faithfully, under the guidance of a competent teacher, these techniques will expand your consciousness.

Introduction to Yoga

Yoga is not an ancient myth buried in oblivion. It is the most valuable inheritance of the present. It is the essential need of today and the culture of tomorrow.

—*Swami Satyananda Saraswati*

Yoga is the science of right living and, as such, is intended to be incorporated in daily life. It works on all aspects of the person: the physical, vital, mental, emotional, psychic and spiritual.

The word *yoga* means 'unity' or 'oneness' and is derived from the Sanskrit word *yuj*, which means 'to join'. This unity or joining is described in spiritual terms as the union of the individual consciousness with the universal consciousness. On a more practical level, yoga is a means of balancing and harmonizing the body, mind and emotions. This is done through the practice of asana, pranayama, mudra, bandha, shatkarma and meditation, and must be achieved before union can take place with the higher reality.

The science of yoga begins to work on the outermost aspect of the personality, the physical body, which for most people is a practical and familiar starting point. When imbalance is experienced at this level, the organs, muscles and nerves no longer function in harmony; rather they act in opposition to each other. For instance, the endocrine system might become irregular and the efficiency of the nervous system decrease to such an extent that a disease will manifest. Yoga aims at bringing the different bodily functions into perfect coordination so that they work for the good of the whole body.

1

From the physical body, yoga moves on to the mental and emotional levels. Many people suffer from phobias and neuroses as a result of the stresses and interactions of everyday living. Yoga cannot provide a cure for life, but it does present a proven method for coping with it.

Swami Sivananda Saraswati of Rishikesh explained yoga as an ". . . integration and harmony between thought, feeling and deed, or integration between head, heart and hand". Through the practices of yoga, awareness develops of the interrelation between the emotional, mental and physical levels, and how a disturbance in any one of these affects the others. Gradually, this awareness leads to an understanding of the more subtle areas of existence.

There are many branches of yoga: raja, hatha, jnana, karma, bhakti, mantra, kundalini and laya, to name but a few, and many texts explain them in detail. Each individual needs to find those yogas most suited to his or her particular personality and need. In the last half of the twentieth century, hatha yoga had become the most well-known and widely practised of the systems. However, the concept of what constitutes yoga is broadening as more people take it up, and this knowledge is spreading. In the ancient texts, hatha yoga consists of the sha'karmas, cleansing practices, only. Today, however, hatha yoga commonly embraces the practices of asana, pranayama, mudra and bandha as well.

History of yoga

The yoga we know today was developed as a part of the tantric civilization which existed in India and all parts of the world more than ten thousand years ago. In archaeological excavations made in the Indus Valley at Harappa and Mohenjodaro, now in modern Pakistan, many statues have been found depicting deities resembling Lord Shiva and Shakti (in the form of Parvati) performing various asanas and practising meditation. These ruins were once the dwelling place of people who lived in the pre-vedic age before the Aryan civilization started to flourish in the Indus subcontinent. According to mythical tradition, Shiva is said to be the founder of yoga, and Parvati, his first disciple.

Lord Shiva is considered to be the symbol or embodiment of supreme consciousness. Parvati represents supreme knowledge, will and action, and is responsible for all creation. This force or energy is also known as *kundalini shakti,* the cosmic force which lies dormant in all beings. Parvati is regarded as the mother of the whole universe. The individual soul is embodied and bound to the world of name and form, and also liberated from the bondage of the world and united with supreme consciousness through her grace. Out of love and compassion for her children, she imparted her secret knowledge of liberation in the form of tantra. The techniques of yoga have their source in tantra and the two cannot be separated, just as consciousness, Shiva, cannot be separated from energy, Shakti.

Tantra is a combination of two words, *tanoti* and *trayati,* which mean 'expansion' and 'liberation' respectively. Therefore, it is the science of expanding the consciousness and liberating the energy. Tantra is the way to attain freedom from the bondage of the world while still living in it. The first step in tantra is to know the limitations and capacities of the body and mind. Next it prescribes techniques for the expansion of consciousness and the liberation of energy whereby individual limitations are transcended and a higher reality experienced.

Yoga arose at the beginning of human civilization when humankind first realized their spiritual potential and began to evolve techniques to develop it. The yogic science was slowly developed by ancient sages all over the world. The essence of yoga has often been shrouded in or explained by different symbols, analogies and languages. Some traditions believe that yoga was a divine gift revealed to the ancient sages so that humankind could have the opportunity to realize its divine nature.

In ancient times, yoga techniques were kept secret and were never written down or exposed to public view. They were passed on from teacher or guru to disciple by word of mouth. In this way there was a clear understanding of their meaning and aim. Through personal experience, realized yogis and sages were able to guide sincere aspirants along the correct path, removing any confusion, misunderstanding and excessive intellectual contemplation.

3

The first books to refer to yoga were the ancient Tantras and later the Vedas, which were written about the time the Indus Valley culture was flourishing. Although they do not give specific practices, they allude to yoga symbolically. In fact, the verses of the Vedas were heard by the *rishis*, seers, in states of deep yogic meditation or *samadhi*, and are regarded as revealed scriptures. It is, however, in the Upanishads that yoga begins to take a more definable shape. These scriptures collectively form *Vedanta*, the culmination of the Vedas, and are said to contain the essence of the Vedas.

Sage Patanjali's treatise on raja yoga, the *Yoga Sutras*, codified the first definitive, unified and comprehensive system of yoga. Often called the eight-fold path, it is comprised of *yama*, self-restraints, *niyama*, self-observances, *asana*, *pranayama*, *pratyahara*, disassociation of consciousness from the outside environment, *dharana*, concentration, *dhyana*, meditation, and *samadhi*, identification with pure consciousness.

In the 6th century BC, Buddha's influence brought the ideals of meditation, ethics and morality to the fore and the preparatory practices of yoga were ignored. However, Indian thinkers soon realized the limitations of this view. The yogi Matsyendranath taught that before taking to the practices of meditation, the body and its elements need purifying. He founded the Nath cult and the yogic pose matsyendrasana was named after him. His chief disciple, Gorakhnath, wrote books on hatha yoga in the local dialect and in Hindi.

Indian tradition previously required that original texts be written in Sanskrit. In some cases they clothed their writings in symbolism so that only those qualified to receive a teaching would be able to understand it. One of the most outstanding authorities on hatha yoga, Swami Swatmarama, wrote the *Hatha Yoga Pradipika*, or 'Light on Yoga', in Sanskrit, collating all extant material on the subject. In doing so, he reduced the emphasis on yama and niyama, thereby eliminating a great obstacle experienced by many beginners. In the *Hatha Yoga Pradipika*, Swatmarama starts with the body and only later, when the mind has become stable and balanced, are the yamas and niyamas (self-control and self-discipline) introduced.

4

The relevance of yoga today

Today, in the 21st century, a spiritual heritage is being reclaimed of which yoga is very much a part. While yoga's central theme remains the highest goal of the spiritual path, yogic practices give direct and tangible benefits to everyone regardless of their spiritual aims.

Physical and mental cleansing and strengthening is one of yoga's most important achievements. What makes it so powerful and effective is the fact that it works on the holistic principles of harmony and unification. According to medical scientists, yoga therapy is successful because of the balance created in the nervous and endocrine systems which directly influences all the other systems and organs of the body.

For most people in the 20th century, yoga was simply a means of maintaining health and wellbeing in an increasingly stressful society. Asanas do remove the physical discomfort accumulated during a day at the office sitting in a chair, hunched over a desk. Relaxation techniques help to maximize the effectiveness of ever-diminishing time off. In an age of mobile phones, internet and twenty-four hour shopping, yogic practices make great personal and even business sense.

In the 21st century, beyond the needs of individuals, the underlying principles of yoga provide a real tool to combat social malaise. At a time when the world seems to be at a loss, rejecting past values without being able to establish new ones, yoga provides a means for people to find their own way of connecting with their true selves. Through this connection with their real selves, it is possible for people to manifest harmony in the current age, and for compassion to emerge where hitherto there has been none.

In this respect, yoga is far from simply being physical exercises. It is an aid to establishing a new perception of what is real, what is necessary, and how to become established in a way of life which embraces both inner and outer realities. This way of life is an experience which cannot be understood intellectually and will only become living knowledge through practice and experience. However, the renaissance has begun.

Asana

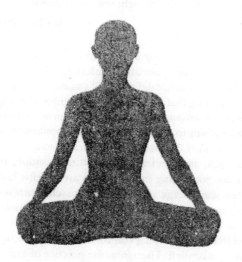

हठस्य प्रथमांगत्वादासनं पूर्वमुच्यते ।
कुर्यात्तदासनं स्थैर्यमारोग्यं चांगलाघवम् ॥ 1:17 ॥

Hathàsya prathamaangatvaadaasanam poorvamuchyate.
Kuryaattadaasanam sthairyamaarogyam chaangalaaghavam.

Prior to everything, asana is spoken of as the first part of
hatha yoga.
Having done asana, one attains steadiness of body and mind,
freedom from disease and lightness of the limbs.

Hatha Yoga Pradipika

Asana means a state of being in which one can remain physically and
mentally steady, calm, quiet and comfortable. In the *Yoga Sutras* of
Patanjali there is a concise definition of yogasanas: "Sthiram sukham
aasanam", meaning that position which is comfortable and steady. So,
we can see that yogasanas in this context are practised to develop the
practitioner's ability to sit comfortably in one position for an extended
length of time, as is necessary during meditation.

In raja yoga, asana refers to the sitting position, but in hatha
yoga it means something more. Asanas are specific body positions
which open the energy channels and psychic centres. They are
tools to higher awareness and provide the stable foundation for our
exploration of the body, breath, mind and beyond. The hatha yogis
also found that by developing control of the body through asana, the
mind is also controlled. Therefore, the practice of asana is foremost
in hatha yoga.

Introduction to Yogasana

In the *Yoga Sutras* of Patanjali there is a concise definition of yogasana: *"Sthiram sukham aasanam"*, meaning 'that position which is comfortable and steady'. In this context, asanas are practised to develop the ability to sit comfortably in one position for an extended period of time, an ability necessary for meditation. Raja yoga equates yogasana to the stable sitting position.

The hatha yogis, however, found that certain specific body positions, asanas, open the energy channels and psychic centres. They found that developing control of the body through these practices enabled them to control the mind and energy. Yogasanas became tools to higher awareness, providing the stable foundation necessary for the exploration of the body, breath, mind and higher states. For this reason, asana practice comes first in hatha yoga texts such as *Hatha Yoga Pradipika*.

In the yogic scriptures it is said that there were originally 8,400,000 asanas, which represent the 8,400,000 incarnations every individual must pass through before attaining liberation from the cycle of birth and death. These asanas represented a progressive evolution from the simplest form of life to the most complex: that of a fully realized human being. Down through the ages the great rishis and yogis modified and reduced the number of asanas to the few hundred known today. Of these few hundred, only the eighty-four most useful are discussed in detail. Through their practice, it is possible to side-step the karmic process and bypass many evolutionary stages in one lifetime.

Animal postures

Many of the yogasanas described in this book are named after and reflect the movements of animals. Through observation, the rishis understood how animals live in harmony with their environment and with their own bodies. They understood, through experience, the effects of a particular posture and how the hormonal secretions could be stimulated and controlled by it. For example, by imitating the rabbit or hare in shashankasana they could influence the flow of adrenaline responsible for the 'fight or flight' mechanism. Through imitating animal postures, the rishis found they could maintain health and meet the challenges of nature for themselves.

Yogasanas and prana

Prana, vital energy, which corresponds to *ki* or *chi* in Chinese medicine, pervades the whole body, following flow patterns, called *nadis*, which are responsible for maintaining all individual cellular activity. Stiffness of the body is due to blocked prana and a subsequent accumulation of toxins. When prana begins to flow, the toxins are removed from the system, ensuring the health of the whole body. As the body becomes supple, postures which seemed impossible become easy to perform, and steadiness and grace of movement develop. When the quantum of prana is increased to a great degree, the body moves into certain postures by itself and asanas, mudras and pranayamas occur spontaneously.

Yogasanas and kundalini

The ultimate purpose of yoga is the awakening of *kundalini shakti*, the evolutionary energy in man. Practising asanas stimulates the chakras, distributing the generated energy of kundalini all over the body. About thirty-five asanas are specifically geared to this purpose: chakrasana for manipura chakra, sarvangasana for vishuddhi, sirshasana for sahasrara and so on. The other asanas regulate and purify the nadis, facilitating the conduction of prana throughout the body. The main object of hatha yoga is to create balance between the interacting activities and processes of the pranic and mental

10

forces. Once this has been achieved, the impulses generated give a call of awakening to *sushumna nadi*, the central pathway in the spine, through which the kundalini energy ascends to sahasrara chakra, thereby illumining the higher centres of human consciousness.

Hatha yoga, therefore, not only strengthens the body and improves health, but also activates and awakens the higher centres responsible for the evolution of human consciousness.

Yogasanas and the body-mind connection

The mind and body are not separate entities, although there is a tendency to think and act as though they are. The gross form of the mind is the body and the subtle form of the body is the mind. The practice of asana integrates and harmonizes the two. Both the body and the mind harbour tensions or knots. Every mental knot has a corresponding physical, muscular knot and vice versa.

The aim of asana is to release these knots. Asanas release mental tensions by dealing with them on the physical level, acting somato-psychically, through the body to the mind. For example, emotional tensions and suppression can tighten up and block the smooth functioning of the lungs, diaphragm and breathing process, contributing to debilitating illnesses in the form of respiratory disorders.

Muscular knots can occur anywhere in the body: tightness of the neck as cervical spondylitis, the face as neuralgia, etc. A well chosen set of asanas, combined with pranayama, shatkarmas, meditation and yoga nidra, is most effective in eliminating these knots, tackling them from both the mental and physical levels. The result is the release of dormant energy; the body becomes full of vitality and strength, and the mind becomes light, creative, joyful and balanced.

Regular practice of asana maintains the physical body in an optimum condition and promotes health even in an unhealthy body. Through asana practice, the dormant energy potential is released and experienced as increased confidence in all areas of life.

11

Yogasana and exercise

Yogasanas have often been thought of as a form of exercise. They are not exercises, but techniques which place the physical body in positions that cultivate awareness, relaxation, concentration and meditation. Part of this process is the development of good physical health by stretching, massaging and stimulating the pranic channels and internal organs, so asana is complementary to exercise. Before the difference between the two can be understood, it is necessary to know that exercise imposes a beneficial stress on the body. Without it the muscles waste, the bones become weak, the capacity to absorb oxygen decreases, insulin insensitivity can occur, and the ability to meet the physical demands of sudden activity is lost.

There are several differences in the way asana and exercise affect body mechanisms. When yogasanas are performed, respiration and metabolic rates slow down, the consumption of oxygen and the body temperature drop. During exercise, however, the breath and metabolism speed up, oxygen consumption rises, and the body gets hot. Yoga postures tend to arrest catabolism whereas exercise promotes it. In addition, asanas are designed to have specific effects on the glands and internal organs, and to alter electrochemical activity in the nervous system.

Yogasanas classified

The asanas are classified into three groups: beginners, intermediate and advanced. It is not necessary to perform all the asanas in a particular group. Regular practice of a balanced program, tailored to individual needs, is recommended for maximum benefit.

The beginners group should be performed by those who have never practised yogasanas before. Only a selection from this group, tailored to individual needs, should be practised by those who are infirm in any way, weak or sick. They will give greater benefits than more difficult practices. This group consists of elementary techniques designed to prepare the body and mind for major and meditation asanas. These practices are in no way inferior to the advanced asanas and are very useful in improving physical health. Experienced practitioners in particular will notice the profound yet subtle balancing effect. Included in this group are the pawanmuktasana series, eye exercises, relaxation, pre-meditation and meditation poses, asanas performed from vajrasana, standing asanas, surya and chandra namaskara.

The intermediate group consists of asanas which are reasonably difficult and are recommended for people who can perform the beginners group without discomfort or strain. These asanas require a greater degree of steadiness, concentration and coordination with the breath. Included in this group are asanas performed from padmasana, backward and forward bending, spinal twisting, inverted and balancing asanas.

The advanced group is intended for people with extensive control over their muscles and nervous system, who have already mastered the middle group of asanas. Practitioners should not be too eager to start these asanas. It is preferable to practise them under the guidance of a competent teacher.

Dynamic and static yogasanas
Dynamic practices often involve energetic movements of the body. They are intended to increase flexibility, improve circulation, tone the muscles and joints, release energy blocks and remove stagnant waste from different parts of the body. These asanas strengthen the lungs and improve the digestive and excretory systems. Dynamic practices are particularly useful for beginners. They include the pawanmuktasana series, surya namaskara, chandra namaskara, dynamic paschimottanasana and dynamic halasana.

Static practices of intermediate and advanced asanas are performed by experienced practitioners. They have a more subtle and powerful effect on the pranic and mental bodies. They are performed with little or no movement, the body often remaining in one position for a few minutes. These asanas are intended to gently massage the internal organs, glands and muscles as well as to relax the nerves throughout the body. They are specifically concerned with bringing

13

tranquillity to the mind and preparing the practitioner for the higher practices of yoga, such as meditation. Some of them are particularly useful for inducing the state of sense withdrawal, *pratyahara*.

General notes for the practitioner

The following practice notes should be thoroughly understood before going any further. Although anybody can practise asanas, they become more efficacious and beneficial when performed in the proper manner after correct preparation.

Breathing: Always breathe through the nose unless specific instructions are given to the contrary. Coordinate the breath with the asana practice.

Awareness: This is as essential to the practice of asana as it is to all yoga practices. The purpose of asana practice is to influence, integrate and harmonize all the levels of being: physical, pranic, mental, emotional, psychic and spiritual. At first it may appear that asanas are merely concerned with the physical level because they deal with the movement of different parts of the body, but they have profound effects at every level of being if they are combined with awareness.

Awareness in this context may be understood as consciously noting sensations in the body, the physical movement, the posture itself, breath control and synchronization, movement of prana, concentration on an area of the body or chakra and, most importantly, witnessing any thoughts or feelings that may arise during the practice. Implicit in the concept of awareness is the acceptance of any thought or feeling which comes uninvited to the mind. This awareness is essential in order to receive optimum benefits from the practices.

Right or left side: An example of the necessity for continual awareness is that most right-handed people will find it easier to commence an asana on the right side, which is more developed due to habitual patterns of behaviour. Once the asana is learned, however, it is better to lead with the left side and promote its development.

Relaxation: Shavasana may be performed at any point during asana practice, especially when feeling physically or mentally tired. It should also be practised on completion of the asana program.

Sequence: After completing shatkarma, asana should be done, followed by pranayama, then pratyahara and dharana which lead to meditation.

Counterpose: When practising the middle and advanced group of asanas particularly, it is important that the program is structured so that backward bends are followed by forward bends and vice versa, and that whatever is practised on one side of the body is repeated on the other side. This concept of counterpose is necessary to bring the body back to a balanced state. Specific counterposes are recommended for certain asanas described in this book.

Time of practice: Asanas may be practised at any time of day except after meals. The best time, however, is the two hours before and including sunrise. This period of the day is known in Sanskrit as *brahmamuhurta*, the most conducive time for higher yogic practices, when the atmosphere is pure and quiet, the activities of the stomach and intestines have stopped, the mind has no deep impressions on the conscious level and is empty of thoughts in preparation for the day ahead. The practitioner will probably find that the muscles are stiffest early in the morning compared to the late afternoon when they become more supple. Nevertheless this time is recommended for practice. In the evening the two hours around sunset is also a favourable time.

Pregnancy: Many asanas are helpful during pregnancy, but it is important to check with a midwife, doctor, or competent yoga teacher prior to practising. Do not strain. Do not use inverted asanas in the later stages of pregnancy.

Age limitations: Asanas may be practised by people of all age groups, male and female.

Place of practice: Practise in a well-ventilated room where it is calm and quiet. Asanas may also be practised outdoors, but the surroundings should be pleasant, a beautiful garden with trees and flowers, for example. Do not practise in a strong wind, in the cold, in air that is dirty, smoky or which carries an unpleasant odour. Do not practise in the vicinity of furniture, a fire or anything that prevents free fall to the ground, especially while performing asanas such as sirshasana. Many accidents occur because people fall against an object. Do not practise under an electric fan unless it is extremely hot.

Blanket: Use a folded blanket of natural material for the practices as this will act as an insulator between the body and the earth. Do not use a mattress which is spongy or filled with air as this does not give sufficient support to the spine.

Clothes: During practice it is better to wear loose, light and comfortable clothing. Before commencing, remove spectacles, wristwatches and any jewellery.

Bathing: Try to take a cold shower before starting. This will greatly improve the effect of the asanas.

Emptying the bowels: Before commencing the asana program, the bladder and intestines should preferably be empty. If constipated, drink two or three glasses of warm, slightly salted water and practise the asanas given in the chapter on shankhaprakshalana, namely tadasana, tiryaka tadasana, kati chakrasana, tiryaka bhujangasana and udarakarshanasana. This should relieve the constipation. If not, practising pawan-muktasana part 2 should help. Choose one time daily to go to the toilet before doing asanas. Do not strain; try to relax the whole body. After some weeks the bowels will automatically evacuate at the set time every day. Try to avoid using laxative drugs.

Empty stomach: The stomach should be empty while doing asanas and to ensure this, they should not be practised until at least three or four hours after food. One reason why early morning practice is recommended is that the stomach is sure to be empty.

Diet: There are no special dietary rules for asana practitioners, although it is better to eat natural food and in moderation. Contrary to popular belief, yoga does not say that a vegetarian diet is essential, although in the higher stages of practice it is recommended. At meal times it is advised to half fill the stomach with food, one quarter with water and leave the remaining quarter empty. Eat only to satisfy hunger and not so much that a feeling of heaviness or laziness occurs. Eat to live rather than live to eat.

Foods which cause acidity or gas in the digestive system, which are heavy, oily and spicy, should be avoided, especially when asanas are practised with a spiritual aim.

No straining: Never exert undue force while doing asanas. Beginners may find their muscles stiff at first, but after several weeks of regular practice they will be surprised to find that their muscles are more supple.

Contra-indications: People with fractured bones or who are suffering from acute infections or backache, or chronic ailments and diseases such as stomach ulcer, tuberculosis, cardiac problems or hernia, and those recuperating from operations, should consult a competent yoga teacher or doctor before commencing asanas. Carefully observe the contra-indications given in the introductions to each section, and those given for individual asanas.

Inverted asana: People with heart problems, high blood pressure, arteriosclerosis, glaucoma, an active ear infection or any disease of the brain should refrain from inverted postures. Those with cervical problems should not practise postures where the neck is weight bearing.

For any asana where the head is lower than the trunk of the body (semi-inverted), the general cautions given in the section for Inverted Asana apply.

Termination of asana: If there is excessive pain in any part of the body, the asana should be terminated immediately and, if necessary, medical advice sought. Do not stay in an asana if discomfort is felt.

Asana

Beginners Group

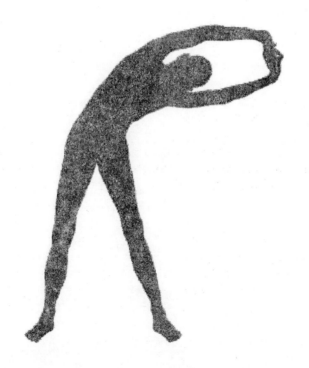

Pawanmuktasana Series

The pawanmuktasana series is one of the most important groups of practices that has a very profound effect on the human body and mind and is thus a most useful tool for the yogic management of various disorders and maintenance of health. It is one of the special contributions of the teachings of Swami Satyananda Saraswati. It is essential for laying a firm foundation for the perfection of yogic asanas.

Pawanmuktasana is valuable for understanding the meaning of asana by developing awareness of the body's movements and the subtle effects they have at the various levels of being. It is very useful as a preparatory practice as it opens up all the major joints and relaxes the muscles of the body. The series may be practised by anyone: beginner or advanced, young or elderly. It should never be ignored and treated casually just because the practices are simple, gentle and comfortable.

In Sanskrit these practices are referred to as *sukshma vyayama*, which means 'subtle exercise'. The word *pawan* means 'wind' or 'prana'; *mukta* means 'release' and *asana* means 'pose'. Therefore, pawanmuktasana means a group of asanas that remove any blockages preventing the free flow of energy in the body and mind.

Sometimes, due to bad posture, disturbed bodily functions, psychological or emotional problems or an unbalanced lifestyle, the energy becomes blocked. This initially results in stiffness, muscular tension, lack of proper blood flow and minor functional defects. However, if these blockages become chronic, a limb, joint or physical organ may malfunction, fail or become diseased. Regular practice of pawanmuktasana removes energy blockages from the body and prevents new ones from forming. In this way, it promotes total health, regulating and stabilizing the flow of energy throughout the body.

Mind-body aspect

Most modern day diseases are psychosomatic in nature. Drug treatment of these ailments is only symptomatic and fails to touch the roots of the disease. These asanas, if done correctly, in a non-competitive and relaxed atmosphere, not only relax the muscles of the body, but these relaxing impulses travel back to the brain and relax the mind. By integrating the breath synchronization and awareness, the attentive faculty of the mind is made active and is not allowed to wander into tension and stress. The nature of these asanas is thus more mental than physical. If asanas are performed correctly they relax the mind, tune up the autonomic nerves, hormonal functions and the activities of internal organs. Right-handed people will generally find that these asanas are easily learned with the right side leading. They should then be performed with the left side leading to counterbalance the effects of habitual behaviour patterns.

Three groups

Pawanmuktasana is divided into three distinct groups of asanas: the anti-rheumatic group, the digestive/abdominal group and the shakti bandha group to release energy blocks. All three groups supplement each other, stimulating and encouraging a free flow of energy throughout the body. Practitioners are advised to perfect each group before attempting the major asanas. Daily practice of pawanmuktasana parts 1, 2 and 3 over a period of months brings about a profound relaxation and toning of the entire psycho-physiological structure which is necessary for the practice of advanced techniques. The asanas in each group should be performed in the order given.

Advanced yogasanas are frequently physically demanding and have a powerful effect on the body and mind. It is essential to respect this and prepare correctly.

Pawanmuktasana Part 1

ANTI-RHEUMATIC GROUP

This group of asanas is concerned with releasing tensions from the joints of the body. It is excellent for those debilitated by rheumatism, arthritis, high blood pressure, heart problems or other ailments where vigorous physical exercise is not advised. It is particularly useful for eliminating energy blockages in the joints of the physical body, and for improving coordination, self-awareness and self-confidence.

Awareness

The practices may be performed in three ways:

1. With awareness of the actual physical movement, the interaction between the various components of the body, i.e. bones, joints, ligaments, muscles, etc.; the movement in relation to other parts of the body; with mental counting of each completed round; and with awareness of thoughts arising in the mind. This method of practice induces peace, balance and one-pointedness, which in turn brings about harmony in the physical body.

2. With awareness and integrated breathing. In addition to the awareness of physical movement described above, individual movements are synchronized with the breath. The movements become slower, which in turn slows the brain waves, further enhancing relaxation and awareness. This method of practice has a greater influence at the physical and pranic levels and is especially useful for harmonizing and revitalizing the body and improving

the function of the internal organs. Breathing should be practised as indicated in the description of each asana. In addition, experienced students may find greater benefit gained if ujjayi pranayama is used as a breathing technique. This effectively stimulates and balances the pranic energy flowing through the nadis.

3. With awareness of the movement of prana. Prana may be experienced as a tingling sensation in the body to which one becomes sensitized with practice. Mentally, one may feel light, yet one-pointed, emotionally fresh and receptive.

Periodic rest

After every two or three practices, sit quietly in the base position with the eyes closed and be aware of the natural breath, of the part or parts of the body that have just been moved, and of any thoughts or feelings that come into the mind. After a minute or so continue the practice. This will not only rest the body, but will also develop awareness of the internal energy patterns, and the mental and emotional processes. This rest period is almost as important as the asanas themselves and should not be neglected.

If tiredness is experienced at any point during the asana program, rest in shavasana. Shavasana should be performed for three to five minutes at the end of the program.

Base position

All the practices of pawanmuktasana part 1 are performed while sitting on the floor in the base position (see the diagram on page 25). The body should be relaxed, and only those muscles associated with the asana being executed should be used. Full awareness should be given to performance of the asana as per the notes above. For maximum benefit the eyes can remain closed. Do not practise mechanically, be aware throughout the practice.

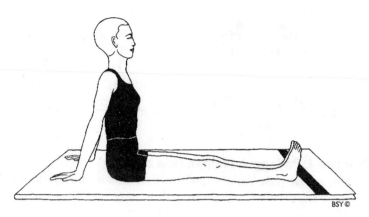

Prarambhik Sthiti (base position)

Sit with the legs outstretched, feet close together but not touching.

Place the palms of the hands on the floor to the sides, just behind the buttocks.

The back, neck and head should be comfortably straight.

Straighten the elbows.

Lean back slightly, taking the support of the arms.

Close the eyes and relax the whole body in this position.

PADANGULI NAMAN & GOOLF NAMAN

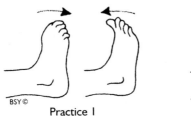
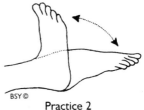

Practice 1   Practice 2

Practice 1: Padanguli Naman (toe bending)

Sit in the base position with the legs outstretched and the feet together. Place the hands beside and slightly behind the buttocks.

Lean back a little, using the arms to support the back.

Keep the spine straight.

Be aware of the toes. Move only the toes of both feet slowly backward and forward, keeping the feet upright and the ankles relaxed and motionless.

Hold each position for a few seconds.

Repeat 10 times.

Breathing: Inhale as the toes move backward.

Exhale as the toes move forward.

Awareness: On the stretching produced by the movement and the breath.

Practice 2: Goolf Naman (ankle bending)

Remain in the base position.

Slowly move both feet backward and forward, bending them from the ankle joints. Try to stretch the feet forward to touch the floor and then draw them back towards the knees. Hold each position for a few seconds.

Repeat 10 times.

Breathing: Inhale as the feet move backward.

Exhale as the feet move forward.

Awareness: On the stretch in the foot, ankle, calf and leg, and the breath.

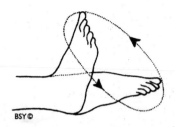

BSY©

Practice 3: Goolf Chakra (ankle rotation)

Remain in the base position.

Keep the legs shoulder-width apart and straight.

Keep the heels on the ground throughout the practice.

Stage 1: Slowly rotate the right foot clockwise from the ankle 10 times and then repeat 10 times anti-clockwise.

Repeat the same procedure with the left foot.

Stage 2: Slowly rotate both feet together in the same direction.

Focus on rotating the feet and not the knees.

Practise 10 times clockwise and then 10 times anti-clockwise.

Stage 3: Keep the feet separated.

Slowly rotate both feet from the ankles together, but in opposite directions.

Do 10 rotations in one direction and then 10 rotations in the opposite direction.

Breathing: Inhale on the upward movement.

Exhale on the downward movement.

Awareness: On the rotation of the ankle and the breath.

GOOLF GHOORNAN

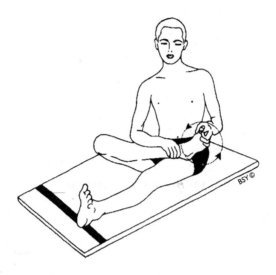

Practice 4: Goolf Ghoornan (ankle crank)

Remain in the base position.

Bend the right knee and bring the foot towards the groin. Turn the knee out to the side and if there is no strain, gently place the foot on the left thigh.

Make sure the ankle is far enough over the thigh to be free for rotation.

Hold the right ankle with the right hand.

Hold the toes of the right foot with the left hand.

With the aid of the left hand, slowly rotate the right foot 10 times clockwise, then 10 times anti-clockwise.

Change the leg and repeat with the left foot placed on the right thigh.

Breathing: Inhale on the upward movement.

Exhale on the downward movement.

Awareness: On the rotation and the breath.

Benefits: All the foot and calf asanas help in returning the stagnant lymph and venous blood. They thus relieve tiredness and cramp, and help prevent venous thrombosis, especially in bedridden, post-operative patients.

Practice 5: Janufalak Akarshan (kneecap contraction)
Stay in the base position.
Gently contract the muscle surrounding the right knee, drawing the kneecap back towards the thigh.
Hold the contraction for 3 to 5 seconds, counting mentally.
Release the contraction and let the kneecap return to its normal position.
Practise 10 times. Repeat with the left kneecap 10 times, then with both kneecaps together.
Breathing: Inhale while contracting.
Exhale while relaxing the knee muscles.
Awareness: On the contraction and the breath.

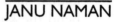

JANU NAMAN

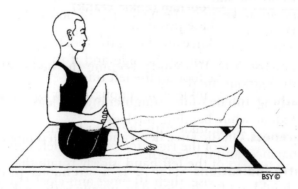

BSY©

Practice 6: Janu Naman (knee bending)
Stage I: Stay in the base position. Bend the right knee, bringing the thigh near the chest and clasp the hands under the right thigh.
Straighten the right leg, pulling up the kneecap.
Keep the hands under the thigh, but straighten the arms.
Keep the heel about 10 cms off the floor.
Again bend the right knee so that the thigh comes close to the chest and the heel near the groin.
Keep the head and spine straight.

29

This is one round.

Practise 10 rounds with the right leg and then 10 rounds with the left leg.

Stage 2: Bend both knees together, bringing the thighs near the chest and place the feet on the floor in front of the groin.

Hold the backs of the thighs.

Raise the feet slightly from the floor and balance on the buttocks.

Straighten the legs as much as you can without straining.

The arms straighten naturally while the hands continue to support the thighs.

Point the toes forward.

The hands and arms should support and maintain the stability of the body. Keep the head and spine upright.

Remain in the position for a few seconds.

Bend the knees and bring the legs back to the starting position, keeping the heels slightly above the floor.

Draw the toes back towards the shins.

This is one round.

Practise 5 to 10 rounds, keeping the heels off the floor throughout the practice.

Breathing: Inhale while straightening the legs.

Exhale while bending the legs.

Awareness: On the knee bend and associated movement and balance, and the breath.

Contra-indications: Stage 2 is a strenuous practice and should not be attempted by people with weak abdominal muscles, back conditions, high blood pressure or heart conditions.

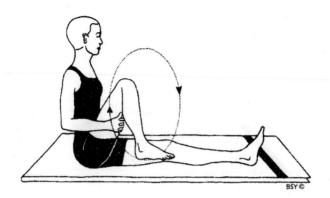

BSY©

Practice 7: Janu Chakra (knee crank)

Sit in the base position.

Bend the right knee and bring the thigh near the chest.

Place the hands under the right thigh and interlock the fingers or cross the arms holding the elbows.

Raise the right foot from the ground.

Rotate the lower leg from the knee in a large circular movement; try to straighten the leg at the top of the upward movement.

The upper leg and trunk should be completely still.

Rotate 10 times clockwise and then 10 times anti-clockwise.

Repeat with the left leg.

Breathing: Inhale on the upward movement.

Exhale on the downward movement.

Awareness: On the movement and perfection of circular rotation, and the breath.

Benefits: Since the knee joint bears the whole weight of the body and has no strong muscles for support, it is most vulnerable to injuries, sprains and osteoarthritis. All the knee asanas strengthen the quadriceps muscle and the ligaments around the knee joint. These asanas rejuvenate the joint by activating the healing energies.

ARDHA TITALI ASANA

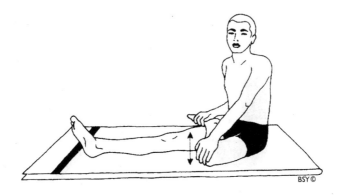

Practice 8: Ardha Titali Asana (half butterfly)

Sit in the base position.

Bend the right leg and place the right foot comfortably on the left thigh.

Place the right hand on top of the bent right knee.

Hold the toes of the right foot with the left hand.

This is the starting position.

Stage 1: with breath synchronization

While breathing in, gently move the right knee up towards the chest. Breathing out, gently push the knee down and try to touch the knee to the floor.

The trunk should not move.

Do not force this movement in any way.

The leg muscles should be passive, the movement being achieved by the exertion of the right arm.

Slowly practise 10 up and down movements.

Awareness: On the movement of the knee, ankle and hip joints, relaxation of the inner thigh muscles, and the breath.

Stage 2: without breath synchronization

Remain in the same position with the right leg on the left thigh.

Relax the right leg muscles as much as possible.

Push the right knee down with the right hand and try to touch the knee to the floor.

Do not strain.

Let the knee spring up by itself.

The movement is achieved by use of the right arm only.

Practise 30 up and down movements in quick succession. Breathing should be normal and unrelated to the practice.

Repeat stages 1 and 2 and the unlocking procedure (see note below) with the left leg.

Awareness: On the movement of the knee, ankle and hip joints and relaxation of the inner thigh muscles.

Benefits: This is an excellent preparatory practice for loosening up the knee and hip joints for meditative poses. Those people who cannot sit comfortably in cross-legged positions should practise ardha titali asana daily, both morning and evening.

Practice note: Gently straighten the leg after completing the practice, then again slowly and carefully bend it once, bringing the heel near the groin, then stretch the leg in front fully.

This procedure will ensure that the knee joint is realigned correctly.

SHRONI CHAKRA

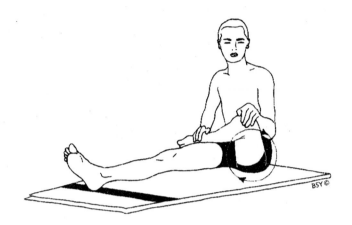

Practice 9: Shroni Chakra (hip rotation)

Sit in the same starting position as for ardha titali asana with the right foot on the left thigh.

Use the right hand to rotate the right knee in a circle and make the circular movement as large as possible.

The index finger may be pointed out and used as a guide to perfection of the circular movement.

Practise 10 rotations clockwise and then 10 rotations anti-clockwise.

Straighten the leg slowly.

Repeat with the left leg.

Breathing: Inhale on the upward movement.

Exhale on the downward movement.

Awareness: On the rotation of the knee, ankle and hip joint, and the breath.

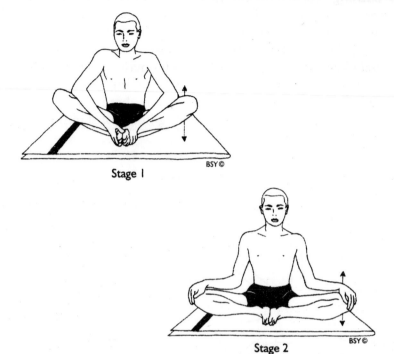

Stage 1

BSY©

Stage 2

BSY©

Practice 10: Poorna Titali Asana (full butterfly)

Sit in the base position.

Bend the knees and bring the soles of the feet together,
keeping the heels as close to the perineum as possible.

Fully relax the inner thigh muscles.

Stage 1: Clasp the feet with both hands.

Gently move the knees up and then down towards the
floor, but do not use any force.

Practise up to 30 up and down movements.

Stage 2: Keep the soles of the feet together.

Place the hands on the knees.

Using the hands, gently push the knees down towards the
floor, allowing them to spring up again.

Do not force this movement.

Repeat 10 to 30 times. Straighten the legs and relax.

35

Breathing: Normal breathing, unrelated to the practice.
Awareness: On the hip joint, movement and relaxation.
Contra-indications: People with sciatica and sacral conditions
  should avoid this asana.
Benefits: Both stages prepare the legs for mastery of padmasana
  and other meditative asanas. The inner thigh muscles hold
  a lot of tension which is relieved by these asanas. They
  also remove tiredness due to long hours of standing and
  walking.

MUSHTIKA BANDHANA

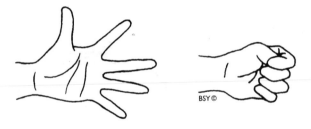

Practice 11: Mushtika Bandhana (hand clenching)
  Sit in the base position or a cross-legged pose.
  Hold both arms straight in front of the body at shoulder
  level.
  Open the hands, palms down, and stretch the fingers as
  wide apart as possible.
  Close the fingers to make a tight fist with the thumbs
  inside.
  The fingers should be slowly wrapped around the thumbs.
  Again open the hands and stretch the fingers.
  Repeat 10 times.
Breathing: Inhale on opening the hands.
  Exhale on closing the hands.
Awareness: On the stretching sensation and movement, and
  the breath.

36

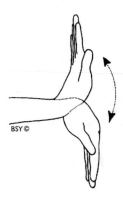

BSY©

Practice 12: Manibandha Naman (wrist bending)
Remain in the base position or a cross-legged pose.
Stretch the arms in front of the body at shoulder level.
Keep the palms open and fingers straight throughout the entire practice.
Bend the hands backward from the wrists as if pressing the palms against a wall with the fingers pointing toward the ceiling.
Bend the hands forward from the wrists so that the fingers point toward the floor.
Keep the elbows straight throughout the practice.
Do not bend the knuckle joints or fingers.
Bend the hands up again for the next round.
Repeat 10 times.
Breathing: Inhale with the backward movement.
Exhale with the forward movement.
Awareness: On the movement in the wrist joint and stretching of the forearm muscles, and the breath.

MANIBANDHA CHAKRA

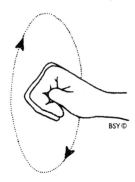

BSY©

Practice 13: Manibandha Chakra (wrist joint rotation)
Remain in the base position or a comfortable cross-legged pose, but keep the back straight.

Stage 1: Extend the right arm forward at shoulder level.
Make a loose fist with the right hand, with the thumb inside.
This is the starting position.
Slowly rotate the fist about the wrist, ensuring that the fist faces downward throughout the rotation.
The arms and elbows should remain perfectly straight and still. Make as large a circle as possible.
Practise 10 times clockwise and 10 times anti-clockwise.
Repeat the same with the left fist.

Stage 2: Extend both arms in front of the body with the fists loosely clenched.
Keep the arms straight and at shoulder level.
Rotate the fists together in the same direction.
Practise 10 times in each direction.

Stage 3: Practise as in stage 2.
Rotate the fists in opposite directions.
Practise 10 times in each direction.

Benefits: The hand and wrist asanas are beneficial for the related joints. They also relieve tension caused by prolonged writing, typing and so on.

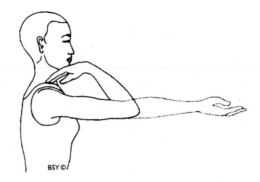

BSY ©

Practice 14: Kehuni Naman (elbow bending)

Stage 1: Remain in the base position or a cross-legged pose. Stretch the arms in front of the body at shoulder level. The hands should be open with the palms facing up. Bend the arms at the elbows and touch the fingers to the shoulders. Keep the upper arm parallel to the floor. Straighten the arms again.
This is one round.
Repeat 10 times.

Stage 2: Extend the arms sideways at shoulder level, hands open and palms facing the ceiling. Bend the arms at the elbows and touch the fingers to the shoulders. Keep the upper arms parallel to the floor. Again straighten the arms sideways.
Repeat 10 times.

Breathing: Inhale while straightening the arms. Exhale while bending the arms.

Awareness: On the movement of the elbow joint and arm muscles, and the breath.

KEHUNI CHAKRA

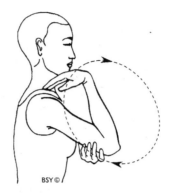

Practice 15: Kehuni Chakra (elbow rotation)

Remain in the base position or a cross-legged pose.
Stretch the right arm in front of the body at shoulder level.
The right hand can be open, or loosely closed.
Support the right upper arm with the left hand.
Bend the right arm at the elbow, rotating the elbow joint so that the lower arm and hand move clockwise.
Keep the upper arm steady and parallel to the floor.
The movement should be smooth. The fingers should almost touch the right shoulder as they move past.
Practise slowly 10 times clockwise and then 10 times anti-clockwise.
Gently lower the right arm.
Repeat on the other side.

Breathing: Inhale on the upward stroke.
Exhale on the downward stroke.

Awareness: On the rotation of the elbow joint with the breath and on keeping the upper arm steady.

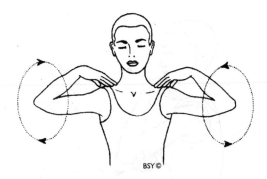

BSY ©

Practice 16: Skandha Chakra (shoulder socket rotation)
Stage 1: Remain in the base position or a cross-legged pose.
Place the fingers of the right hand on the right shoulder.
Keep the left hand on the left knee and the back straight.
Rotate the right elbow in a large circle.
Practise 10 times clockwise and 10 times anti-clockwise.
Repeat with the left elbow.
Make sure that the head, trunk and spine remain straight
and still.
Stage 2: Place the fingers of the left hand on the left shoulder
and the fingers of the right hand on the right shoulder.
Fully rotate both elbows at the same time in a large circle.
Try to touch the elbows in front of the chest on the forward
movement and touch the ears while moving up. Stretch
the arms back in the backward movement and touch the
sides of the trunk while coming down.
Practise slowly 10 times clockwise and then 10 times anti-
clockwise.
Breathing: Inhale on the upward stroke.
Exhale on the downward stroke.
Awareness: On the stretching sensation around the shoulder
joint and the breath.
Benefits: The shoulder asanas relieve the strain of driving and
office work, and also help relieve the pressure in cervical
spondylitis and frozen shoulder. They maintain the shape
of the shoulders and chest.

41

GREEVA SANCHALANA

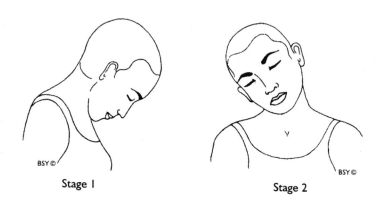

Stage 1   Stage 2

Practice 17: Greeva Sanchalana (neck movements)

Stage 1: Sit in a cross-legged pose with the hands resting on the knees in jnana or chin mudra. Close the eyes.
Slowly move the head forward and try to touch the chin to the chest.
Move the head as far back as is comfortable. Do not strain. Feel the stretch of the muscles in the front and back of the neck, and the loosening of the vertebrae in the neck.
Practise 10 times.

Breathing: Inhale on the backward movement.
Exhale on the forward movement.

Stage 2: Remain in the same position, keeping the eyes closed.
Face directly forward.
Relax the shoulders.
Slowly move the head to the right, bringing the right ear close to the right shoulder without raising the shoulders.
Move the head to the left side and bring the left ear close to the left shoulder.
Do not strain; touching the shoulder is not necessary.
This is one round. Practise 10 rounds.

Breathing: Inhale on the upward movement.
Exhale on the downward movement.

Awareness: On the stretching sensation of the muscles in the sides of the neck, and the breath.

42

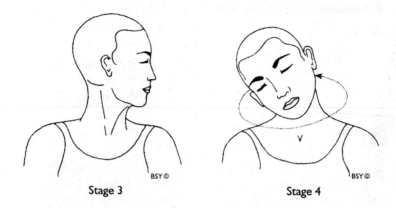

Stage 3　　　　　　　　　　Stage 4

Stage 3: Remain in the same sitting position.
　　Keep the head upright and the eyes closed.
　　Gently turn the head to the right so that the chin is in line with the right shoulder.
　　Feel the release of tension in the neck muscles and the loosening of the neck joints.
　　Slowly turn the head to the left as far as is comfortable.
　　Do not strain.
　　Practise 10 times on each side.
Breathing: Inhale while turning to the front.
　　Exhale while turning to the side.
Stage 4: Remain in the same position with the eyes closed.
　　Slowly rotate the head downward, to the right, backward and then to the left side in a relaxed, smooth, rhythmic, circular movement.
　　Feel the shifting stretch around the neck and the loosening up of the joints and muscles of the neck.
　　Practise 10 times clockwise and then 10 times anti-clockwise.
　　Do not strain.
　　If dizziness occurs, open the eyes and discontinue the practice for that day.
　　After the practice, keep the neck straight and the eyes closed. Be aware of the sensations in the head and neck.
Breathing: Inhale as the head moves up.
　　Exhale as the head moves down.

43

Awareness: On the movement and the breath.

Contra-indications: These four neck movements should not be performed by elderly people and those suffering from low blood pressure, high blood pressure, vertigo or extreme cervical spondylosis. Expert advice should be sought for any of these problems. Cervical spondylosis patients should strictly avoi forward bending of the neck.

Benefits: All the nerves connecting the different organs and limbs of the body pass through the neck. Therefore, the muscles of the neck and shoulders accumulate tension, especially after prolonged work at a desk. These asanas release tension, heaviness and stiffness in the head, neck and shoulder region.

Pawanmuktasana Part 2

DIGESTIVE/ABDOMINAL GROUP

This group of asanas is concerned specifically with strengthening the digestive system. It is excellent for people with indigestion, constipation, acidity, excess wind or gas, lack of appetite, diabetes, disorders of the male or female reproductive systems and varicose veins. It also eliminates energy blockages in the abdominal area.

Awareness
Throughout the practice become aware of the following:
1. Movement
2. Intra-abdominal pressure
3. The stretch of the muscles
4. Breathing

Periodic rest
Before starting the practice, the body and mind should be calm and relaxed. This is best achieved through the practice of shavasana. In addition, a short rest should be taken between asanas, lying in shavasana. One minute or thirty seconds should be sufficient, but a more reliable guide is to rest until the breathing returns to normal.

No strain
When starting this series, it is not advisable to attempt all the practices in one go, especially the ones which involve using both legs together. It is better to choose one practice at a time

45

and incorporate that into the previous practices. The pawan-muktasana part 2 series requires a great deal of effort and may put a strain on the lower back. Therefore, be aware of physical limitations and do not strain.

Contra-indications

These practices should not be performed by people suffering from high blood pressure, serious heart conditions, back conditions such as sciatica and slipped disc, or soon after abdominal surgery. If there is any doubt, please consult a competent therapist. In asanas where the feet are raised above the head, consult the cautions for inverted asanas as well as observing the contra-indications given for individual practices.

Starting position

All these asanas are performed by lying flat on the back with the legs together and straight. The arms should be by the sides, palms down, and the head, neck and spine in a straight line. Be sure to use a thin mat or a blanket, particularly with asanas such as supta pawanmuktasana and jhulana lurhakanasana where the body is balanced on the spinal vertebrae.

Right-handed people will find these asanas are easily learned with the right side leading. They should then be practised with the left side leading to balance development of the limbs, nerves and behaviour patterns.

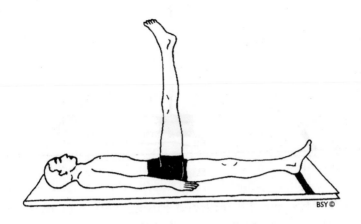

Practice 1: Padotthanasana (raised legs pose)

Stage 1: Lie in the starting position with the palms flat on
the floor.

Inhale and raise the right leg as high as is comfortable,
keeping it straight and the foot relaxed.

The left leg should remain straight and in contact with
the floor.

Hold the posture for 3 to 5 seconds while retaining the
breath.

Exhale and slowly lower the leg to the floor.

This is one round.

Practise 10 rounds with the right leg and then 10 rounds
with the left leg.

If the back is weak, the left leg can be bent so that the foot
is flat on the floor and the knee is up.

Breathing: Inhale while raising the leg(s). Hold the posture
and the breath.

Exhale while lowering the leg(s).

Awareness: On the stretch in the legs and synchronizing the
movement with the breath.

Contra-indications: Not to be performed by persons suffering
from high blood pressure or serious back conditions such
as sciatica and slipped disc.

47

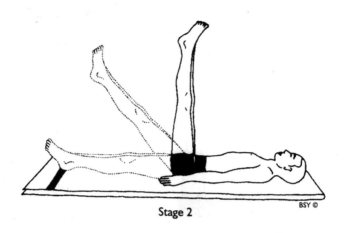

Stage 2

Stage 2: This may be repeated raising both legs together, but do not strain. Be aware that this is a more strenuous practice. Do not lift the buttocks off the floor.

Breathing: Inhale in the starting position. Hold the breath in while raising the legs.

Exhale while lowering the legs.

Awareness: On the stretch in the legs, the muscular effort in the back and abdomen, and synchronizing the movement with the breath.

Benefits: This asana strengthens the abdominal muscles and massages the organs. It strengthens the digestive system, lower back, pelvic and perineal muscles and helps correct prolapse.

Practice note: Padotthanasana may be repeated raising the legs to progressive heights in each round.

48

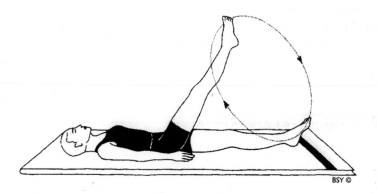

BSY ©

Practice 2: Padachakrasana (leg rotation)
Stage I: Lie in the starting position and relax.

Raise the right leg 5 cm from the ground, keeping the knee straight.

Rotate the entire leg clockwise 10 times in as large a circle as comfortable.

The heel should not touch the floor at any time during the rotation.

Rotate 10 times anti-clockwise.

Repeat with the left leg, first clockwise, then anti-clockwise. Do not strain.

Rest and practise abdominal breathing until the respiration returns to normal.

Stage 2: This may be repeated raising both legs together, but do not strain. Be aware that this is a more strenuous practice. Keep the legs together and straight throughout the practice.

Rotate both legs clockwise and then anti-clockwise 3 to 5 times.

The circular movement should be as large as possible.

Breathing: Inhale while moving the leg(s) upwards.

Exhale while lowering the leg(s).

Awareness: On the rotation of the leg(s), the effects of the asana on the hips and abdomen, and synchronizing the movements with the breath.

Contra-indications: Not to be performed by persons suffering from high blood pressure or serious back conditions such as sciatica and slipped disc.

Benefits: Good for the hip joints, obesity, toning of the abdominal and spinal muscles.

PADA SANCHALANASANA

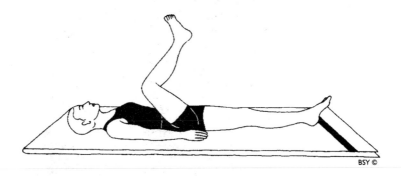

Practice 3: Pada Sanchalanasana (cycling)

Stage 1: Lie in the starting position and relax.

Raise the right leg.

Bend the knee and bring the thigh to the chest.

Raise and straighten the leg completely. Then lower the straight leg in a forward movement.

Bend the knee and bring it back to the chest to complete the cycling movement.

The heel should not touch the floor during the movement. Practise 10 times in a forward direction and then 10 times in reverse. Repeat with the left leg.

Breathing: Inhale while straightening the leg.

Exhale while bending the knee and bringing the thigh to the chest.

Stage 2: Raise both legs. Practise alternate cycling movements as though peddling a bicycle.

Practise 10 times forward and then 10 times backward.

Breathing: Breathe normally throughout.

Stage 3: Raise both legs and keep them together throughout the practice.

Bring the knees as close as possible to the chest on the backward movement and straighten the legs fully on the forward movement. Slowly lower the legs together, keeping the knees straight, until the legs are just above the floor. Then bend the knees and bring them back to the chest.

Practise 3 to 5 forward cycling movements and the same in reverse.

Do not strain.

Breathing: Inhale while straightening the legs.

Exhale while bending the legs to the chest.

Awareness: On the smoothness of the movement and proper coordination, especially while reverse cycling. When relaxing, be aware of the abdomen, hip, thighs and lower back, and the breath.

Contra-indications: Not to be performed by persons suffering from high blood pressure or serious back conditions such as sciatica and slipped disc.

Benefits: Good for hip and knee joints. Strengthens abdominal and lower back muscles.

Practice note: Keep the rest of the body, including the head, flat on the floor throughout the practice. After completing each stage remain in the base position and relax until the respiration returns to normal. If cramping is experienced in the abdominal muscles, inhale deeply, gently pushing out the abdomen, and then relax the whole body with exhalation. Do not strain; this applies especially to stage 3, which is a more strenuous practice.

SUPTA PAWANMUKTASANA

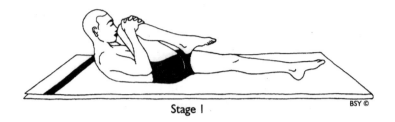

Stage 1   BSY ©

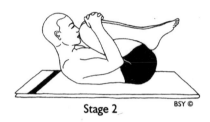

Stage 2   BSY ©

Practice 4: Supta Pawanmuktasana (leg lock pose)

Stage 1: Lie in the starting position and relax.

Bend the right knee and bring the thigh to the chest.

Interlock the fingers and clasp the hands on the shin just below the right knee.

Keep the left leg straight and on the ground.

Inhale deeply, filling the lungs as much as possible.

Exhaling, raise the head and shoulders off the ground and without straining bring the right knee to the nose.

Remain in the final position for a few seconds.

While slowly inhaling, return to the base position.

Relax the body.

Repeat 3 times with the right leg and then 3 times with the left leg.

Practice note: Ensure that the straight leg remains in contact with the ground.

It is important to start with the right leg because it presses the ascending colon directly.

Follow with the left leg which presses the descending colon directly.

Stage 2: Remain in the starting position.

Bend both knees and bring the thighs to the chest.

Interlock the fingers and clasp the hands on the shin bones just below the knees.

Inhale deeply.

Exhaling, raise the head and shoulders and try to place the nose in the space between the two knees.

Hold the raised position for a few seconds, counting mentally.

Slowly lower the head, shoulders and legs while inhaling.

Practise this 3 times.

Awareness: On the movement, the abdominal pressure, and the breath.

Contra-indications: Not to be performed by persons suffering from high blood pressure or serious back conditions such as sciatica and slipped disc.

Benefits: Supta pawanmuktasana strengthens the lower back muscles and loosens the spinal vertebrae. It massages the abdomen and the digestive organs and is therefore very effective in removing wind and constipation. By massaging the pelvic muscles and reproductive organs, it is also useful for impotence, sterility and menstrual problems.

JHULANA LURHAKANASANA

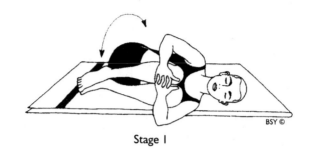

Stage 1

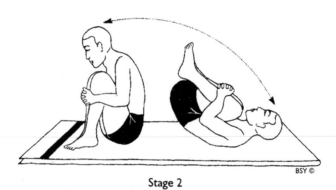

Stage 2

Practice 5: Jhulana Lurhakanasana (rocking and rolling)

Stage 1: Lie flat on the back. Bend both legs to the chest.
Interlock the fingers of both hands and clasp them around
the shins just below the knees.
This is the starting position.
Roll the body from side to side 5 to 10 times, touching the
side of the legs on the floor.

Breathing: Exhale while rolling to one side.
Inhale while returning to the centre.
Exhale rolling to the other side.

Stage 2: Sit in the squatting position with the buttocks just
above the floor.
Interlock the fingers of both hands and clasp them around
the shins just below the knees.

Rock the whole body backwards and forwards on the spine. Try to come up into the squatting pose on the feet when rocking forward. If it is difficult to perform with the hands clasped on the shins, then hold the side of the thighs adjacent to the knees.

Practise 5 to 10 backward and forward movements.

Breathing: Inhale as you roll backwards.
Exhale as you come forward.

Awareness: On the coordination of movement.

Contra-indications: Not to be performed by persons with serious back conditions.

Benefits: This asana massages the back, buttocks and hips. It is most useful if done first thing in the morning after waking.

Practice note: Use a folded blanket for this practice so that there is no possibility of causing damage to the spine. While rocking back, the head should remain forward. Be careful not to hit the head on the floor.

SUPTA UDARAKARSHANASANA

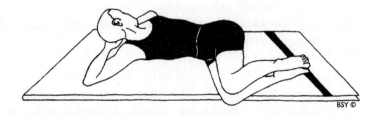

Practice 6: Supta Udarakarshanasana (sleeping abdominal stretch pose)

Lie in the starting position and relax.

Bend the knees and place the soles of both feet flat on the floor, directly in front of the buttocks.

Keep the knees and feet together throughout the practice. Interlock the fingers of both hands, place the palms under the back of the head and let the elbows touch the floor.

Breathe in, and while breathing out, slowly lower the legs to the right, trying to bring the knees down to the floor. The feet should remain in contact with each other, although the left foot will move slightly off the floor. At the same time, gently turn the head and neck in the opposite direction to the legs. This will give a uniform twisting stretch to the entire spine. Hold the breath in the final position while mentally counting three seconds.

While breathing in, raise both legs to the upright position. Keep the shoulders and elbows on the floor throughout.

Repeat on the left side to complete one round.

Practise 5 complete rounds.

Variation: Bend the knees and bring the thighs up to the chest. Interlock the fingers and place them behind the head. Roll the body from side to side, keeping the elbows on the floor.

Breathing: Exhale while lowering the legs to the sides.

Hold the breath in the final position.

Inhale while raising the legs.

Awareness: On the twisting stretch of the paraspinal and abdominal muscles, and the breath.

Benefits: This asana gives an excellent stretch to the abdominal muscles and organs, and thereby helps to improve digestion and eliminate constipation. The twisting stretch of the spinal muscles relieves the strain and stiffness caused by prolonged sitting.

The distance of the feet from the buttocks determines the placement of the spinal twist. If the feet are about 60 cm from the buttocks, the adjustment is in the lower area of the spine. As the feet approach the buttocks, the adjustment rises up the spine. When the feet are next to the buttocks, the adjustment is in the area of the cardiac plexus. Therefore, moving the feet about 3 cm each time works on each vertebra, bringing suppleness to the whole spinal column.

SHAVA UDARAKARSHANASANA

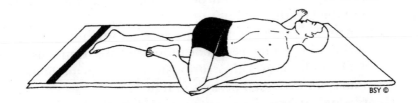

Practice 7: Shava Udarakarshanasana (universal spinal twist)
Lie in the starting position with the legs and feet together.
Stretch the arms out to the sides at shoulder level with the
palms of the hands facing down.
Bend the right leg and place the sole of the foot beside the
left kneecap. Place the left hand on top of the right knee.
This is the starting position.
Gently bring the right knee down towards the floor on the
left side of the body, keeping the leg bent and the foot in
contact with the left knee.
Turn the head to the right, looking along the straight arm,
and gaze at the middle finger of the right hand.
The left hand should be on the right knee and the right arm
and shoulder should remain in contact with the floor.
In the final position, the head should be turned in the
opposite direction to the folded knee and the other leg
should remain straight.
Hold the position for as long as is comfortable.
Return to the starting position, bringing the head and
knee to the centre. Stretch the right arm out to the side
and straighten the right leg.
Repeat on the opposite side.
Practise once to each side, gradually extending the holding
time.
Breathing: Inhale in the starting position.
Exhale while pushing the knee towards the floor and
turning the head.

Breathe deeply and slowly in the final position.
Inhale while centring the body and exhale while straightening the leg.

Awareness: On the relaxation of the back, arms and shoulders, and the breath.

Sequence: This asana should be performed after forward and backward bending asanas or those that are strenuous on the lower back, and after sitting in chairs or in meditation asanas for extended periods of time.

Contra-indications: This asana can realign the hip joint. It should be stopped if the practice is painful.

Benefits: Tightness and tiredness are relieved, especially in the lower back. The pelvic and abdominal organs are toned through its massaging action.

NAUKASANA

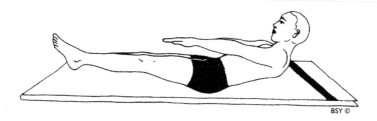

Practice 8: Naukasana (boat pose)
Lie in the starting position.

Keep the eyes open throughout.

Breathe in deeply. Hold the breath and then raise the legs, arms, shoulders, head and trunk off the ground.

The shoulders and feet should be no more than 15 cm off the floor. Balance the body on the buttocks and keep the spine straight.

The arms should be held at the same level and in line with the toes. The hands should be open with the palms down. Look towards the toes.

Remain in the final position and hold the breath. Count to 5 mentally (or for longer if possible).

Return to the supine position and then breathe out. Be careful not to injure the back of the head while returning to the floor.

Relax the whole body.

This is one round.

Practise 3 to 5 rounds.

Relax in shavasana after each round, gently pushing out the abdomen with inhalation to relax the stomach muscles.

Variation: Repeat the same process as above, but clench the fists and tense the whole body as much as possible in the raised position.

Breathing: Inhale before raising the body.

Retain the breath while raising, tensing and lowering the body.

Exhale in the supine position.

Awareness: On the movement, mental counting and tensing of the body (especially the abdominal muscles) in the final position, and the breath.

Benefits: This asana stimulates the muscular, digestive, circulatory, nervous and hormonal systems, tones all the organs and removes lethargy. It is especially useful for eliminating nervous tension and bringing about deep relaxation. It may be performed before shavasana in order to attain a deeper state of relaxation. If practised upon waking, it immediately restores freshness.

It is also useful for women preparing for childbearing and may be practised during the second trimester of pregnancy.

Pawanmuktasana Part 3

SHAKTI BANDHA ASANAS
(ENERGY BLOCK POSTURES)

This group of asanas is concerned with improving the energy flow within the body and breaking down neuro-muscular knots. They also eliminate energy blockages in the spine, activate the lungs and heart, and improve endocrine function. The series is useful for those with reduced vitality and a stiff back and is especially useful for menstrual problems and toning the pelvic organs and muscles. It can be practised after pregnancy for retoning flaccid muscles.

The shakti bandha series may be started straight away if good health and fitness prevail. However, if there are any serious ailments, a therapist should be consulted. Also take care to observe the contra-indications given for individual practices.

Right-handed people will find these asanas are easily learned with the right side leading. They should then be practised with the left side leading to balance development of the limbs, nerves and behaviour patterns.

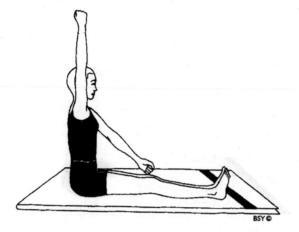

Practice 1: Rajju Karshanasana (pulling the rope)

Sit on the floor with the legs straight and together.

Keep the eyes open.

Imagine that there is a rope hanging in front of the body.

Breathe in while reaching up with the right hand as though to grasp the rope at a higher point.

Keep the elbow straight.

Look upward.

While breathing out, slowly pull the right arm down, putting power into it as though pulling the rope downwards. Let the eyes follow the downward movement of the hand.

Repeat with the left hand and arm to complete the first round.

Both arms do not move at the same time.

Practise 10 rounds.

Breathing: Inhale while raising the arm.

Exhale while lowering the arm.

Awareness: On the movement and stretch of the upper back and shoulder muscles, and the breath.

Benefits: This asana loosens the shoulder joints and stretches the upper back muscles. It firms the breast and develops the muscles of the chest.

61

GATYATMAK MERU VAKRASANA

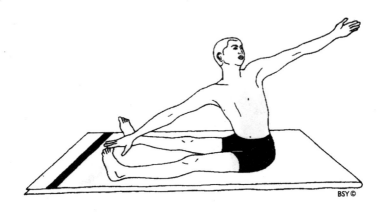

Practice 2: Gatyatmak Meru Vakrasana (dynamic spinal twist)

Sit on the floor with both legs outstretched.

Separate the legs as far apart as comfortable.

Do not allow the knees to bend.

Stretch the arms sideways at shoulder level.

Keeping the arms straight, twist to the left and bring the right hand down towards the left big toe.

Stretch the straight left arm behind the back as the trunk twists to the left.

Keep both arms in one straight line.

Turn the head to the left and gaze at the left outstretched hand.

Twist in the opposite direction and bring the left hand down towards the right big toe.

Stretch the straight right arm behind the back. Turn the head to the right and gaze at the right outstretched hand. This is one round.

Practise 10 rounds.

Start slowly and then gradually increase the speed.

Breathing: To give maximum flexion of the spine: exhale when twisting and inhale when returning to the centre.

Awareness: On the twisting movement and the effect on the spinal vertebrae and muscles, and the breath.

Contra-indications: People with back conditions should avoid this asana.

Benefits: This asana removes stiffness of the back and increases flexibility of the spine.

CHAKKI CHALANASANA

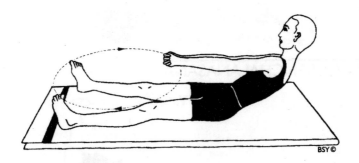

Practice 3: Chakki Chalanasana (churning the mill)

Sit with the legs stretched out in front of the body with the feet widely separated. Interlock the fingers of both hands and hold the arms out straight in front of the chest.

Keep the arms straight and horizontal throughout the practice; do not bend the elbows.

Bend forward as far as possible without straining. Imagine the action of churning a mill with an old-fashioned stone grinder.

Swivel to the right so that the hands pass above the right toes and as far to the right as possible without straining.

Lean back as far as possible on the backward swing.

Try to move the body from the waist. On the forward swing, bring the arms and hands to the left side, over the left toes and then back to the centre position.

One rotation is one round.

Practise 5 to 10 rounds clockwise and then the same number of rounds anti-clockwise.

Breathing: Inhale while leaning back.
Exhale while moving forward.

Awareness: On the movement and sensations in the lower back, hips and pelvic area, and the breath.

Benefits: This asana is excellent for toning the nerves and organs of the pelvis and abdomen. It is very useful for regulating the menstrual cycle and may be performed during the first three months of pregnancy. It is also an excellent exercise for postnatal recovery.

NAUKA SANCHALANASANA

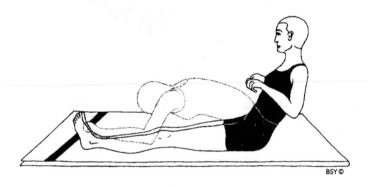

BSY©

Practice 4: Nauka Sanchalanasana (rowing the boat)
Sit with both legs straight in front of the body.
Imagine the action of rowing a boat.
Clench the hands as though grasping oars, with the palms facing down.
Breathe out and bend forward from the waist as far as is comfortable, straightening the arms.
Breathing in, lean back as far as possible, drawing the hands back towards the shoulders.
This is one round.
The hands should make a complete circular movement in every round, moving up the sides of the legs and trunk.
The legs should be kept straight throughout.

Practise 5 to 10 rounds.
Reverse the direction of the rowing movement as though going in the opposite direction.
Practise 5 to 10 times.

Breathing: Inhale while leaning back.
Exhale while bending forward.

Awareness: On the movement and sensations in the lower back, hips and pelvic area, and the breath.

Benefits: This asana has a positive effect on the pelvis and abdomen and releases energy blockages in these areas. It is especially useful for gynaecological disorders and post-natal recovery. It also removes constipation.

KASHTHA TAKSHANASANA

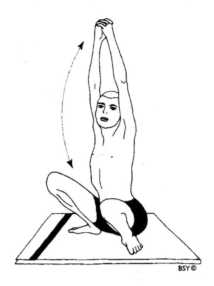

Practice 5: Kashtha Takshanasana (chopping wood)

Squat with the feet flat on the floor about 45 cm apart.
The knees should be fully bent and separated.
Clasp the fingers of both hands together and place them just above the floor between the feet. Straighten the arms and keep them straight throughout the practice.
The elbows should be inside the knees.
The eyes should remain open.
Imagine the action of chopping wood. Raise the arms above and behind the head, stretching the spine upward. Look up towards the hands.
Make a downward stroke with the arms, as if chopping wood. Expel the breath making a 'Ha!' sound. The hands should return near the floor in between the feet.
This is one round.
Practise 5 to 10 rounds.

Breathing: Inhale while raising the arms.
Exhale while lowering the arms.

Awareness: On the movement and stretch of the shoulder and upper back muscles, and the breath.

Contra-indications: Not for people with knee problems or sciatica.

Benefits: This asana loosens up the pelvic girdle and tones the pelvic muscles. It also has a special effect on the usually inaccessible muscles of the back between the shoulder blades, as well as the shoulder joints and upper back muscles. It helps to release frustration and lighten the mood.

Practice note: Those people who find the squatting pose too difficult should practise in the standing position. The benefits, however, will be less.

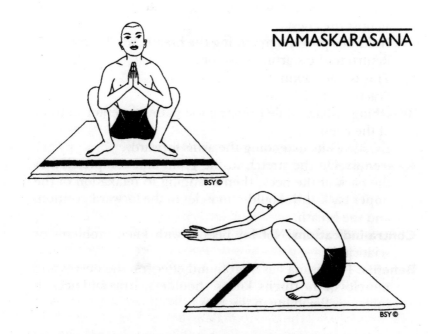

NAMASKARASANA

Practice 6: Namaskarasana (salutation pose)

Squat with the feet flat on the floor about 60 cm apart. The knees should be wide apart and the elbows pressing against the insides of the knees.

Bring the hands together in front of the chest in a gesture of prayer.

This is the starting position.

The eyes may be open or closed.

Inhale and bend the head backwards. Feel the pressure at the back of the neck.

Simultaneously, use the elbows to push the knees as wide apart as comfortable.

Hold this position for 3 seconds while retaining the breath.

Exhale and straighten the arms directly in front of the body.

At the same time, push in with the knees, pressing the upper arms inward.

The head should be bent forward with the chin pressed against the chest.

Hold this position, retaining the breath, for 3 seconds.

Return to the starting position.

This is one round.

Practise 5 to 10 rounds.

Breathing: Inhale while bringing the palms together in front of the chest.

Exhale while extending the arms forward.

Awareness: On the stretch in the groin and compression at the back of the neck, then changing to relaxation of the upper back and shoulder muscles in the forward position, and the breath.

Contra-indications: Not for people with knee problems or sciatica.

Benefits: This asana has a profound effect on the nerves and muscles of the thighs, knees, shoulders, arms and neck. It increases flexibility in the hips.

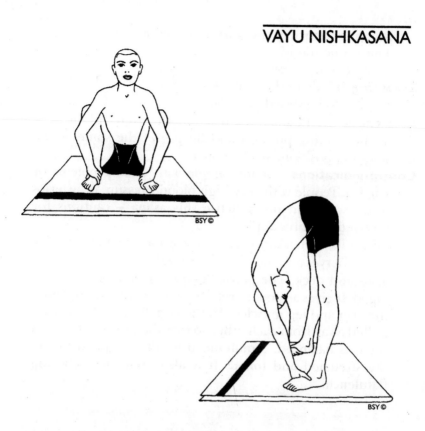

Practice 7: Vayu Nishkasana (wind releasing pose)

Squat with the feet about 60 cm apart.

Grasp the insteps of the feet, placing the fingers under the soles with the thumbs above.

The upper arms should be pressing against the insides of the knees with the elbows slightly bent.

The eyes should be open throughout the practice.

Inhale while moving the head back. Direct the gaze upward. This is the starting position.

Hold the breath for 3 seconds, accentuating the backward movement of the head.

While exhaling, straighten the knees, raise the buttocks and bring the head forward towards the knees.

Hold the breath for 3 seconds, accentuating the spinal bend. Do not strain.

Inhaling, return to the starting position.

This is one round.

Practise 5 to 10 rounds.

Breathing: Inhale in the squatting position.

Exhale in the raised position.

Awareness: On the squatting position, the stretch of the neck in the starting position and flexing of the spine in the standing position, and the breath.

Contra-indications: Not for people with knee problems or sciatica. People with very high blood pressure or arteriosclerosis should not practise this asana – cautions for inverted postures apply.

Benefits: Like namaskarasana, this pose has a beneficial effect on the nerves and muscles of the thighs, knees, shoulders, arms and neck. The pelvic organs and muscles are massaged. It gives an equal stretch to the whole spine and both the arm and leg muscles. All the vertebrae and joints are pulled away from each other so that the pressure between them is balanced. Simultaneously, all the spinal nerves are stretched and toned. It is also useful for relieving flatulence.

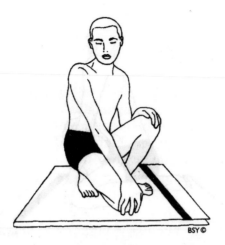

BSY©

Practice 8: Kauva Chalasana (crow walking)

Squat with the feet apart and the buttocks above the heels.

Place the palms of the hands on the knees.

Take small steps in the squatting position.

Try to keep the knees flexed so that the buttocks are not moved away from the heels. Walk either on the toes or the soles of the feet, whichever is most difficult.

As you take a step forward, bring the opposite knee to the floor.

Take as many steps as possible, up to 50, and then relax in shavasana.

Breathing: Breathe normally throughout.

Awareness: While walking: on smoothness of movement.

While resting in shavasana: on the effects of the asana on the lower back, hips, knees and ankles, and on the heartbeat or breath.

Contra-indications: People suffering from disorders of the knees, ankles or toes should not practise this asana.

Benefits: This asana prepares the legs for meditation asanas and improves blood circulation in the legs. It also helps to remove constipation.

71

UDARAKARSHANASANA

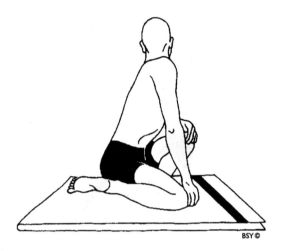

BSY©

Practice 9: Udarakarshanasana (abdominal stretch pose)
Squat with the feet apart and the hands on the knees.
Inhale deeply.
Exhale, bringing the right knee to the floor near the left foot.
Using the left hand as a lever, push the left knee towards the right, simultaneously twisting to the left.
Keep the inside of the right foot on the floor.
Try to squeeze the lower abdomen with the combined pressure of both thighs.
Look over the left shoulder.
Hold the breath out for 3 to 5 seconds in the final position.
Inhale when returning to the starting position.
Repeat on the other side of the body to complete one round.
Practise 5 to 10 rounds.
Awareness: On the movement and the alternate stretch and compression of the lower abdomen, and on the synchronized breath.
Contra-indications: Not for people with knee problems or sciatica.

72

Benefits: This pose is very useful for abdominal ailments because it alternately compresses and stretches the organs and muscles of this region. It also relieves constipation.

Note: *This is one of the asanas practised in shankhaprakshalana. Take care not to overstretch the back as the body begins to feel lighter and more flexible.*

73

Yoga Exercises for the Eyes

Many people wear spectacles or contact lenses to improve their vision. Glasses, however, do not actually cure bad eyesight. In fact, eye problems frequently get worse through their use, necessitating ever more powerful lenses.

Factors which contribute to bad eyesight are: artificial and bad lighting, prolonged computer use, television or video watching, poor diet, muscle inefficiency due to prolonged hours of office work and study, mental and emotional tension, toxic condition of the body and ageing.

Solving the problem of lighting is fairly straightforward. Diet, however, is more complex and it affects not only the health of the eyes, but of the whole body. Simplifying the diet and avoiding heavy, indigestible, oily, spicy foods as well as tinned, processed, pre-packed and junk foods will help rectify poor vision. A vegetarian diet is also recommended or, at least, a reduction in non-vegetarian food.

Contrary to popular belief, long periods of reading do not damage the eyes, providing the mind and eyes are relaxed while doing so. If there is tension, then even a short period of reading can strain the eyes. Try to develop the ability to read with relaxed awareness and a good posture. Before starting to read, if mental or muscular tension is experienced in the eyes, perform shashankasana for a few minutes. This asana will do much to calm the mind and relax the eyes.

Try to depend less on the use of glasses. Use them only when it is absolutely necessary. Leave them off during leisure time whenever possible. This will help the eyes to adjust and start functioning normally.

The habit of walking with bare feet on the grass, sand or bare earth, either early in the morning or around sunset, is claimed to have a relaxing and beneficial effect on the eyes. This is due to the reflex connections between the soles of the feet and the visual areas of the brain. It is especially recommended where the feet are often in restrictive footwear.

A simple sun bath may also be taken while facing the rising or setting sun. The eyes should be closed. Feel the ultra-violet rays soothing and relaxing the eyes.

Eye exercises: Excluding diseases such as glaucoma, trachoma and cataract, the most common eye disorders today are related to functional defects in the ocular muscles exacerbated by chronic mental and emotional tension. The following simple exercises help to alleviate various disorders related to the malfunctioning of the eye muscles, such as short and long-sightedness, presbyopia and squint.

The eye exercises should be practised regularly with patience and perseverance. Do not expect instant cure or improvement. It takes years for the eyes to become defective; it will also take time, a few months or more, before noticeable progress will be made. However, improvement will come, as it has to many people who have adopted a yogic way of life and gradually reduced the power of their glasses.

Preparation: Before starting, it is a good idea to splash pure, cold water on to the eyes a few times. Hold a little water in the palms above a water basin and splash it on to the eyelids. Do this about 10 times and then begin the exercises. This procedure will help stimulate the blood supply and generally tone up the eyes.

Contra-indications: Those who suffer from major eye diseases or disorders such as glaucoma, trachoma, cataract, retinal detachment, retinal artery or vein thrombosis, iritis, keratitis or conjunctivitis should only perform yoga practices after consulting an eye specialist. Inverted asanas and kunjal kriya should be avoided altogether while the condition lasts. Adopting a yogic lifestyle and a simple vegetarian diet, however, may be of great benefit.

Practice notes: Eye exercises should be performed one after the other in the sequence given. The series should be practised in its entirety, once early in the morning and/or once in the evening.

The most important thing to remember during practice is to be totally relaxed. Do not strain as this will lead to fatigue and tiredness of the eyes. The facial muscles, eyebrows and eyelids should remain totally relaxed. After each exercise the eyes should be closed and rested for at least half a minute. The practice of palming may be performed at this time.

Glasses should not be worn while performing the eye exercises.

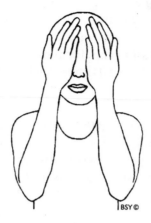

Exercise 1: Palming

Sit quietly and close the eyes.

Rub the palms of the hands together vigorously until they become warm. Place the palms gently over the eyelids, without any undue pressure.

Feel the warmth and energy being transmitted from the hands into the eyes and the eye muscles relaxing.

The eyes are being bathed in a soothing darkness.

Remain in this position until the heat from the hands has been absorbed by the eyes.

Then lower the hands, keeping the eyes closed.

Again rub the palms together until they become hot and place them over the closed eyes. (Make sure the palms and not the fingers cover the eyes.)

Repeat this procedure at least 3 times.

Benefits: Palming relaxes and revitalizes the eye muscles, and stimulates the circulation of the aqueous humour, the liquid that runs between the cornea and the lens of the eye, aiding the correction of defective vision.

Practice note: The benefits are enhanced if the exercise is practised in front of the rising or setting sun. Be aware of the warmth and light on the closed lids. Never look directly at the sun, except for a few initial moments when it is just rising or when it is about to set.

Exercise 2: Blinking

Sit with the eyes open.

Blink the eyes 10 times quickly.

Close the eyes and relax for 5 or 6 relaxed breaths.

Repeat the blinking 10 times quickly and then again close the eyes and relax.

Repeat 5 times.

Benefits: Many people with defective eyesight blink irregularly and unnaturally. This is related to the state of habitual tension in the eyes. This exercise encourages the blinking reflex to become spontaneous, inducing relaxation of the eye muscles.

SIDEWAYS VIEWING

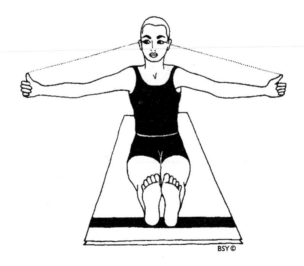

BSY©

Exercise 3: Sideways viewing

Assume a sitting position with the legs straight in front of the body.

Raise the arms to the sides at shoulder level, keeping them straight, make a loose fist and point the thumbs upwards. The thumbs should be just in the peripheral vision when the head is facing forward. If they are not clearly visible, bring them slightly forward until they come into view. The head should not move. Look at a fixed point directly in front and on a level with the eyes. Fix the position of the head in this neutral position. Then, without moving the head sideways, focus the eyes on the following, one after the other:

a) left thumb
b) space between the eyebrows, bhrumadhya
c) right thumb
d) space between the eyebrows
e) left thumb.

Repeat this cycle 10 times, keeping the head and spine straight throughout.

Finally, close and rest the eyes.

Palming may be performed several times.

Breathing: Inhale in the neutral position.
Exhale while looking to the sides.
Inhale and come to the centre.

Benefits: Sideways viewing relaxes the tension of the muscles strained by constant reading and close work. It also prevents and corrects squint.

Practice note: If the arms become tired they should be supported on two stools.

FRONT AND SIDEWAYS VIEWING

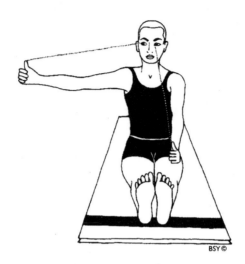

Exercise 4: Front and sideways viewing

Maintain the same body position as in exercise 3, but place the left fist on the left knee so that the thumb points upward.

Hold the right thumb to the right of the body so that it points upward.

Without moving the head, focus the eyes on the left thumb, then on the right thumb and then return to the left thumb.

Repeat this process 10 times, then rest and close the eyes.

Repeat the same procedure on the left side of the body.

Keep the head and spine straight throughout.

Finally, close and rest the eyes.

Palming may be performed several times.

Breathing: Inhale in the neutral position.

Exhale while looking forward.

Inhale while looking to the side.

Benefits: Front and sideways viewing improves coordination of the medial and lateral muscles of the eyeball.

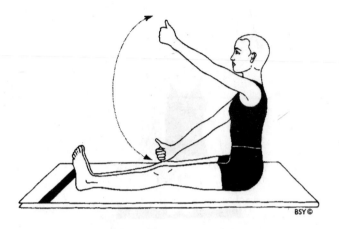

Exercise 5: Up and down viewing

Maintain the same position as in exercise 4.

Place both fists on the knees with both thumbs pointing upward.

Keeping the arms straight, slowly raise the left thumb while following the motion of the thumb with the eyes.

Once the thumb is raised to the maximum, slowly return to the starting position, all the time keeping the eyes focused on the thumb without moving the head.

Practise the same movement with the right thumb.

Repeat 10 times with each thumb.

Keep the head and spine straight throughout.

Finally, close and rest the eyes.

Palming may be performed several times.

Breathing: Inhale while raising the eyes.

Exhale while lowering the eyes.

Benefits: Up and down viewing balances the upper and lower eyeball muscles.

ROTATIONAL VIEWING

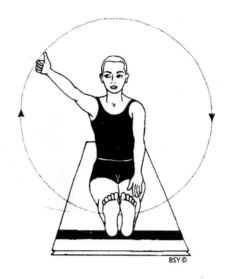

Exercise 6: Rotational viewing

Maintain the same body position as in exercise 5.

Place the right hand on the right knee.

Hold the left fist above the left leg with the left thumb pointing upward and the elbow straight.

Make a large circular movement with the left arm to the left, then upward, curving to the right, and finally returning to the starting position. Keep the eyes focused on the thumb without moving the head.

Perform 10 times clockwise and then 10 times anti-clockwise.

Repeat with the right thumb.

Keep the head and spine straight throughout.

Finally, close and rest the eyes.

Palming may be performed several times.

Breathing: Inhale while completing the upper arc of the circle. Exhale while completing the lower arc.

The breath should be smooth and synchronized with the forming of a perfect circle.

Benefits: Rotational viewing improves the coordinated activities of all the eye muscles.

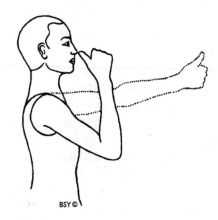

BSY©

Exercise 7: Preliminary Nasikagra Drishti (preliminary nosetip gazing)

Sit with the legs straight in front or in a cross-legged pose.

Hold the left arm straight directly in front of the nose.

Make a fist with the left hand, keeping the thumb pointing upward.

Focus both eyes on the tip of the thumb.

Bend the arm and slowly bring the thumb to the nosetip, keeping the eyes focused on the tip of the thumb.

Remain for a few seconds with the thumb held at the nosetip and the eyes focused there.

Slowly straighten the arm, continuing to gaze at the thumb tip.

This is one round.

Practise 10 rounds.

Keep the head and spine straight throughout.

Finally, close and rest the eyes.

Palming may be performed several times.

Breathing: Inhale as the thumb is drawn towards the nose. Exhale as the arm is straightened.

Benefits: This exercise improves the accommodating and focusing power of the eye muscles.

Exercise 8: Near and distant viewing

Stand or sit at an open window, preferably with a clear view of the horizon, with the arms by the sides.

Focus the eyes on the nosetip, nasikagra drishti, for 5 seconds.

Then focus on a distant object on the horizon for 5 seconds.

Repeat this process 10 times.

Close the eyes and relax.

Palming may be performed at this time.

Breathing: Inhale during near viewing.

Exhale during distant viewing.

Benefits: Same as for exercise 7, but the range of movements in these eye muscles is further increased.

Practice note: Lie in shavasana for a few minutes after completing all 8 exercises.

Relaxation Asanas

The importance of this series of relaxation poses cannot be overemphasized. They should be performed before and after the asana session and at any time when the body becomes tired. The asanas in this group appear very easy at first, yet to do them properly is quite difficult as the tension in all the muscles of the body must be consciously released. The muscles often seem to be completely relaxed but, in fact, tightness still remains. Even during sleep, relaxation is elusive.

The asanas in this chapter give the body the rest it so badly needs. Constant postural abnormalities put excess strain on the muscles of the back and just lying down does not relieve it. These relaxation practices, which are done in the prone position, are very relaxing to the spine and related structures. They are especially recommended for any back or spinal problem. These postures can be adopted during any time of the day for any comfortable duration. They can be combined with relaxing daily activities as well.

SHAVASANA

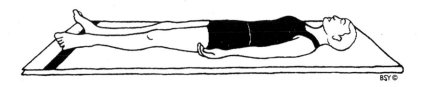

Shavasana (corpse pose)
Lie flat on the back with the arms about 15 cm away from
the body, palms facing upward. A thin pillow or folded cloth
may be placed behind the head to prevent discomfort. Let
the fingers curl up slightly.
Move the feet slightly apart to a comfortable position and
close the eyes.
The head and spine should be in a straight line.
Make sure the head does not fall to one side or the other.
Relax the whole body and stop all physical movement.
Become aware of the natural breath and allow it to become
rhythmic and relaxed.
After some time, again become aware of the body and
surroundings, and gently and smoothly release the posture.

Breathing: Natural and relaxed, or begin to count the breaths
from number 27 backwards to zero. Mentally repeat, "I am
breathing in 27, I am breathing out 27, I am breathing in
26, I am breathing out 26", and so on, back to zero.
If the mind wanders and the next number is forgotten,
bring it back to the counting and start again at 27. If the
mind can be kept on the breath for a few minutes, the
body will relax.

Duration: According to time available. In general, the longer
the better, although a minute or two is sufficient between
asana practices.

Awareness: Physical – first on relaxing the whole body, then
on the breath.
Spiritual – on ajna chakra.

Benefits: This asana relaxes the whole psycho-physiological system. It should ideally be practised before sleep; before, during and after asana practice, particularly after dynamic exercises such as surya namaskara; and when the practitioner feels physically and mentally tired. It develops body awareness. When the body is completely relaxed, awareness of the mind increases, developing pratyahara.

Practice note: Do not move the body at all during the practice as even the slightest movement disturbs the practice.

A personal mantra may be repeated with every inhalation and exhalation.

For maximum benefit, this technique should be performed after a hard day's work, before evening activities, or to refresh the body and mind before sitting for meditation, or just before sleep.

Note: *This asana is also known as* mritasana, *the dead man's pose.*

ADVASANA

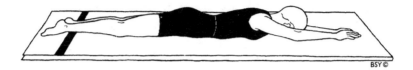

Advasana (reversed corpse pose)

Lie on the stomach.

Stretch both arms above the head with the palms facing downward. The forehead should be resting on the floor.

Relax the whole body in the same way as described for shavasana.

If there is difficulty breathing or a sense of suffocation is experienced, a pillow may be placed under the chest.

After some time, again become aware of the body and surroundings, and gently and smoothly release the posture.

Breathing: Natural and rhythmic. The number of breaths may be counted as in shavasana while gently pushing the abdomen against the floor.

Duration: For relaxation in the treatment of ailments, it should be performed for as long as is comfortable. Before or during an asana session, a few minutes is sufficient.

Awareness: Physical–on relaxing the whole body, and on the breath.

Spiritual–on ajna or manipura chakra.

Benefits: Recommended for those with slipped disc, stiff neck and stooping figure.

Practice note: Mantra may also be synchronized with the breath as in shavasana.

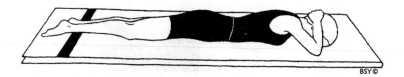

BSY©

Jyestikasana (superior posture)

Lie flat on the stomach with the legs straight and the forehead resting on the floor.

Interlock the fingers and place the palms on the back of the head or neck.

Allow the elbows to rest on the floor.

Relax the whole body and become aware of the breathing process as described for shavasana.

After some time, again become aware of the body and surroundings, and gently and smoothly release the posture.

Breathing: Natural and rhythmical.

Awareness: Physical–on relaxing the whole body, feeling the soothing warmth of the palms melting away the tensions in the neck and related areas, and feeling the breath.
Spiritual–on ajna or manipura chakra.

Benefits: This asana is helpful for all spinal complaints, especially cervical spondylitis and stiff neck or upper back.

Variation: This asana may also be performed with the fingers of both hands interlocked and placed under the forehead, palms facing up.

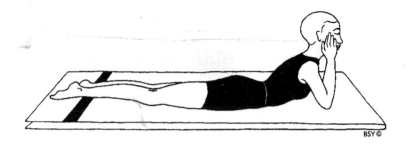

Makarasana (crocodile pose)

Lie flat on the stomach.

Raise the head and shoulders and rest the chin in the palms of the hands with the elbows on the floor.

Keep the elbows together for a more pronounced arch to the spine. Separate the elbows slightly to relieve excess pressure on the neck.

In makarasana the effect is felt at two points: the neck and the lower back. If the elbows are too far in front, tension will be felt in the neck; if they are drawn too close to the chest, tension will be felt more in the lower back. Adjust the position of the elbows so that these two points are equally balanced. The ideal position is when the whole spine is equally relaxed.

Relax the whole body and close the eyes.

After some time, again become aware of the body and surroundings, and gently and smoothly release the posture.

Breathing: Natural and rhythmic, or practise inhaling, moving the awareness up along the spine from the tail bone to the neck and exhaling, bringing the awareness back down from the neck to the tail bone. Feel the breath moving up and down the spine. This will quickly activate the healing energies in this area.

For lower back pain due to tension, concentrate on this area and feel it expanding and relaxing with every inhalation and exhalation.

Duration: For as long as is comfortable.

Awareness: Physical–with concentration on the lower back, and relaxing the whole body, and on the breathing process. Spiritual–on manipura chakra.

Contra-indications: Those with back conditions, such as exaggerated lumbar curve, should not practise this asana if any pain is experienced.

Benefits: This asana is very effective for people suffering from slipped disc, sciatica, and certain types of lower back pain. They should remain in this asana for extended periods of time as it encourages the vertebral column to resume its normal shape and releases compression of the spinal nerves. Asthmatics and people who have any other lung ailments should practise this simple asana regularly with breath awareness as it allows more air to enter the lungs.

MATSYA KRIDASANA

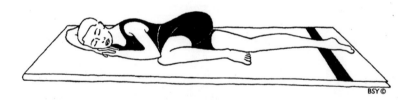

Matsya Kridasana (flapping fish pose)

Lie on the stomach with the fingers interlocked under the head. Bend the left leg sideways and bring the left knee close to the ribs.

The right leg should remain straight.

Swivel the arms to the left and rest the left elbow near the left knee.

Rest the right side of the head on the crook of the right arm, or a little further down the arm for more comfort.

Relax in the final pose and, after some time, change sides.

This position resembles a flapping fish.

91

After some time, again become aware of the body and surroundings, and gently and smoothly release the posture.

Breathing: Normal and relaxed in the static pose.

Duration: Practise this asana for as long as comfortable on both sides. It may also be used for sleeping and resting.

Awareness: Physical – on relaxing the whole body, and on the breath.

Spiritual – on manipura chakra.

Benefits: This asana stimulates digestive peristalsis. It relieves sciatic pain by relaxing the nerves in the legs. People for whom the practice of forward bending asanas is not recommended may practise matsya kridasana as a counterpose after backward bending asanas. It relaxes tension in the perineum. In the later months of pregnancy, lying on the back may cause pressure over major veins and block the circulation. In such circumstances, this posture is ideal for relaxing, sleeping or practising yoga nidra. The bent knee and the head may be supported on a pillow for further comfort.

Meditation Asanas

The main purpose of the meditation asanas is to allow the practitioner to sit for extended periods of time without moving the body and without discomfort. Only when the body has been steady and still for some time will meditation be experienced. Deep meditation requires the spinal column to be straight and very few asanas can satisfy this condition. Furthermore, in high stages of meditation the practitioner loses control over the muscles of the body. The meditation asana, therefore, needs to hold the body in a steady position without conscious effort. Why not lie in shavasana, then, for meditation since it satisfies all the requirements? Because in shavasana there is a tendency to drift into sleep. It is essential to remain awake and alert while going through the various stages which lead to successful meditation.

Swami Sivananda of Rishikesh said the following about asanas and meditation: "You must be able to sit in one of the meditation asanas for a full three hours at a stretch without the body shaking. Then only will you gain true *asana siddhi,* mastery over the asana, and be able to practise the higher stages of pranayama and dhyana. Without securing a steady asana, you cannot progress well in meditation. The more steady you are in your asana, the more you will be able to concentrate with a one-pointed mind. If you can be steady in a posture even for one hour, you will be able to acquire a one-pointed mind and feel the *atmic anandam,* infinite peace and soulful bliss inside you."

Initially, most people will find it difficult to sit in one asana for a long time. However, through regular practice of the pre-meditation poses listed here, the legs and hips will become flexible enough to comfortably maintain a steady posture.

Pre-meditation asanas: The following selected practices from the pawanmuktasana series are most useful for preparing the body for the meditation asanas:

1. Goolf chakra (ankle rotation)
2. Janu chakra (knee crank)
3. Ardha titali asana (half butterfly)
4. Shroni chakra (hip rotation)
5. Poorna titali (full butterfly)
6. Vayu nishkasana (wind releasing pose)
7. Udarakarshan asana (abdominal stretch pose)
8. Shaithalyasana (animal relaxation pose), refer to chapter on forward bending asanas.

Stillness: When sitting in meditation postures, program the mind with suggestions like, "I am as steady as a rock" or "I am becoming motionless like a statue." This way the asana will quickly become steady and, after a while, will be comfortable for extended periods of time. This is the practice of *kaya sthairyam*, complete body stillness.

Alternative postures: Apart from the postures mentioned in this chapter, there are four other asanas which are useful for meditation. These are described in the chapter on the vajrasana group of asanas. They are:

1. Vajrasana (thunderbolt pose)
2. Ananda madirasana (intoxicating bliss pose)
3. Padadhirasana (breath balancing pose)
4. Bhadrasana (gracious pose).

Other asanas, such as gorakhshasana or moola bandhasana, may also be used for meditation, but they are advanced practices and not comfortable for prolonged periods of time. These are described in the advanced asanas chapter.

Precautions: If there is discomfort or pain in the legs after sitting for some time in a meditation asana, slowly unlock the legs and massage them. When the blood circulation has returned to normal and there is no pain, resume the asana.

94

However, be aware that the knee is a very delicate and much abused joint of the body and be careful not to strain it, especially while moving into or out of these meditation asanas. Do not on any account use undue force or strain to sit in a meditation asana. Carefully observe the contra-indications given for individual asanas.

Right or left leg: In all the asanas discussed in this chapter, either the left or the right leg may be placed uppermost. It is a matter of personal preference and depends on whichever is the more comfortable. Ideally, the leg position should be alternated so that the balance on both sides of the body is maintained.

Practice note: A useful suggestion to make the following postures more comfortable is to place a small cushion under the buttocks.

Note: Padmasana may seem out of place in the beginners group. It has been included because a series of asanas in the intermediate group is performed using it as the base position.

SUKHASANA

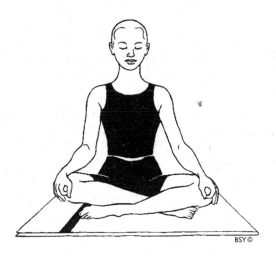

Sukhasana (easy pose)

Sit with the legs straight in front of the body.

Bend one leg and place the foot under the opposite thigh.

Bend the other leg and place the foot under the opposite thigh.

Place the hands on the knees in chin or jnana mudra.

Keep the head, neck and back upright and straight, but without strain. Close the eyes.

Relax the whole body. The arms should be relaxed and not held straight.

Benefits: Sukhasana is the easiest and most comfortable of the meditation postures. It can be utilized without ill effect by persons who are unable to sit in the more difficult meditation postures. It facilitates mental and physical balance without causing strain or pain.

Practice note: Sukhasana is a relaxing posture which may be used after extended periods of sitting in siddhasana or padmasana.

Although sukhasana is said to be the simplest meditation posture, it is difficult to sustain for long periods of time unless the knees are close to the ground or on the ground. Otherwise most of the body weight is supported by the buttocks and backache develops. The other meditation asanas create a larger and therefore steadier area of support.

Variation: For those who are extremely stiff, sukhasana may be performed sitting cross-legged with a belt or cloth tied around the knees and lower back.

Hold the spine upright.

Concentrate on the physical balance and equalizing the weight on the right and left side of the body. A light, spacey feeling may be experienced.

While maintaining the posture, place the hands on the knees in chin or jnana mudra.

ARDHA PADMASANA

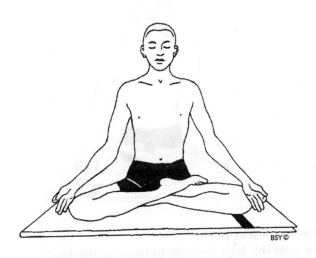

Ardha Padmasana (half lotus pose)

Sit with the legs straight in front of the body.

Bend one leg and place the sole of the foot on the inside of the opposite thigh.

Bend the other leg and place the foot on top of the opposite thigh.

Without straining, try to place the upper heel as near as possible to the abdomen. Adjust the position so that it is comfortable.

Place the hands on the knees in either chin or jnana mudra. Keep the back, neck and head upright and straight. Close the eyes and relax the whole body.

Contra-indications: Those who suffer from sciatica or knee problems should not perform this asana.

Benefits: The same benefits as given for padmasana but at a reduced level.

PADMASANA

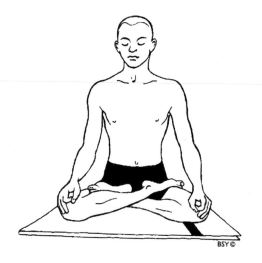

BSY©

Padmasana (lotus pose)

Sit with the legs straight in front of the body.

Slowly and carefully bend one leg and place the foot on top of the opposite thigh.

The sole should face upward and the heel should be close to the pubic bone.

When this feels comfortable, bend the other leg and place the foot on top of the opposite thigh.

Both knees should, ideally, touch the ground in the final position.

The head and spine should be held upright and the shoulders relaxed.

Place the hands on the knees in chin or jnana mudra.

Relax the arms with the elbows slightly bent and check that the shoulders are not raised or hunched.

Close the eyes and relax the whole body.

Observe the total posture of the body. Make the necessary adjustments by moving forward or backward until balance and alignment are experienced. Perfect alignment indicates the correct posture of padmasana.

Contra-indications: Those who suffer from sciatica or weak or injured knees should not perform this asana. This asana should not be attempted until flexibility of the knees has been developed through practice of the pre-meditation asanas. It is not advisable during pregnancy as the circulation in the legs is reduced.

Benefits: Padmasana allows the body to be held completely steady for long periods of time. It holds the trunk and head like a pillar with the legs as the firm foundation. As the body is steadied, the mind becomes calm. This steadiness and calmness is the first step towards real meditation. Padmasana directs the flow of prana from mooladhara chakra in the perineum to sahasrara chakra in the head, heightening the experience of meditation.

This posture applies pressure to the lower spine, which has a relaxing effect on the nervous system. The breath becomes slow, muscular tension is decreased and blood pressure is reduced. The normally large blood flow to the legs is redirected to the abdominal region. This activity also stimulates the digestive process.

SIDDHASANA

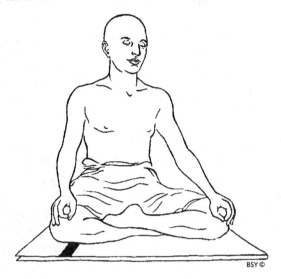

Siddhasana (accomplished pose for men)

Sit with the legs straight in front of the body.

Bend the right leg and place the sole of the foot flat against the inner left thigh with the heel pressing the perineum (the area midway between the genitals and anus).

Bend the left leg. Push the toes and the outer edge of the left foot into the space between the right calf and thigh muscles. If necessary, this space may be enlarged slightly by using the hands or temporarily adjusting the position of the right leg.

Place the left ankle directly over the right ankle so that the ankle bones are touching and the heels are one above the other.

Press the pubis with the left heel directly above the genitals. The genitals will therefore lie between the two heels.

If this last position is too difficult, simply place the left heel as near as possible to the pubis.

Grasp the right toes and pull them up into the space between the left calf and thigh.

Again adjust the body so that it is comfortable.

Sit on top of the right heel. This is an important aspect

of siddhasana. Adjust the body until it is comfortable and the pressure of the heel is firmly applied.

The legs should now be locked, with the knees touching the ground and the left heel directly above the right heel.

Make the spine erect and feel as though the body is fixed on the floor.

Place the hands on the knees in jnana, chin or chinmaya mudra.

Close the eyes and relax the whole body.

Contra-indications: Siddhasana should not be practised by those with sciatica or sacral infections.

Benefits: Siddhasana directs the energy from the lower psychic centres upward through the spine, stimulating the brain and calming the entire nervous system. The position of the lower foot at the perineum presses mooladhara chakra, stimulating moola bandha, and the pressure applied to the pubic bone presses the trigger point for swadhisthana, automatically activating vajroli/sahajoli mudra. These two psycho-muscular locks redirect sexual nervous impulses back up the spinal cord to the brain, establishing control over the reproductive hormones which is necessary in order to maintain brahmacharya for spiritual purposes.

Prolonged periods in siddhasana result in noticeable tingling sensations in the mooladhara region, which may last for ten to fifteen minutes. This is caused by a reduction in the blood supply to the area and by a rebalancing of the pranic flow in the lower chakras.

This posture redirects blood circulation to the lower spine and abdomen, toning the lumbar region of the spine, the pelvis and the abdominal organs, and balancing the reproductive system and the blood pressure.

Practice note: Siddhasana may be performed with either leg uppermost. Many people experience discomfort due to the pressure applied where the ankles cross each other. If necessary, place a folded cloth or piece of sponge between the legs at this point. At first the pressure at the perineum may be uncomfortable to maintain, but with practice this will be eased.

Note: *The Sanskrit word* siddha *means 'power' and 'perfection'. The word* siddhi *is derived from siddha and refers to a psychic power or faculty developed through yogic practices. Siddhis include clairvoyance and telepathy as well as many other lesser known powers such as the ability to disappear at will. Siddhasana, or siddha yoni asana for women, is believed to be the asana that helps develop these powers.*

SIDDHA YONI ASANA

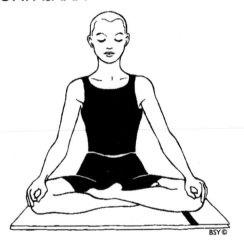

BSY©

Siddha Yoni Asana (accomplished pose for women)
Sit with the legs straight in front of the body.
Bend the right leg, placing the sole of the foot flat against the inner left thigh and the heel firmly against the groin.
Adjust the body position so that there is comfortable pressure of the right heel.
Bend the left leg and wedge the left toes down into the space between the right calf and thigh.
Grasp the toes of the right foot and pull them up into the space between the left calf and thigh.
The left heel is above the right heel and may exert a light pressure against the pubic bone.

Again adjust the position so that it is comfortable.
Ensure that the knees are firmly on the ground.
Make the spine fully erect and straight as though it were planted solidly in the earth.
Place the hands on the knees in chin or jnana mudra.
Close the eyes and relax the whole body.

Contra-indications: As for siddhasana.

Benefits: As for siddhasana.

Note: *The Sanskrit word* yoni *means 'womb' or 'source'.*

SWASTIKASANA

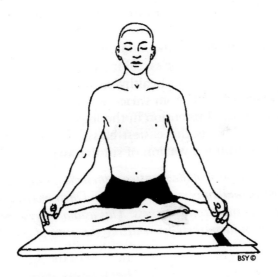

BSY©

Swastikasana (auspicious pose)
Sit with the legs straight in front of the body.
Bend the left knee and place the sole of the left foot against the inside of the right thigh so there is no contact between the heel and the perineum.
Bend the right knee and place the right foot in the space between the left thigh and calf muscle so that there is no contact between the heel and the pubis.

Grasp the toes of the left foot and pull them up into the space between the right calf and thigh.

Adjust the position so that it is comfortable. The knees should be firmly on the floor.

Straighten the spine. Place the hands on the knees in chin, jnana or chinmaya mudra.

Variation: Sit with the legs straight in front of the body.

Bend the left leg and place the sole against the inside of the right thigh.

Similarly, bend the right leg and place the heel of the right foot on the floor in front of the left foot with the sole resting against the left shin. The heels will now be one in front of the other.

The hands may be placed on the knees in jnana, chin or chinmaya mudra, or they may be placed in the lap.

Close the eyes and relax the whole body.

Contra-indications: Swastikasana should not be performed by people with sciatica or sacral infections.

Benefits: Swastikasana is a healthy position to sit in, especially for those suffering from varicose veins, tired and aching muscles or fluid retention in the legs.

Practice note: This is the easiest classical meditation asana and is a simplified version of siddhasana.

Note: *Here the symbol of the swastika represents the different corners of the earth and universe, the spokes, and their meeting point and common centre of consciousness. This asana may be regarded as the one most favourable for realizing the unity of existence.*

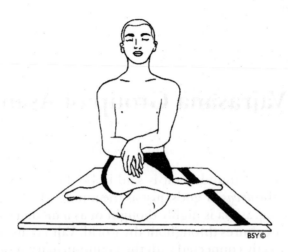

BSY ©

Dhyana Veerasana (hero's meditation pose)

Sit with both legs straight in front of the body.

Bend the left leg underneath the right leg so that the left heel is touching the right buttock.

Bring the right leg over the top of the bent left leg so that the right heel touches the left buttock.

Adjust the right knee so that it is above the left knee.

Place the hands either on the right knee, one on top of the other, or on top of each foot, whichever is comfortable.

Hold the head, neck and back straight.

Close the eyes and relax the whole body.

Be aware of the breath at the nosetip.

Benefits: This asana is quite easy and comfortable to sustain for long periods of time as a comparatively large area of the body is in contact with the floor. It is a useful alternative to other meditation asanas. The legs and hips are not rotated outwards as in the other meditation postures, rather the knees are brought to the centre. This affects the pelvic structure and stretches the outer rather than the inner muscles of the thigh. This position also massages and tones the pelvic and reproductive organs.

105

Vajrasana Group of Asanas

The *vajra* or thunderbolt is said to be the weapon of Indra, king of the *devas* or gods, just as the mind is the king of all the senses. Vajrasana is highly thought of as a meditation posture in many cultures throughout the world. Vajra is also the major nadi directly connected with the genito-urinary system, which regulates the sexual energy in the body. Control of vajra nadi leads to sublimation and control of sexual energy. The vajrasana series is therefore very beneficial for the reproductive as well as digestive organs and is also reasonably easy to perform.

Right-handed people will generally find that these asanas are easily learned with the right side leading. They should then be performed with the left side leading to counter balance the effects of habitual behaviour patterns.

Precautions: Do not practise vajrasana and other static asanas in this series until the ankles and knees are sufficiently flexible. Vajrasana is not advisable in osteoarthritis, or in pregnancy when extra weight can overload the knee joints. Carefully observe the contra-indications given for individual asanas.

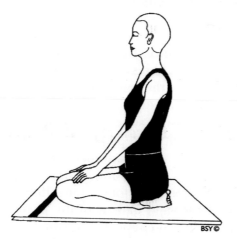

Vajrasana (thunderbolt pose)

Kneel on the floor with the knees close together.
Bring the big toes together and separate the heels.
Lower the buttocks on to the inside surface of the feet with the heels touching the sides of the hips.
Place the hands on the knees, palms down.
The back and head should be straight but not tense.
Avoid excessive backward arching of the spine.
Close the eyes, relax the arms and the whole body.
Breathe normally and fix the attention on the flow of air passing in and out of the nostrils.

Duration: For extended periods of time if performed for spiritual aims. A few minutes daily is sufficient to loosen up the legs. If any strain is experienced, stop the asana. Practise vajrasana directly after meals, for at least 5 minutes to enhance the digestive function. In cases of acute digestive disorder, sit in vajrasana and practise abdominal breathing for 100 breaths before and after food. Do not strain.

Awareness: Physical – on the sensations in the legs, buttocks and spine. When comfortable in the asana become aware of the normal breathing process. This will bring tranquillity to the mind if practised with the eyes closed.
Spiritual – on manipura chakra.

107

Benefits: Vajrasana alters the flow of blood and nervous impulses in the pelvic region and strengthens the pelvic muscles. It is a preventative measure against hernia and also helps to relieve piles. It reduces the blood flow to the genitals and massages the nerve fibres which feed them, making it useful in dilated veins of the testicles and hydrocele in men. It alleviates menstrual disorders. It increases the efficiency of the entire digestive system, relieving stomach ailments such as hyperacidity and peptic ulcer.

Vajrasana is a very important meditation posture because the body becomes upright and straight with no effort. It is the best meditation asana for people suffering from sciatica. It stimulates the vajra nadi, activates prana in sushumna and redirects sexual energy for spiritual purposes.

Practice note: If there is pain in the thighs, the knees may be separated slightly while maintaining the posture.

Beginners may find that their ankles ache after a short time in vajrasana. To remedy this, release the posture, sit with the legs stretched forward and shake the feet vigorously one after the other until the stiffness disappears. Then resume the posture.

Note: *Vajrasana is used by Muslims and Zen Buddhists as a position for prayer and meditation. People who cannot perform padmasana or siddhasana, or find them uncomfortable, may sit in vajrasana for meditation practice.*

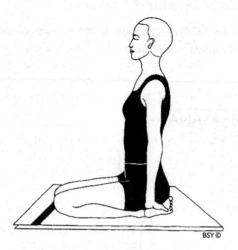

Ananda Madirasana (intoxicating bliss pose)

Sit in vajrasana.

Place the palms on top of the heels so that the fingers are pointing towards each other. If this is uncomfortable, place the palms just above the heels.

Keep the head and spine erect, close the eyes and relax the whole body.

Fix the attention at bhrumadhya, the eyebrow centre.

Breathing: Slow and deep. Imagine that the breath is moving in and out of the eyebrow centre. Inhale from the eyebrow centre to ajna chakra and exhale from ajna to the eyebrow centre.

Duration: For extended periods of time if performed for spiritual aims.

A few minutes daily is sufficient to loosen up the legs.

If any strain is experienced, stop the asana.

Awareness: Physical – in the early stages of the practice, awareness should be on the physical sensation, then on the breathing process. When sufficient relaxation has been achieved, awareness may be transferred to the eyebrow centre.

Spiritual – on ajna chakra.

Benefits: This asana is used primarily to awaken ajna chakra. It also calms the mind, relaxes the nervous system and gives all the benefits of vajrasana.

Note: *Ananda madirasana may be performed as an alternative to classical meditation postures.*

PADADHIRASANA

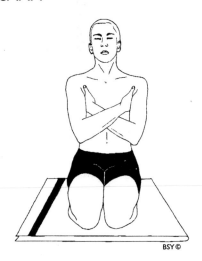

BSY©

Padadhirasana (breath balancing pose)

Sit in vajrasana.

Cross the arms in front of the chest, placing the hands under the opposite armpits with the thumbs pointing upward, or, for a stronger effect, make fists of the hands and place them under the armpits.

Close the eyes and become aware of the breathing process.

Breathing: Slow, deep and rhythmical. Practise until the flow of the breath in both nostrils becomes equalized.

Duration: To prepare for pranayama, practise until the flow of the breath equalizes, or for 5 to 10 minutes.

Awareness: Physical – on the breathing process in the nose. Spiritual – on ajna chakra.

Benefits: The pressure under both the armpits helps to open the nostrils to facilitate the practice of pranayama. Since the breath flow in the right and left nostrils influences the activities of the sympathetic and parasympathetic nervous systems respectively, opening of the two nostrils induces a state of autonomic balance.

Practice note: Padadhirasana may be used as a preparation for pranayama. It is specially useful when one or both nostrils are blocked.

If only one nostril is blocked, or partially blocked, place the hand of that side underneath the opposite armpit. Maintain the pressure for a minute or two, although changes may sometimes occur within a few seconds.

BHADRASANA

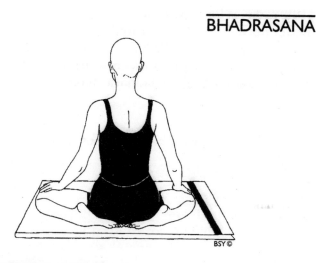

Bhadrasana (gracious pose)

Sit in vajrasana.

Separate the knees as far as possible, while keeping the toes in contact with the floor.

Separate the feet just enough to allow the buttocks and perineum to rest flat on the floor between the feet.

Try to separate the knees further, but *do not strain*.

Place the hands on the knees, palms downward.

When the body is comfortable, practise nasikagra drishti, concentration on the nosetip. As the eyes become tired, close them for a short time and then resume nosetip gazing.

Breathing: Slow and rhythmic with awareness of the breath at the nosetip.

Duration: For extended periods of time if performed for spiritual aims.

A few minutes daily is sufficient to loosen up the legs.

If any strain is experienced, stop the asana.

Awareness: Physical – sensations of opening and relaxing the perineum, and on the natural breath or the nosetip.

Spiritual – on mooladhara chakra.

Benefits: This is predominantly a pose for spiritual aspirants as it has a stimulating influence on mooladhara chakra. It is an excellent meditation pose. The benefits are basically the same as for vajrasana.

Practice note: If necessary, a folded blanket may be placed under the buttocks. Whether a blanket is used or not, it is important that the buttocks rest firmly on the ground in order to stimulate mooladhara chakra.

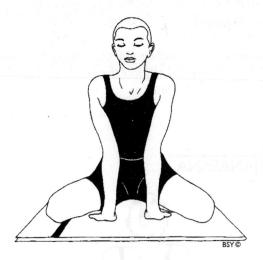

Simhasana (lion pose)

Sit in vajrasana with the knees about 45 cm apart.

The toes of both feet should remain in contact with each other.

Lean forward and place the palms of the hands on the floor between the knees, with the fingers pointing towards the body.

Straighten the arms fully and arch the back.

Rest the body on the straight arms.

Tilt the head back so that there is a comfortable amount of tension in the neck.

Close the eyes and focus the inner gaze at the eyebrow centre, performing shambhavi mudra.

The eyes may also be kept open, in which case gaze at a point on the ceiling.

The mouth should be closed.

Relax the whole body and mind.

Benefits: In this posture there is a very definite extension of the spinal cord and the body is absolutely fixed. There is total physical stability.

113

Note: *Generally, simhasana is associated with the roaring lion posture, but the scriptures give that posture as a variation of simhasana (see* simhagarjanasana, *the roaring lion, given in the following practice).*

In this asana the lion is sitting quietly, waiting for something to happen. This is the mental attitude the mind has to adopt in order to enter deep meditative states.

SIMHAGARJANASANA

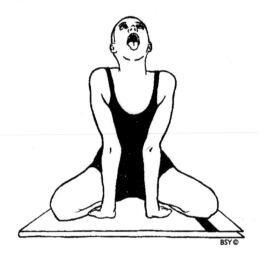

Simhagarjanasana (roaring lion pose)

Sit in simhasana.

Open the eyes and gaze at the eyebrow centre, adopting shambhavi mudra.

Relax the whole body.

Keep the mouth closed.

Inhale slowly and deeply through the nose.

At the end of inhalation, open the mouth and extend the tongue out as far as possible towards the chin.

While slowly exhaling, produce a clear, steady 'aaa' sound from the throat, keeping the mouth wide open. Do not

114

strain or force the sound in any way.

At the end of exhalation, close the mouth and breathe in. This is one round.

Breathing: Inhale slowly through the nose and then slowly exhale through the mouth with the 'aaah' sound.

Duration: To maintain general health practise 5 to 10 rounds daily.

The eyes, tongue and mouth may be relaxed for a few moments between each round.

This asana may be performed at any time.

Awareness: Physical – on opening the chest, and the sensation in the eyes and tongue. While inhaling, on the breath. While exhaling, on the sound produced, the feeling of emotional release, and the effect on the throat area.

Spiritual – on vishuddhi or ajna chakra.

Benefits: This is an excellent asana for the throat, nose, ears, eyes and mouth, especially if performed facing the healing rays of the early morning sun. It relieves frustration and releases emotional tension. Tension is removed from the chest and diaphragm. Simhagarjanasana is useful for people who stutter or who are nervous and introverted. It develops a strong and beautiful voice.

Other benefits are as for shambhavi mudra.

Variation: Move the tongue slowly from side to side, while making a long 'aaa' sound.

VEERASANA

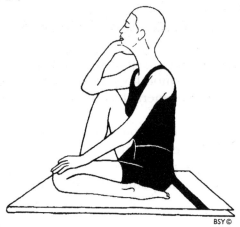

BSY©

Veerasana (hero's pose)

Sit in vajrasana.

Raise the right knee and place the right foot flat on the floor beside the inside of the left knee.

Put the right elbow on the right knee and rest the chin on the palm of the right hand.

Rest the left palm on the left knee.

Close the eyes and relax.

Keep the body completely motionless and the spine and head straight.

Hold for some time, then release the pose and relax the knees.

Repeat with the left foot placed beside the right knee.

Breathing: Slow, deep breathing, feeling that the energy synchronized with the breath is flowing in and out of bhrumadhya, the eyebrow centre.

Duration: Practise for a minimum of two minutes. Repeat on the other side with the left elbow on the left knee.

Awareness: Physical – on keeping the head and spine straight, on the sense of balance, and on the breath.

Spiritual – on ajna chakra.

Benefits: This asana balances the mind, increases the power of concentration, allows more awareness of the unconscious realms and induces physical and mental relaxation quickly.

The thinking process becomes very clear and precise. It is useful for those who think too much or who have disturbed or uncontrollable thoughts. It is very good for the kidneys, liver, reproductive and abdominal organs.

Note: *Veerasana is also known as the thinker's or philosopher's pose.*

Variation 1: This asana may also be practised by sitting on the heel so that it stimulates mooladhara chakra.

Variation 2: Sit on the heels in vajrasana.
Place the right foot on top of the left thigh as in the half lotus posture. The foot should come up on the thigh as near to the lower abdomen as is comfortable, and the right knee should rest on the floor.
Relax the whole body.
Slowly rise on to the knees, using the hands and left leg as levers and the right knee as a support.
The movement should be controlled without any jerking.
Place the palms together in front of the chest at the heart centre in the prayer position.
Straighten the spine.
When balanced, raise the hands above the head, keeping the palms together and the fingers pointing upward.
Hold the final position for as long as is comfortable.
Bring the hands back to the heart centre, feel the balance, then gently and evenly lower the body down to the floor.
Repeat with the left foot on top of the right thigh.
Practise up to 3 times on each side.

Breathing: Inhale while raising the body from the floor.
Breathe normally in the final position.
Exhale while lowering the body.

Awareness: Physical – on maintaining balance and steadiness in the upright position.
Spiritual – on swadhisthana chakra.

Contra-indications: Variation 2 should not be performed by people with weakness in the knees or inflammatory conditions such as arthritis, osteoarthritis, etc.

Benefits: This is a preliminary balancing pose which aids in stabilizing the nervous system.

MARJARI-ASANA

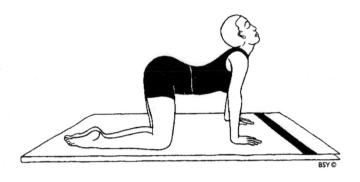

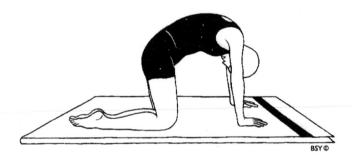

Marjari-asana (cat stretch pose)

Sit in vajrasana.

Raise the buttocks and stand on the knees.

Lean forward and place the hands flat on the floor beneath the shoulders with the fingers facing forward.

The hands should be in line with the knees; the arms and thighs should be perpendicular to the floor.

The knees may be slightly separated so that they are well aligned under the hips.

This is the starting position.

Inhale while raising the head and depressing the spine so that the back becomes concave.

Expand the abdomen fully and fill the lungs with the maximum amount of air. Hold the breath for 3 seconds.

Exhale while lowering the head and stretching the spine upward.

At the end of exhalation, contract the abdomen and pull in the buttocks.

The head will now be between the arms, facing the thighs. Hold the breath for 3 seconds, accentuating the arch of the spine and the abdominal contraction.

This is one round.

Breathing: Perform the movement breathing as slowly as is comfortable. Aim at taking at least 5 seconds for both inhalation and exhalation.

Duration: Perform 5 to 10 full rounds for general purposes.

Awareness: Physical – on the flexion of the spine from top to bottom, and on the breath synchronized with the movement.

Spiritual – on swadhisthana chakra.

Benefits: This asana improves the flexibility of the neck, shoulders and spine. It gently tones the female reproductive system, giving relief from menstrual cramps and leucorrhea. It may be safely practised during pregnancy; forceful contraction of the abdomen, however, should be avoided.

Practice note: Do not bend the arms at the elbows. Keep the arms and thighs vertical throughout.

VYAGHRASANA

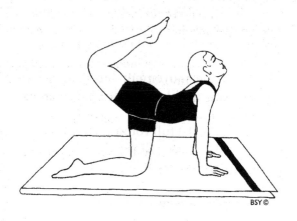

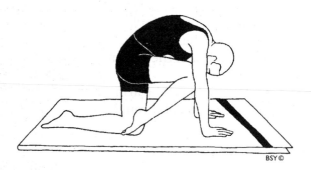

Vyaghrasana (tiger pose)

Assume the starting position for marjari-asana and look forward.

Relax the whole body.

Arching the back downwards, straighten the right leg, stretching it up and back.

Bend the right knee.

Look up and bring the toes towards the back of the head. Hold the breath for a few seconds in this position.

Straighten the right leg, bend the knee and swing the leg under the hips.

Simultaneously, arch the back up and bend the head down, bringing the knee towards the nose.

The right foot should not touch the floor.

The thigh presses against the chest.

Hold for a few seconds while retaining the breath outside.

Move the foot straight back and again stretch the leg.

Bend the knee and continue with the slow swinging movements.

After practising on one side, relax in marjari-asana.

Repeat with the other leg.

Breathing: Inhale while stretching the leg backward.

Retain in the final position.

Exhale while swinging the knee to the chest.

Duration: Perform this asana 5 times with each leg.

Awareness: Physical – on the forward and backward stretching of the spine and legs, and on the alternate compression and stretching of the abdomen and chest. Be aware of the balance, and the movement synchronized with the breath. Spiritual – on swadhisthana chakra.

Benefits: This asana exercises and loosens the back by bending it alternately in both directions and tones the spinal nerves. It relaxes the sciatic nerves, relieving sciatica, and loosens up the legs and hip joints. It tones the female reproductive organs and is especially beneficial for women after child-birth and those who have given birth to many children. It stretches the abdominal muscles, promotes digestion and stimulates blood circulation. Weight is reduced from the hips and thighs.

Note: *This asana is so called because it emulates the stretching movement made by a tiger.*

SHASHANKASANA

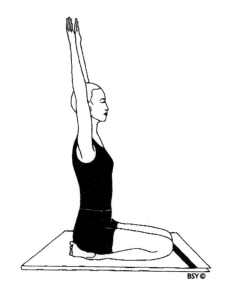

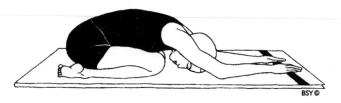

Shashankasana (pose of the moon or hare pose)

Sit in vajrasana, placing the palms on the thighs just above the knees.

Close the eyes and relax, keeping the spine and head straight.

While inhaling, raise the arms above the head, keeping them straight and shoulder width apart.

Exhale while bending the trunk forward from the hips, keeping the arms and head straight and in line with the trunk.

At the end of the movement, the hands and forehead should rest on the floor in front of the knees.

If possible, the arms and forehead should touch the floor at the same time.

Bend the arms slightly so that they are fully relaxed and let the elbows rest on the floor.

Retain the breath for up to 5 seconds in the final position. Then simultaneously inhale and slowly raise the arms and trunk to the vertical position. Keep the arms and head in line with the trunk.

Breathe out while lowering the hands to the knees.

This is one round.

Practise 3 to 5 rounds.

Duration: Beginners should slowly increase the length of time in the final position until they are able to hold it comfortably for at least 3 minutes with normal breathing. Those who wish to calm anger and frayed nerves should further increase the time to 10 minutes, breathing normally.

Awareness: Physical – in the final position, on the pressure of the abdomen against the thighs; on the alignment of arms, neck and head moving into and out of the asana; on the breath synchronized with the physical movement.

Spiritual – on manipura or swadhisthana chakra in the final position.

Contra-indications: Not to be performed by people with very high blood pressure, slipped disc or those who suffer from vertigo.

Benefits: This asana stretches and strengthens the back muscles and separates the individual vertebrae from each other, releasing pressure on the discs. Often nerve connections emanating from the spinal cord are squeezed by these discs, giving rise to various forms of backache.

This posture helps to relieve this problem in some cases and encourages the discs to resume their correct position. It also regulates the functioning of the adrenal glands. It tones the pelvic muscles and the sciatic nerves and is beneficial for both the male and female reproductive organs. Regular practice relieves constipation.

Note: *The Sanskrit word* shashank *means 'moon'. It is derived from two words:* shash *meaning 'hare' and* ank *meaning 'lap'. People in India have seen the dark patches on the full moon as resembling the shape of a hare with the moon in its lap. Furthermore, the moon symbolizes peace and calm; it emits soothing and tranquillizing vibrations. Shashankasana has a similar calming and cooling effect. More simply, it is the position frequently adopted by hares and rabbits.*

Variation 1: Sit in vajrasana and close the eyes.
Hold the right wrist with the left hand behind the back.
Relax the whole body and close the eyes.
Inhale and then, while exhaling, slowly bend the trunk forward from the hips so that the forehead rests on the floor. Remain in the final position for a comfortable length of time while breathing normally or deeply or in ujjayi.
Return to the starting position while inhaling.
Benefits: Gives the benefits of shashankasana. This variation is more advisable for people with back problems.
Variation 2: Sit in vajrasana.
Place the fists in front of the lower abdomen.
Inhale and then, while exhaling, slowly bend forward until the forehead touches the floor.
The fists will exert pressure on the lower abdominal organs.
Retain the breath out in the final position for as long as is comfortable.
Inhale while raising the trunk and head.
Practise 2 to 3 rounds.
Awareness: Physical – on the pressure of the fists in the abdomen in the final position.
Benefits: This variation massages and improves the efficiency of the intestines and digestive organs, relieving ailments such as constipation and excessive wind in addition to the benefits derived from the basic form of the practice.
Variation 3: Sit in vajrasana.
Interlock the fingers of both hands behind the back.
Inhale deeply. Then exhaling, move the head and trunk forward and rest the head on the floor.

Simultaneously, raise the arms up and bring them as far forward as possible.

Inhaling, raising the head and trunk and lowering the arms.

This is one round. Practise 2 to 3 rounds.

Benefits: This variation releases tension in the upper back and neck muscles, bringing great relief to those who experience stiffness in this area. It also gives the benefits of the basic practice.

Variation 4: If the forehead does not comfortably reach the floor, make two fists and place one vertically on top of the other. Rest the forehead on this support.

Benefits: This variation gives basically the same benefits as shashankasana and can be practised by people who are overweight or who have slightly raised blood pressure.

SHASHANK BHUJANGASANA

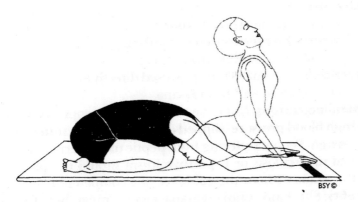

BSY©

Shashank Bhujangasana (striking cobra pose)

Assume the starting position for marjari-asana.

Lower the buttocks on to the heels, moving into shashankasana with the arms outstretched in front of the shoulders.

Then, to come into bhujangasana without moving the position of the hands, slowly move the chest forward,

125

sliding it just above the floor until it is in line with the hands. Move the chest further forward and then upward, as the arms straighten, and lower the pelvis to the floor.

Ideally, the nose and chest should just brush the surface of the floor as the body moves forward like the movement of a snake. Do not strain to achieve this.

In the final position, the arms should be straight, the back arched and the head raised as in bhujangasana, even if the navel does not touch the floor.

Hold this position for a few seconds.

Slowly raise the buttocks and move backwards, keeping the arms straight, returning to shashankasana.

This is one round.

Relax the whole body for a short time before starting another round.

Practise 5 to 7 rounds.

Breathing: Inhale on the forward movement.

Hold the breath for a few seconds in the final position.

Exhale while returning to shashankasana.

Awareness: Physical – on the flexibility of the spine and the sensation in the arms, shoulders, chest and abdomen; on synchronizing the movement with the breath.

Spiritual – on swadhisthana chakra.

Sequence: This asana may be practised directly after shashank-asana and followed by tadasana.

Contra-indications: Not to be performed by people with very high blood pressure, slipped disc or those who suffer from vertigo. People suffering from peptic ulcer, hernia, intestinal tuberculosis or hyperthyroidism should not practise this asana without the guidance of a competent teacher.

Benefits: Shashank bhujangasana gives similar benefits to bhujangasana and shashankasana. However, the benefits of the latter postures come from maintaining the final position, whereas shashank bhujangasana acts mainly by alternately flexing the spine backward and forward.

This asana gently tones the male and female reproductive organs, alleviates menstrual disorders and is an excellent post-natal asana, strengthening and tightening the abdominal and pelvic region. It tones and improves the functioning of the liver, kidneys and other visceral organs. It also strengthens the back muscles.

Practice note: The hand position should not change throughout the entire practice.

NAMAN PRANAMASANA

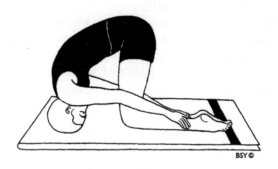

BSY©

Naman Pranamasana (prostration pose)

Sit in vajrasana. Grasp the lower calves just above the ankles, keeping the thumbs uppermost.

Slowly bend forward and place the crown of the head on the floor in front of the knees. (Place a small folded blanket under the head.)

Raise the buttocks as high as possible, allowing the chin to press against the chest, until the thighs are as vertical as comfortable.

Remain in the final position for 5 to 20 seconds.

Lower the buttocks and come back into shashankasana for a short time before returning to vajrasana.

Practise this asana 5 times.

Breathing: Inhale in vajrasana.

Exhale while lowering the head to the floor.

Inhale while raising the buttocks.

Hold the breath in the final position or breathe normally if remaining in the position for more than a few seconds.

Exhale while sitting the buttocks back on the heels.

Rest in shashankasana, breathing normally.

Inhale while raising the trunk and head and returning to vajrasana.

Awareness: Physical – on the increased pressure on the crown of the head in the final position, and on the synchronization of the breath with the physical movement.

Spiritual – on sahasrara chakra.

Contra-indications: Not to be performed by people with vertigo, weak neck or high blood pressure. Cautions for inverted postures apply.

Benefits: As a preparatory practice for sirshasana (the head-stand pose) it allows the brain to gradually adapt to the extra pressure in the head when the body is inverted. It gives many of the benefits of sirshasana, but to a lesser degree.

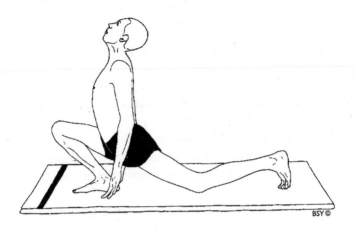

Ashwa Sanchalanasana (equestrian pose)

Sit in vajrasana.

Stand up on the knees with the knees and ankles slightly apart and the arms by the sides.

Starting with the right side, take a big step forward, placing the right foot firmly on the floor so that the thigh is horizontal and the ankle is before or directly under the knee.

This is the starting position. Centre yourself and inhale deeply.

Exhale and lunge forward smoothly, transferring the body weight on to the right foot.

The left leg becomes stretched back fully as the trunk comes forward, with the back straight.

Do not strain. Depending on flexibility, the fingertips or palms may touch the floor, or bend forward slightly so that the fingertips reach the floor.

In the final posture, the right foot, both hands, left knee and toes support the body. The back is slightly arched and the head faces forward.

To release the posture, inhale and roll the body weight back smoothly, centering in the starting position.

This is one round. Continue with the forward and backward lunges on this side.

After practising on one side, again stand on both knees, return to vajrasana and relax.

Stand on both knees, take a big step forward with the left foot into the starting position and practise an equal number of rounds on this side.

Practise up to 10 rounds on each side.

Breathing: Breathe normally in vajrasana and while coming into the starting position.

Inhale deeply in the starting position.

Exhale while moving forward into the posture.

Hold the breath for a few seconds while feeling the balance.

Inhale while returning to the starting position.

Breathe normally returning to vajrasana.

Awareness: Physical – on the back, thigh muscles, knees, ankles and Achilles tendons; on the balance and synchronizing the movement with the breath.

Spiritual – on swadhisthana chakra.

Contra-indications: Not for people with injured knees or ankles.

Benefits: This asana tones the abdominal organs and gives a good stretch to the lower back. It strengthens the hips, legs, ankles and feet, and induces balance in the nervous system.

Note: *This is the fourth asana practised in surya namaskara and chandra namaskara.*

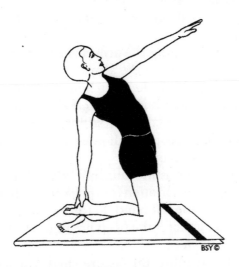

Ardha Ushtrasana (half camel pose)

Sit in vajrasana. Move the knees apart and the ankles to the side of the buttocks.

Stand up on the knees with the arms at the sides.

Keep the feet flat behind the body.

Stretch the arms sideways and raise them to shoulder level.

Do not strain in any way.

Twist to the right, reach back with the right hand and hold the left heel or ankle.

Simultaneously, stretch the left arm in front of the head so that the hand is at eyebrow level.

The head should be slightly back with the eyes gazing at the raised hand.

Push the hips forward in the final position and keep the thighs vertical.

Hold this position while comfortable, retaining the gaze on the left hand.

Return to the starting position.

Repeat on the other side to complete one round.

Practise 3 to 5 rounds.

Breathing: Inhale while stretching the arms sideways.
Exhale while twisting to the side.
Hold the breath out or breathe normally in the final position.
Inhale while bringing the arms back to shoulder level.
Exhale while releasing the arms.

Awareness: Physical–on the stretch in the back and neck, or on the normal breath if holding the posture.
Spiritual–on anahata or vishuddhi chakra.

Contra-indications: People with severe back ailments should not practise this asana.

Benefits: As given for ushtrasana, but at a reduced level.

Variation 1: A simpler variation is to place the right hand on the right heel and the left hand on the left heel. This posture also becomes easier if the heels are raised by balancing on the balls of the feet.

Variation 2: After twisting, the outstretched arm may be raised above the head to a vertical position. The head should be held back with the eyes gazing at the raised hand.

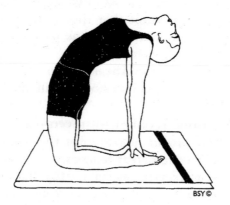

BSY©

Ushtrasana (camel pose)

Sit in vajrasana.

Stand on the knees with the arms at the sides.

The knees and feet should be together, but may be separated if this is more comfortable.

Lean backward, slowly reaching for the right heel with the right hand and then the left heel with the left hand.

Do not strain.

Push the hips forward, keeping the thighs vertical, and bend the head and spine backward as far as is comfortable.

Relax the whole body, especially the back muscles, into the stretch.

The weight of the body should be evenly supported by the legs and arms.

The arms should anchor the shoulders to maintain the arch of the back.

Remain in the final position for as long as is comfortable.

Return to the starting position by slowly releasing the hands from the heels one at a time.

Breathing: Normal. Do not try to breathe deeply because the chest is already stretched.

Duration: Practise up to 3 times as a dynamic asana.

Hold the final position up to 3 minutes as a static pose.

133

Awareness: Physical – on the abdomen, throat, spine or natural breathing.

Spiritual – on swadhisthana or vishuddhi chakra.

Sequence: It is important that this asana is followed by a forward bending asana, such as paschimottanasana, to release any tension in the back. The most convenient counterpose is shashankasana since it may be performed immediately from vajrasana without unnecessary body movement.

Contra-indications: People with severe back ailments such as lumbago should not attempt this asana without the guidance of a competent teacher.

Benefits: This asana is beneficial for the digestive and reproductive systems. It stretches the stomach and intestines, alleviating constipation. The backward bend loosens up the vertebrae and stimulates the spinal nerves, relieving backache, rounded back and drooping shoulders. The posture is improved. The front of the neck is fully stretched, toning the organs in this region and regulating the thyroid gland. It is helpful for people suffering from asthma.

Variation 1: To begin with this asana may be practised with the balls of the feet on the floor.

Variation 2: To accentuate the asana, the right heel may be grasped with the left hand and the left heel with the right hand.

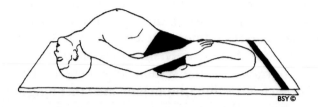

Supta Vajrasana (sleeping thunderbolt pose)

Sit in vajrasana. Slowly bend back, taking the support of first the right elbow and arm and then the left.

Bring the top of the head to the ground, arching the back. Find the balance in this position, then place the hands on the thighs.

Try to keep the knees in contact with the floor. If necessary, separate the knees. Care should be taken not to strain the muscles and ligaments of the thighs and knees by forcing the knees to touch the ground in the final position.

Close the eyes and relax the body.

Breathe deeply and slowly in the final position.

Return to the starting position by breathing in and taking the support of the elbows and arms to return to vajrasana.

Breathing: Deep and slow.

Duration: Beginners should start with only a few seconds in the final position, increasing the duration slowly. For physical benefits, up to one minute is sufficient.

For spiritual benefits, practise for longer periods.

Awareness: Physical – on the crown of the head, neck, lower back, abdomen or breath.

Spiritual – on swadhisthana, anahata or vishuddhi chakra.

Sequence: Follow supta vajrasana with a forward bending asana. The most convenient counterpose is shashankasana since it may be performed immediately from vajrasana without unnecessary body movement.

Contra-indications: This posture should not be practised by people suffering from neck problems, sciatica, slipped disc, sacral ailments or knee complaints.

Benefits: This asana massages the abdominal organs, alleviating digestive ailments and constipation. It tones the spinal nerves, makes the back flexible and realigns rounded shoulders. The nerves in the neck and the thyroid gland are particularly influenced. The chest is stretched and expanded to full capacity, filling the lungs and bringing more oxygen into the system. It is beneficial for those suffering from asthma, bronchitis and other lung ailments. It loosens up the legs in preparation for sitting in meditation asanas. It redirects sexual energy to the brain for spiritual purposes.

Practice note: Never leave the final position by straightening the legs first, as this may dislocate the knee joints. Return to vajrasana first and then straighten the legs.

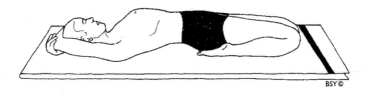

Variation: The back of the head, instead of the top, is placed on the floor in the final position.

Join the hands together and place them under the back of the head, or fold the arms comfortably above the head.

Try to keep the knees on the floor.

Close the eyes and relax the whole body.

Breathing: Deep and slow in the final position.

Benefits: This is an important variation which intensifies the stretch of the abdominal region, without placing pressure on the neck.

Practice note: Never leave the final position by straightening the legs first, as this may dislocate the knee joints. Return to vajrasana first and then straighten the legs.

Note: *The Sanskrit word* supta *means 'sleeping' and* vajra *refers to the nerve and energy pathway which connects the sexual organs to the brain.*

Standing Asanas

This series of asanas has a stretching and strengthening effect on the back, shoulders and leg muscles. They are particularly useful for those who spend a lot of time sitting down or who have stiffness or pain in the back. They improve posture, balance and muscular coordination. They also strengthen the muscles used to keep the back straight during meditation and increase oxygenation and lung capacity. Those who suffer from sciatica or slipped disc may practise bandha hasta utthanasana, akarna dhanurasana and tadasana, but should not practise any of the other standing asanas except under the guidance of a competent teacher. Carefully observe the specific contra-indications for each practice.

Right-handed people will find these asanas are easily learned with the right side leading. They should then be practised with the left side leading to counterbalance the effect of habitual behaviour patterns.

BANDHA HASTA UTTHANASANA

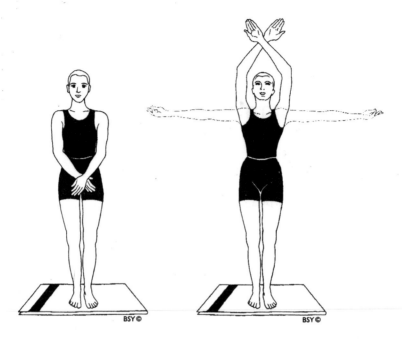

Bandha Hasta Utthanasana (locked hand raising pose)

Stand erect with the feet together and the arms by the sides. Relax the whole body and balance the body weight equally on both feet.

Cross the wrists in front of the body.

Slowly raise the arms above the head, keeping the wrists crossed, and at the same time bend the head slightly backward and look up at the hands.

Spread the arms out to the sides so that they form a straight line at shoulder level.

Hold the position, then reverse the movement, re-crossing the wrists above the head.

Lower the arms straight down so that they are once again in the starting position, and look forward.

Repeat the process 10 times.

Breathing: For beginners – inhale raising the arms, exhale while spreading them out to the sides, inhale while re-crossing the wrists above the head, and exhale while lowering the arms.

For more experienced practitioners – inhale while raising the arms and inhale more deeply while spreading them out to the sides. Exhale while re-crossing the wrists above the head and exhale more deeply while lowering the arms.

Awareness: On the stretch in the arms and shoulders, the expansion of the lungs, and on the breath synchronized with the movement.

Benefits: This asana rectifies round shoulders and removes stiffness from the shoulders and upper back. The deep, synchronized breaths improves breathing capacity. This asana also influences the heart and improves blood circulation. The whole body, especially the brain, receives an extra supply of oxygen.

AKARNA DHANURASANA

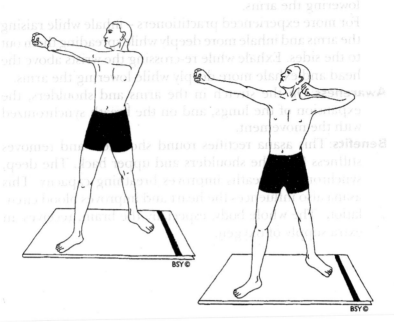

BSY©

BSY©

Akarna Dhanurasana (bow and arrow pose)

Stand erect with the feet shoulder width apart and the arms at the sides.

Take a short step forward with the right leg.

Clench the right fist and raise the arm in front of the body so that it is over the right foot and slightly above eye level.

Clench the left fist and bring it slightly behind the right fist.

Gaze over the right fist as though holding a bow and arrow, and fix the eyes on an imaginary target.

Inhale and slowly pull the left fist back to the left ear, tensing both arms as if drawing the bow. The head should move back slightly with this motion so the neck muscles become taut. Keep the left elbow up at shoulder level.

Exhale and release the imaginary arrow. Relax the neck and bring the left fist forward to the right fist.

Practise 10 times on each side.

Breathing: Inhale while pulling back the bowstring. Exhale while releasing the bowstring and bringing the hand forward.

Awareness: On the tensing of the arms, the imaginary target, and on the breath synchronized with the movement.

Benefits: This asana exercises the shoulders and also uses the short and deep muscles of the neck and shoulder blades. These muscles are not often exercised and can hold a significant amount of postural and subconscious tension which is responsible for stiffness and pain. The alternate tensing and relaxing smoothes out the energy flow and relaxes the muscles. This asana is helpful for people with bad posture, cervical spondylitis, writer's cramp and shoulder or arm stiffness.

TADASANA

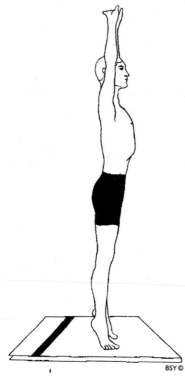

Tadasana (palm tree pose)
Stand with the feet together or about 10 cm apart, and the arms by the sides.
Steady the body and distribute the weight equally on both feet.
Raise the arms over the head.
Interlock the fingers and turn the palms upward.
Place the hands on top of the head.
Fix the eyes at a point on the wall slightly above the level of the head.
The eyes should remain fixed on this point throughout the practice.
Inhale and stretch the arms, shoulders and chest upward.
Raise the heels, coming up on to the toes.
Stretch the whole body from top to bottom, without losing balance or moving the feet.
Hold the breath and the position for a few seconds.
At first it may be difficult to maintain balance, but with practice it becomes easier.
Lower the heels while breathing out and bring the hands to the top of the head.
This is one round.
Relax for a few seconds before performing the next round.
Practise 10 rounds.

Breathing: Inhale while raising the arms, retain or breathe normally in the stretch, and exhale while lowering the arms.

142

Awareness: Physical – on the stretch of the whole body from top to bottom, and on maintaining balance and on the breath.

Spiritual – initially on mooladhara chakra to provide stability. Once balance is achieved, change to ajna chakra.

Sequence: Tadasana can be followed by any inverted asana.

Benefits: This asana develops physical and mental balance. The entire spine is stretched and loosened, helping to clear up congestion of the spinal nerves at the points where they emerge from the spinal column. It helps to increase height by stretching the muscles and ligaments, enabling growing bones to grow longer. Tadasana stretches the rectus abdomini muscles and the intestines, and is useful during the first six months of pregnancy to keep the abdominal muscles and nerves toned.

Variation 1: Tadasana may also be performed while gazing up at the interlocked fingers. It will be slightly more difficult to maintain balance in the final position.

Variation 2: Stand in tadasana with both arms overhead.
While balancing on the toes, lift one leg and extend it either forward or backward.
Repeat with the other leg.
Practise 10 times.

Practice note: Those practitioners who have mastered tadasana with the eyes open may try it with the eyes closed.

Note: *This is one of the asanas for shankhaprakshalana.*

TIRYAKA TADASANA

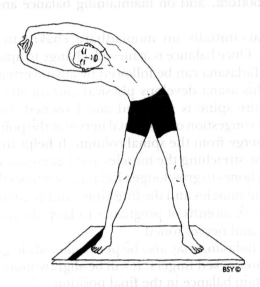

BSY©

Tiryaka Tadasana (swaying palm tree pose)
>   Stand with the feet more than shoulder width apart.
>   Fix the gaze on a point directly in front.
>   Interlock the fingers and turn the palms outward.
>   Raise the arms over the head, stretching upwards.
>   Bend to the right side from the waist.
>   Do not bend forward or backward or twist the trunk.
>   Hold the position for a few seconds, then slowly come back
>   to the upright position.
>   Repeat on the left side. This completes one round.
>   Practise 10 rounds.
>   To end the practice, return to the upright position, release
>   the hands, bringing the arms down to the sides.

Breathing: Inhale raising the arms, exhale while bending to the
>   side, inhale to centre. Exhale while releasing the posture.

Awareness: Physical – on keeping the balance and the stretch
>   along the side of the body. On keeping the body and head
>   facing forward while bending to the sides without twisting.
>   On the breath synchronized with the movement.
>   Spiritual – on mooladhara or manipura chakra.

Benefits: As for tadasana, but it especially massages, loosens and exercises the sides of the waist. It balances the right and left groups of postural muscles.

Variation: Balance on the toes in this practice.

Note: *This is one of the asanas for shankhaprakshalana.*

KATI CHAKRASANA

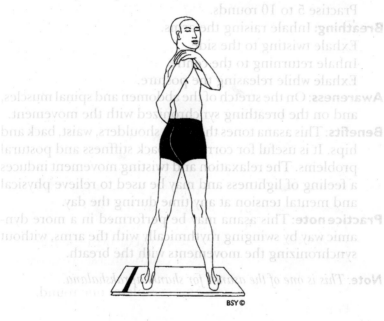

BSY©

Kati Chakrasana (waist rotating pose)

Stand with the feet about shoulder width apart and the arms by the sides.

Raise the arms to shoulder level, then twist the body to the right.

Bring the left hand to the right shoulder and wrap the right arm around the back, bringing the right hand around the left side of the waist. Look over the right shoulder as far as is comfortable.

145

Keep the back of the neck straight and imagine the top of the spine is the fixed point around which the head turns. Hold for two seconds, accentuate the twist, gently stretching the abdomen.

Return to the starting position.

Repeat on the other side to complete one round.

Keep the feet firmly on the ground while twisting.

Relax the arms and back as much as possible throughout the practice. Do not strain. The movement should be relaxed and spontaneous.

Perform the rotation smoothly, without jerking or stiffness.

Practise 5 to 10 rounds.

Breathing: Inhale raising the arms.

Exhale twisting to the side.

Inhale returning to the centre.

Exhale while releasing the posture.

Awareness: On the stretch of the abdomen and spinal muscles, and on the breathing synchronized with the movement.

Benefits: This asana tones the neck, shoulders, waist, back and hips. It is useful for correcting back stiffness and postural problems. The relaxation and twisting movement induces a feeling of lightness and may be used to relieve physical and mental tension at any time during the day.

Practice note: This asana may be performed in a more dynamic way by swinging rhythmically with the arms, without synchronizing the movements with the breath.

Note: *This is one of the asanas for shankhaprakshalana.*

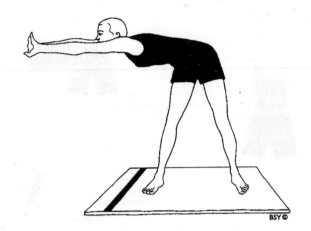

Tiryaka Kati Chakrasana (swaying waist rotating pose)
> Stand erect with the feet about shoulder width apart.
> Interlock the fingers in front of the body.
> Raise the arms over the head and rotate the wrists, turning the palms out.
> Bend forward from the hips to form a right angle between the legs and trunk.
> Watch the back of the hands and keep the back straight.
> Slowly swing the arms and trunk to the right as far as is comfortable, then to the left and then back to the centre.
> Return to the upright position and lower the arms.
> Practise 5 to 10 times.

Breathing: Inhale while raising the arms.
> Exhale while bending forward.
> Hold the breath while swinging from side to side.
> Inhale while raising the trunk and exhale while lowering the arms.

Contra-indications: This asana is quite strenuous and should not be practised by those with back problems, slipped disc or sciatica.

Benefits: As for kati chakrasana. This asana also strengthens the back muscles, and improves balance and coordination.

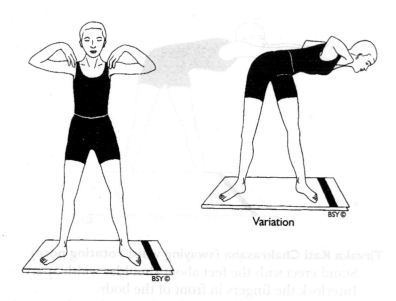

Variation

BSY©

BSY©

Meru Prishthasana (spine and back pose)

Stand erect with the feet shoulder width apart and the toes turned slightly out to the side. Place the fingers of both hands on the shoulders with the elbows pointing sideways. This is the starting position.

Twist the upper torso to the right as far as is comfortable and then return to the centre.

Repeat on the left side.

Practise 5 to 10 times on each side.

Breathing: Inhale while raising the fingers to the shoulders. Exhale while twisting to the sides. Inhale when returning to the centre. Exhale while lowering the arms.

Variation: After twisting to the side, bend from the hips to form a right angle, keeping the legs straight. The head, neck and spine should be in one straight line. The elbows should be level with the shoulders.

Stay in the position for up to 5 seconds.

Return to the upright position and twist to the front.

Repeat on the other side.

Breathing: Inhale while raising the fingers to the shoulders.
Retain the breath inside while twisting.
Exhale when bending forwards.
Inhale while raising the body to the upright position.
Exhale while lowering the arms.
Contra-indications: People with stiff backs or backache should avoid this asana.
Benefits: This asana stretches the spine, tones the back muscles and redistributes excess weight from the waistline.

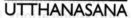

UTTHANASANA

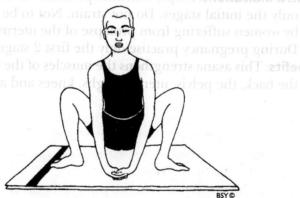

BSY©

Utthanasana (squat and rise pose)

Stand erect with the feet about one metre apart.
Turn the toes out to the sides where they remain throughout the practice.
Interlock the fingers of both hands and let them hang loosely in front of the body.

Stage 1: Slowly bend the knees and lower the buttocks about 20 cm. The knees should bend outward over the toes and the spine should be straight.
Straighten the knees and return to the upright position.

Stage 2: Bend the knees and descend about half a metre. Again return to the upright position.

Stage 3: Bend the knees and lower the buttocks until the hands are about 30 cm above the floor and then rise again.

Stage 4: Finally, lower the buttocks until the hands rest on or as near as possible to the floor.

Keep the arms and shoulders loose and avoid bending forward.

Stay in the final position for a few seconds. Then return to the upright position and relax the body.

Sequence: Beginners should practise only 5 rounds of those stages they can manage comfortably. Practise all the stages one after the other only when there is no strain.

Breathing: Exhale while lowering the body.

Inhale while raising the body.

Contra-indications: People with knee problems should practise only the initial stages. Do not strain. Not to be practised by women suffering from prolapse of the uterus.

During pregnancy practise only the first 2 stages.

Benefits: This asana strengthens the muscles of the middle of the back, the pelvis, uterus, thighs, knees and ankles.

Druta Utkatasana (dynamic energy pose)

Stand erect with both the feet together.

Place the palms together in front of the chest.

While inhaling, raise and straighten the arms above the head. While exhaling, slowly lower the body, bending the knees.

Keep the feet and knees together, and the arms straight throughout the practice.

Stage 1: Lower the body down about 30 cm.

Straighten the legs and return to the upright position.

Stage 2: Repeat the practice, lowering the body about half a metre before returning to the upright position.

Stage 3: Finally, lower the body until the buttocks rest on the floor. Inhale, raising to the upright position.

Breathing: Exhale while lowering the body.

Inhale while raising the body.

Sequence: Beginners should practise only 5 rounds of those stages they can manage comfortably. Practise all the stages one after the other only when there is no strain.

Contra-indications: Not during pregnancy, otherwise as for utthanasana.

Benefits: The muscles of the back and legs are strengthened.

Practice note: This asana stretches the ankles, knees and thighs. At first, therefore, it may be necessary to come on to the toes when squatting until the Achilles' tendons have become more flexible.

151

SAMAKONASANA

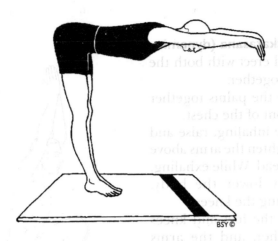

Samakonasana (right angle pose)
Stand with the feet together and the arms by the sides.
Raise the arms straight up above the head. Bend the wrists
so that the fingers are pointing forward.
Allow the hands to hang limp.
Arch the back slightly, pushing the buttocks out a little.
Slowly bend forward at the hips, keeping the legs straight,
until the back is horizontal and forms a right angle with the
legs. Keep the head, neck and spine in a straight line.
Hold the final position for up to 5 seconds.
Slowly return to the upright position, with the arms, head
and back in a straight line. Lower the arms.
Practise 5 to 10 rounds.
Breathing: Inhale while raising the arms above the head.
Exhale while bending forward.
Hold the breath in the final position.
Inhale while raising the trunk.
Exhale while lowering the arms.
Awareness: Physical – on keeping the spine straight and
maintaining balance, and on synchronizing the movement
with the breath.
Spiritual – on anahata chakra.

152

Contra-indications: This asana should not be practised by those suffering from acute sciatica. To avoid strain, people with backache should take care to bend from the hips and not from the waist.

Benefits: This asana works specifically on the shoulders and the back directly behind the chest. It rectifies tension and poor posture.

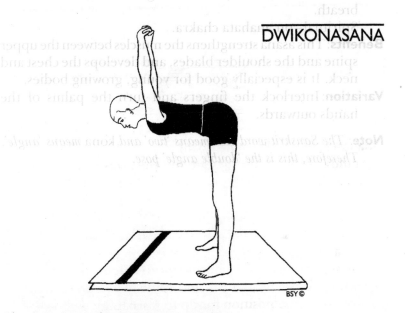

DWIKONASANA

Dwikonasana (double angle pose)

Stand erect with the feet 30 cm apart.

Extend the arms behind the back and interlock the fingers. This is the starting position.

Bend forward from the hips so that the back and face are parallel with the floor.

Raise the arms behind the back as high as possible without strain. The arms act as a lever and accentuate the stretch given to the shoulders and chest.

Remain in the final position for a short time, lower the arms to the back, and then return to the upright position.

Repeat up to 10 times.

Breathing: Inhale while standing erect.

Exhale while bending forward.

Inhale while raising the arms.

Exhale while lowering the arms.

Inhale while returning to the upright position.

Awareness: Physical – on the stretch of the arms, shoulders and upper back, on keeping the back straight and parallel to the floor, and on synchronizing the movement with the breath.

Spiritual – on anahata chakra.

Benefits: This asana strengthens the muscles between the upper spine and the shoulder blades, and develops the chest and neck. It is especially good for young, growing bodies.

Variation: Interlock the fingers and turn the palms of the hands outwards.

Note: *The Sanskrit word* dwi *means 'two' and* kona *means 'angle'. Therefore, this is the 'double angle' pose.*

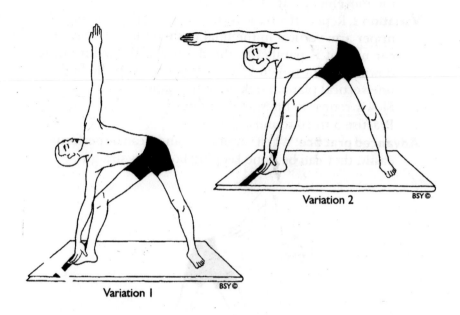

Variation 2 BSY©

Variation I BSY©

Trikonasana (triangle pose)

Variation I: Stand erect with the feet more than shoulder width apart. Turn the right foot to the right side.

Stretch the arms sideways and raise them to shoulder level so that they are in one straight line.

Bend to the right, taking care not to bring the body forward. Simultaneously bend the right knee slightly.

Place the right hand on the right foot, keeping the two arms in line with each other. Turn the left palm forward. Look up at the left hand in the final position.

Return to the upright position with the arms in a straight line.

Repeat on the other side, bending the left knee slightly. This completes one round.

Practise 5 to 10 rounds.

Breathing: Inhale while raising the arms. Exhale while bending. Hold the breath for a few seconds in the final position. Inhale while raising the body to the vertical position.

Awareness: On the stretch along the side of the trunk, legs and arms, on keeping the balance, and on coordinating the movement with the breath.

Variation 2: Repeat the basic form, but instead of keeping the upper arm vertical in the final position, lower it over the ear until it is parallel to the floor with the palm facing down. Try not to bend forward, but to keep the body in one vertical plane. Look up at the hand.

Slowly return to the starting position.

Practise 5 to 10 rounds.

Advanced practice: When variations 1 and 2 can be performed easily, they can be done keeping both legs straight.

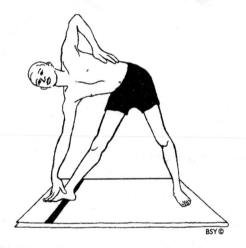

Variation 3: Stand with the feet more than shoulder width apart and the toes facing forward. Gaze directly in front.

Place the palms of the hands on each side of the waist with the fingers pointing downward.

Slowly bend to the right from the hips while sliding the right hand down along the outside of the right thigh as far as is comfortable.

Do not strain and do not bend forward in an effort to achieve the final position in which the right hand reaches the foot. Flexibility will come with practice.

Stay in the final position for a few seconds.

Raise the trunk to the upright position, returning the right hand to the waist.

Repeat on the left side to complete one round.

Practise 10 rounds.

Breathing: Inhale while standing erect with the hands on the waist. Exhale bending to the side.

Hold the breath for a few seconds in the final position. Inhale while returning to the centre.

Awareness: On the stretch along the side of the body, on taking care not to bend forward or strain, and on synchronizing the movement with the breath.

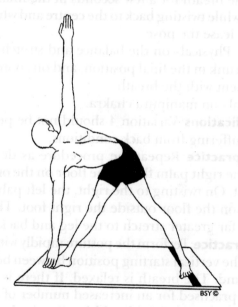

Variation 4: Stand erect with the feet more than shoulder width apart and raise the arms sideways to shoulder level. This is the starting position.

Bend forward.

Twist the trunk to the right, bringing the left hand to the right foot.

The right arm should be stretched vertically so that both arms form a straight line.

Look up at the right hand.

157

Hold the final position for a few seconds, feeling the twist and stretch of the back.

Return to the centre forward position.

Raise the body to the starting position, keeping the arms outstretched to the sides.

Repeat to the other side.

This is one round.

Do not lower the arms. Practise 5 to 10 rounds.

Breathing: Inhale in the starting position.

Exhale while bending forward and twisting.

Hold the breath for a few seconds in the final position.

Inhale while twisting back to the centre and when standing up to release the pose.

Awareness: Physical – on the balance and stretch on the side of the trunk in the final position, and on coordinating the movement with the breath.

Spiritual – on manipura chakra.

Contra-indications: Variation 4 should not be performed by those suffering from back conditions.

Advanced practice: Repeat the procedure as described, but place the right palm flat on the floor on the outside of the left foot. On twisting to the right, the left palm should be placed on the floor outside the right foot. This variation gives a far greater stretch to the leg and back muscles.

Dynamic practice: Perform the posture rapidly without returning to the vertical starting position between both halves of the round. The breath is relaxed. If there is no strain, it can be practised for an increased number of rounds.

Sequence: Each variation should be practised separately to increase flexibility and strength. When each can be practised without strain, they can be combined. This series may be performed daily for a few weeks to tone the entire body.

General benefits: This series affects the muscles on the sides of the trunk, the waist and the back of the legs. It stimulates the nervous system and alleviates nervous depression. It improves digestion. It also strengthens the pelvic area and tones the reproductive organs. Regular practice will help to reduce waistline fat.

158

Practice note: In all variations except 4, it is important not to bend forward, otherwise the benefits of the sideways stretch to the trunk will be lost. To avoid bending forward, pay particular attention to the position of the hips when bending to the side. For example, when bending to the right side, ensure that the left hip stays back and does not move forward.

Increasing the distance between the feet gives a more powerful stretch to the rarely used inner thigh muscles and the top of the thighs.

UTTHITA LOLASANA

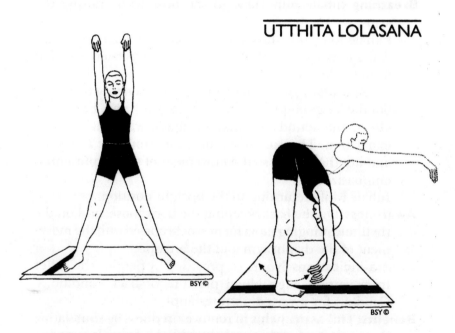

Utthita Lolasana (swinging while standing pose)

Stand erect with the feet a metre apart.

Raise the arms over the head, keeping the elbows straight.

Bend the wrists forward so that the hands hang limp.

Bend forward and swing the trunk down from the hips, allowing the arms and head to swing through the legs.

After this initial major swing, allow the body to swing

159

gently and spontaneously a few times. Then balance for a few moments while the trunk hangs down from the hips. Be tension-free like a rag doll.

Return smoothly to the upright position with the arms raised, then lower the arms to the sides.

Repeat up to 5 times.

Variation: To strengthen the back, after the first major swing downwards, on the subsequent upward swing, raise the trunk so that it is parallel to the floor. On the downward swing bring the hands as far back as comfortable behind the feet.

Breathing: Inhale fully through the nose while raising the arms.

Exhale forcefully through the mouth on each downward swing to make sure all the stagnant air has been expelled from the lungs.

While swinging up, inhalation will be a reflex action only, but the lungs empty totally on the down swing. For added effect, the sound 'ha' may be made with each forced exhalation. This sound should come from the abdomen and not the throat, so the movement of the diaphragm is emphasized.

Inhale while returning to the upright position.

Awareness: On the back, keeping the body loose, and on the rhythmic swinging movement synchronized with the movement of the diaphragm and the breath.

Contra-indications: Not to be practised by people who suffer from vertigo, high blood pressure or back conditions. Cautions for inverted postures apply.

Benefits: This asana helps to remove tiredness by stimulating the circulation and toning the spinal nerves. It stretches the hamstrings and back muscles, loosens the hips and massages the visceral organs. This is an excellent pre-pranayama practice as it opens up all the alveoli and helps drainage of stagnant mucus. It has the added benefits of inverted asanas, especially on the brain.

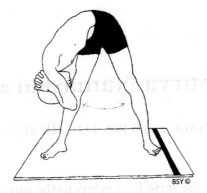

Dolasana (pendulum pose)

Stand with the feet more than shoulder width apart.
Raise the arms and interlock the fingers behind the neck with the elbows pointing sideways.
Turn slightly to the right and bend forward, keeping the feet firmly on the ground.
Bring the head as close as comfortable to the right knee.
The legs should remain straight throughout the practice.
Swing the upper torso from the right to the left knee and back to the right knee. Repeat 3 times.
Return to the centre and stand upright.
Repeat with the swing starting from the left knee.
This is one round, and is usually sufficient.

Breathing: Take a deep breath in while standing.
Exhale while bending forward.
Hold the breath out while swinging from side to side.
Inhale while coming up into the standing position.

Awareness: Physical–on the stretch of the back and the balance.
Spiritual–on swadhisthana chakra.

Contra-indications: Not to be performed by people suffering from vertigo, high blood pressure, sciatica or hiatus hernia.
Cautions for inverted postures apply.

Benefits: This asana strengthens the hamstrings and back muscles, makes the back supple and tones the spinal nerves.
It improves the blood circulation to the head and face.

Surya Namaskara

SALUTATIONS TO THE SUN

The Sanskrit name *surya* here refers to the sun and *namaskara* means 'salutations'. Surya namaskara has been handed down from the enlightened sages of the vedic age. The sun symbolizes spiritual consciousness and in ancient times was worshipped on a daily basis. In yoga the sun is represented by *pingala* or *surya nadi*, the pranic channel which carries the vital, life-giving force.

This dynamic group of asanas is not a traditional part of hatha yoga practices as it was added to the original asana group at a later time. However, it is an effective way of loosening up, stretching, massaging and toning all the joints, muscles and internal organs of the body. Its versatility and application make it one of the most useful methods of inducing a healthy, vigorous and active life, while at the same time preparing for spiritual awakening and the resulting expansion of awareness.

Surya namaskara is a complete *sadhana*, spiritual practice, in itself for it includes asana, pranayama, mantra and meditation techniques. It is an excellent group of asanas with which to start morning practice. Surya namaskara has a direct vitalizing effect on the solar energy of the body which flows through pingala nadi. Regular practice of surya namaskara regulates pingala nadi, whether it is underactive or overactive. Regulation of pingala nadi leads to a balanced energy system at both mental and physical levels.

Surya namaskara generates prana, the subtle energy which activates the psychic body. Its performance, in a steady, rhythmic

162

sequence, reflects the rhythms of the universe; the twenty-four hours of the day, the twelve zodiac phases of the year and the biorhythms of the body. The application of this form and rhythm to the body-mind complex generates the transforming force which produces a fuller and more dynamic life.

Preparation

Before practising surya namaskara, carefully observe the contra-indications for the seven component postures and ensure that they can be performed comfortably. Positions 2 and 3 are combined in the forward bending section as padahastasana variation. Positions 4 and 7 (ashwa sanchalan-asana and bhujangasana) are described independently in the vajrasana and backward bending sections. Positions 8 to 12 repeat the first five postures in reverse order.

General contra-indications

The practice of surya namaskara should be immediately discontinued if a fever, acute inflammation, boils or rashes occur due to excess toxins in the body. When the toxins have been eliminated, the practice may be resumed.

Surya namaskara includes semi-inverted postures, so the cautions for inverted postures apply. It should not be practised by people suffering from high blood pressure, coronary artery diseases, or by those who have had a stroke, as it may overstimulate or damage a weak heart or blood vessel system. It should also be avoided in cases of hernia or intestinal tuberculosis.

People with back conditions should consult a medical expert before commencing this practice. Conditions such as slipped disc and sciatica will be better managed through an alternative asana program.

During the onset of menstruation, this practice should be avoided. If there are no adverse effects, the practice may be resumed towards the end of the period. During pregnancy, it may be practised with care until the beginning of the twelfth week. Following childbirth, it may be commenced approximately forty days after delivery for re-toning the uterine muscles.

163

General benefits

The practice of surya namaskara as a whole gives a great number of benefits. It strengthens the back and helps balance the metabolism. It stimulates and balances all the systems of the body, including the reproductive, circulatory, respiratory and digestive systems. Its influence on the endocrine glands helps to balance the transition period between childhood and adolescence in growing children.

Synchronizing the breath with the physical movements of surya namaskara ensures that the practitioner, at least for a few minutes daily, breathes as deeply and rhythmically as possible, increasing mental clarity by bringing fresh, oxygenated blood to the brain.

Time of practice

The ideal time to practise surya namaskara is at sunrise, the most peaceful time of day, or sunset. Whenever possible, practise in the open air, facing the rising sun. Surya namaskara, however, may be practised at any time provided the stomach is empty.

Awareness

Before commencing the practice, stand with the feet together or slightly apart, and the arms hanging loosely by the sides of the body. Close the eyes gently and become aware of the whole physical body as one homogeneous unit. Minimize swaying movements and balance the body weight equally on both feet.

Take the awareness to the soles of the feet in contact with the floor. Feel that the whole body is being pulled downwards by gravity and that any tensions are being pulled down through the body and into the ground. At the same time, experience the vital force surging up from the earth and flooding the whole being.

Bring the awareness inside the body and mentally begin to relax it. Starting from the top of the head, take the awareness systematically through all the parts, releasing any tension. Intensify, once more, the awareness of the whole physical body and feel in harmony with it.

Finally, take the awareness to the heart or eyebrow centre and visualize a brilliant, red rising sun infusing the whole body and mind with its vitalizing and healing rays.

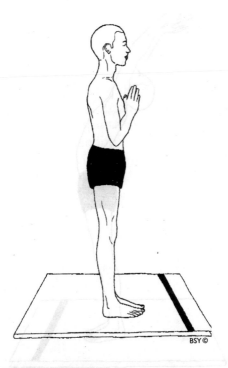

Position 1: Pranamasana (prayer pose)

Keep the eyes closed.

Remain standing upright with the feet together.

Slowly bend the elbows and place the palms together in front of the chest in namaskara mudra, mentally offering homage to the sun, the source of all life.

Relax the whole body.

Breathing: Breathe normally.

Awareness: Physical – on the chest area.

Spiritual – on anahata chakra.

Benefits: This pose establishes a state of concentration and calmness in preparation for the practice to be performed.

Mantra: *Om Mitraya Namaha*, salutations to the friend of all.

HASTA UTTHANASANA

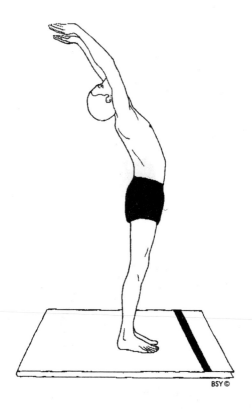

BSY©

Position 2: Hasta Utthanasana (raised arms pose)
Seperate the hands, raise and stretch both arms above the head, keeping them shoulder width apart.

Bend the head, arms and upper trunk slightly backward.

Breathing: Inhale while raising the arms.

Awareness: Physical – on the stretch of the abdomen and expansion of the lungs.

Spiritual – on vishuddhi chakra.

Mantra: *Om Ravaye Namaha*, salutations to the shining one.

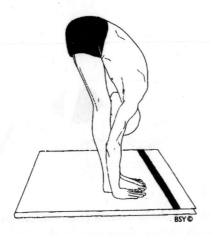

Position 3: Padahastasana (hand to foot pose)

Bend forward from the hips until the fingers or palms of the hands touch the floor on either side of the feet.

Bring the forehead as close to the knees as is comfortable. Do not strain.

Keep the knees straight.

Breathing: Exhale while bending forward.

Contract the abdomen in the final position to expel the maximum amount of air from the lungs.

Awareness: Physical – on the back and pelvic region.

Spiritual – on swadhisthana chakra.

Contra-indications: People with back conditions should not bend forward fully. Bend from the hips, keeping the spine straight, until the back forms a ninety degree angle with the legs, or bend only as far as is comfortable. Cautions for inverted postures apply.

Mantra: *Om Suryaya Namaha,* salutations to he who induces activity.

ASHWA SANCHALANASANA

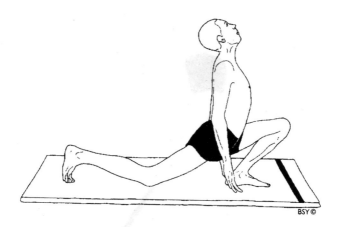

Position 4: Ashwa Sanchalanasana (equestrian pose)
Place the hands on the floor beside the feet.
Stretch the right leg back as far as is comfortable and grasp the floor with the toes.
At the same time, bend the left knee, keeping the left foot on the floor in the same position. Keep the arms straight.
In the final position, the weight of the body should be supported on both hands, the left foot, right knee and toes of the right foot. The head should be tilted backward, the back arched and the inner gaze directed upward to the eyebrow centre.

Breathing: Inhale while stretching the right leg back.

Awareness: Physical – on the stretch from the thigh through the lower back, and on the eyebrow centre while balancing. Spiritual – on ajna chakra.

Contra-indications: The full stretch is not advised for people with knee or ankle problems.

Mantra: *Om Bhanave Namaha,* salutations to he who illumines.

168

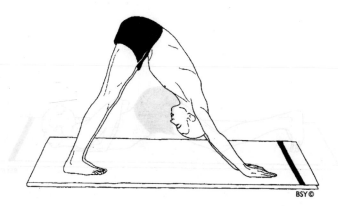

BSY©

Position 5: Parvatasana (mountain pose)

Keep the hands and right foot still, and take the left foot back beside the right foot. Simultaneously, raise the buttocks and lower the head between the arms so that the back and legs form two sides of a triangle.

The legs and arms straighten in the final position and the heels come down towards the floor in the final pose.

Bring the head and shoulders towards the knees.

Do not strain.

Breathing: Exhale while taking the left leg back.

Awareness: Physical – on the stretch through the Achilles' tendons, the back of the legs, shoulders and throat region, and on relaxing the hips.

Spiritual – on vishuddhi chakra.

Contra-indications: Cautions for inverted postures apply.

Benefits: This pose strengthens the nerves and muscles in the limbs and back. It helps to increase height by stretching muscles and ligaments, enabling growing bones to grow longer. Circulation is stimulated, especially in the upper spine between the shoulder blades.

Mantra: *Om Khagaya Namaha*, salutations to he who moves quickly in the sky.

ASHTANGA NAMASKARA

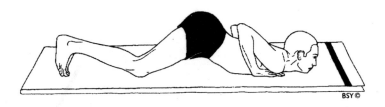

Position 6: Ashtanga Namaskara (salute with eight parts or points)
Keep the hands and feet in place.
Lower the knees, chest and chin to the floor; the feet will come up on to the toes.
In the final position only the toes, knees, chest, hands and chin touch the floor. The knees, chest and chin should touch the floor simultaneously. If this is not possible, first lower the knees, then the chest, and finally the chin.
The buttocks, hips and abdomen should be raised.
Breathing: The breath is held out in this pose. There is no respiration.
Awareness: Physical – on the arch in the lower back and on the abdominal region.
Spiritual – on manipura chakra.
Contra-indications: People with serious back problems, high blood pressure or heart conditions should not do this practice.
Benefits: This pose strengthens the leg and arm muscles, develops the chest and exercises the region of the spine between the shoulder blades.
Mantra: *Om Pushne Namaha,* salutations to the giver of strength.

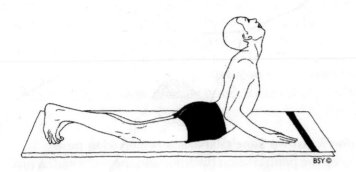

BSY©

Position 7: Bhujangasana (cobra pose)

Keep the hands and feet in place.

Slide the chest forward and raise first the head, the shoulders, then, straightening the elbows, arch the back into the cobra pose. This will lower the buttocks and hips to the floor.

Bend the head back and direct the gaze upward to the eyebrow centre.

The thighs and hips remain on the floor and the arms support the trunk.

Unless the spine is very flexible the arms will remain slightly bent.

Breathing: Inhale while raising the torso and arching the back.

Awareness: Physical – on relaxation of the spine.

Spiritual – on swadhisthana chakra.

Contra-indications: Not advised for people suffering from peptic ulcer, hernia, intestinal tuberculosis or hyperthyroidism.

Mantra: *Om Hiranya Garbhaya Namaha,* salutations to the golden, cosmic self.

171

Position 8: Parvatasana (mountain pose)

The hands and feet do not move from position 7.

From bhujangasana assume parvatasana.

Keep the arms and legs straight, grip the floor with the toes and use the strength of the arms to raise the buttocks and lower the heels to the floor.

Breathing: Exhale while raising the buttocks.

Awareness: As for position 5.

Mantra: *Om Marichaye Namaha,* salutations to the Lord of the Dawn.

Position 9: Ashwa Sanchalanasana (equestrian pose)

Keep the palms flat on the floor and the right foot in place. Bend the left leg and bring the left foot forward between the hands. Simultaneously, lower the right knee so that it touches the floor and push the pelvis forward.

Tilt the head backward, arch the back and gaze at the eyebrow centre.

Breathing: Inhale while assuming the pose.

Awareness: As for position 4.

Mantra: *Om Adityaya Namaha,* salutations to the son of Aditi, the cosmic Mother.

Position 10: Padahastasana (hand to foot pose)

Bring the right foot forward next to the left foot.

Straighten both legs.

Bring the forehead as close to the knees as possible without straining.

Breathing: Exhale while performing the movement.

Awareness: As for position 3.

Mantra: *Om Savitre Namaha,* salutations to the Lord of Creation.

Position 11: Hasta Utthanasana (raised arms pose)

Keep the arms and spine in a straight line.

Raise the torso and stretch the arms above the head.

Keep the arms separated, shoulder width apart.

Bend the head, arms and upper trunk backward slightly.

Breathing: Inhale while straightening the body.

Awareness: As for position 2.

Mantra: *Om Arkaya Namaha,* salutations to he who is fit to be praised.

Position 12: Pranamasana (prayer pose)

Bring the palms together in front of the chest.

Breathing: Exhale while assuming the final position.

Awareness: As for position 1.

Mantra: *Om Bhaskaraya Namaha,* salutations to he who leads to enlightenment.

Positions 13–24: The twelve positions of surya namaskara are practised twice to complete one round. Positions 1 to 12 constitute half a round. In the second half, the positions are repeated with two small changes related to ashwa sanchalanasana:

a) In position 16, instead of stretching the right foot backward, stretch the left foot back.

b) In position 21, bend the right leg and bring the right foot between the hands.

Conclusion: On the completion of each half round, lower the arms to the side, relax the body and concentrate on the breath until it returns to normal. After completing surya namaskara, practise shavasana for a few minutes. This will allow the heartbeat and respiration to return to normal and all the muscles to relax.

Duration: For spiritual benefits, practise 3 to 12 rounds slowly. For physical benefits, practise 3 to 12 rounds more quickly. Beginners should start with 2 or 3 rounds and add one more round every few weeks to avoid fatigue. Advanced students may practise a larger number of rounds; however, strain should be avoided at all times. In special cases, a daily practice of 108 rounds may be undertaken for purification, but only under the guidance of a competent teacher.

Beeja mantras: As an alternative to the twelve names of the sun, there is a series of *bija mantras* or seed syllables. Bija mantras do not have any literal meaning, but set up powerful vibrations of energy within the mind and body.

173

The six bija mantras are repeated consecutively in the following order, four times during a complete round of surya namaskara:

1. *Om Hraam*   4. *Om Hraim*
2. *Om Hreem*   5. *Om Hraum*
3. *Om Hroom*   6. *Om Hrah*

Bija mantras are used when surya namaskara is practised too fast to repeat the sun mantras, or in order to deepen the practice.

Chandra Namaskara

SALUTATIONS TO THE MOON

The word *chandra* means 'moon'. Just as the moon, having no light of its own, reflects the light of the sun, so the practice of chandra namaskara reflects that of surya namaskara. The sequence of asanas is the same as surya namaskara except that *ardha chandrasana*, the half moon pose, is performed after ashwa sanchalanasana. Also, in ashwa sanchalanasana the left leg is extended back in the first half of the round, activating *ida nadi*, the lunar force. In the second half of the round, the right leg is extended back. The inclusion of ardha chandrasana is a significant change. This posture develops balance and concentration, adding another dimension to the practice. A further effect is that the breathing pattern becomes more demanding; inhalation, exhalation and breath retention are all prolonged.

Whereas the twelve positions of surya namaskara relate to the twelve zodiac or solar phases of the year, the fourteen positions of chandra namaskara relate to the fourteen lunar phases. In the lunar calendar the fourteen days before the full moon are known as *shukla paksha*, the bright fortnight, and the fourteen days after the full moon are known as *krishna paksha*, the dark fortnight.

The lunar energy flows within ida nadi. It has cool, relaxing and creative qualities. Ida is the introverted, feminine or mental force which is responsible for consciousness.

Preparation

It is advisable to learn surya namaskara before attempting chandra namaskara as the postures are the same for both,

175

except for one extra pose. In chandra namaskara the added pose, ardha chandrasana, is inserted in the sequence at positions 5 and 11, in the first half of the round, and positions 19 and 25 in the second. Ardha chandrasana is described as an independent practice in the backward bending section. Its insertion as position 5 prolongs the inhalation begun in ashwa sanchalanasana, then prolongs the exhalation and external retention through postions 6 and 7 (parvatasana and ashtanga namaskara). Its insertion as position 11 similarly lengthens inhalation and then exhalation into padahastasana.

Time of practice

Chandra namaskara is best practised in the evening or at night, especially when the moon is visible, or at dawn at the time of the full moon. When practising at night, ensure that the stomach is empty.

Awareness

Before beginning chandra namaskara, a few moments should be given to prepare the body and mind.

Stand in the upright position with the feet together, the eyes closed and the arms at the sides. The weight of the body should be evenly distributed on both feet. Observe any spontaneous movement of the body as it relaxes.

Gradually become more aware of the natural flow of the breath with each inhalation and exhalation. Then include awareness of the movement in the body with the rhythm of the breath. Retain this awareness for a few moments.

Slowly withdraw the awareness from the breath and become aware of *bhrumadhya*, the space between the eyebrows. Within this space, visualize the full moon in a clear night sky, shining brightly upon the waves of the ocean. The full reflection of the moon penetrates the deep waters and the cool shade of moonlight catches the tops of the waves as they dance. See the image clearly and develop awareness of any feelings or sensations that are created in the mind and body.

Slowly let the visualization fade and again become aware of the whole body in the standing position.

ARDHA CHANDRASANA

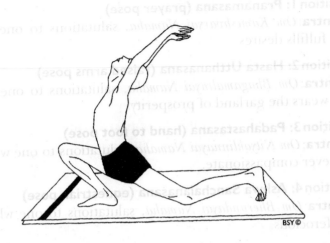

Position 5: Ardha Chandrasana (half-moon pose)

With the left leg extended back, maintain the balance in the full stretch of ashwa sanchalanasana, raise the hands and stretch both arms over the head, keeping the arms shoulder width apart. Arch the back and look up, raising the chin.

There should be a gentle curve from the tips of the fingers to the tips of the toes, resembling a crescent moon.

Hold the pose for a short time.

Lower the arms and place the hands on each side of the front foot as in position 4.

Breathing: Inhale deeply while raising the arms, arching the back and bending the head back.

Retain the breath inside while holding the posture for a few seconds.

Start exhalation while lowering the arms.

Awareness: Physical – on the smooth controlled movement and balance.

Spiritual – on vishuddhi chakra.

177

CHANDRA MANTRAS

Position 1: Pranamasana (prayer pose)
Mantra: *Om Kameshvaryai Namaha*, salutations to one who fulfills desires.

Position 2: Hasta Utthanasana (raised arms pose)
Mantra: *Om Bhagamalinyai Namaha*, salutations to one who wears the garland of prosperity.

Position 3: Padahastasana (hand to foot pose)
Mantra: *Om Nityaklinnayai Namaha*, salutations to one who is ever compassionate.

Position 4: Ashwa Sanchalanasana (equestrian pose)
Mantra: *Om Bherundayai Namaha*, salutations to one who is ferocious.

Position 5: Ardha Chandrasana (half moon pose)
Mantra: *Om Vahnivasinyai Namaha*, salutations to one who resides in fire.

Position 6: Parvatasana (mountain pose)
Mantra: *Om Vajreshvaryai Namaha*, salutations to one who possesses vajra, the thunderbolt, and is adorned with diamond ornaments.

Position 7: Ashtanga Namaskara (salute with 8 parts)
Mantra: *Om Dutyai Namaha*, salutations to one whose messenger is Shiva.

Position 8: Bhujangasana (cobra pose)
Mantra: *Om Tvaritayai Namaha*, salutations to one who is swift.

Position 9: Parvatasana (mountain pose)
Mantra: *Om Kulasundaryai Namaha*, salutations to one who is virtuous, respectable and charming.

Position 10: Ashwa Sanchalanasana (equestrian pose)
Mantra: *Om Nityayai Namaha*, salutations to one who is eternal.

Position 11: Ardha Chandrasana (half moon pose)
Mantra: *Om Nilapatakinyai Namaha*, salutations to one who is adorned with a blue flag.

Position 12: Padahastasana (hand to foot pose)
Mantra: *Om Vijayayai Namaha*, salutations to one who is ever victorious.

Position 13: Hasta Utthanasana (raised arms pose)
Mantra: *Om Sarvamangalayai Namaha*, salutations to one who is the source of all good fortunes.

Position 14: Pranamasana (prayer pose)
Mantra: *Om Jvalamalinyai Namaha*, salutations to one who is fenced with instant flames.

Positions 15–28: Positions 1–14 form the first half of the round and positions 15–28 form the second. In the second half, the same mantras are repeated consecutively and the same positions are repeated with the following changes:
   a) in position 18, ashwa sanchalanasana, instead of stretching the left foot backward, strech the right foot back.
   b) in position 24, the same pose, bend the left knee, bringing the left foot forward between the hands.

Practice: Ardha chandrasana emphasizes the link with the lunar energies set up by the preparatory visualizations. Also, in chandra namaskara the force of each asana is changed subtly by the repetition of mantras related to the lunar energies.

Conclusion: After completing the desired number of rounds, stand upright with the eyes closed, the hands by the sides of the body and again visualize the full moon shining over the waves of the ocean until the body becomes steady. Relax in shavasana.

Duration: For spiritual benefits, slowly practise 3 to 7 rounds.

For physical benefits, practise 3 to 7 rounds more quickly.

Other details: As given for surya namaskara.

Asana

Intermediate Group

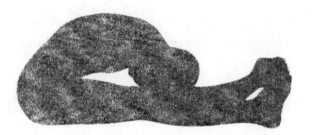

Padmasana Group of Asanas

Padmasana is traditionally regarded as one of the best postures for pranayama and pratyahara as it allows the body to be held completely steady for long periods of time. As the body is steadied, the mind becomes calm and gives a firm foundation for concentration. Padmasana directs the flow of prana from mooladhara chakra in the perineum to sahasrara at the crown of the head, heightening the experience of meditation.

The asanas in this chapter clear physical, emotional and mental blocks, help awaken the energy centres of the body and induce tranquillity. They increase the ability to sit in padmasana for extended periods of time as required for advanced meditation practices, but should only be practised by people who can already sit in padmasana without the slightest difficulty or strain.

Those who suffer from sciatica or weak or injured knees should not perform these asanas until flexibility of the knees has been developed through practice of the pre-meditation asanas. Padmasana is not advisable during pregnancy as the circulation in the legs is reduced. The contra-indications given for individual asanas should also be closely observed.

In all the asanas discussed in this chapter, either the left or the right leg may be placed uppermost. It is a matter of personal preference and depends on whichever is more comfortable. Ideally, the leg position should be alternated so that the balance on both sides of the body is maintained.

YOGAMUDRASANA

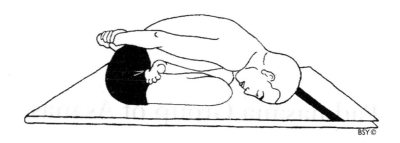

Yogamudrasana (psychic union pose)

Sit in padmasana and close the eyes.

Relax the body for some time, breathing normally.

Hold one wrist behind the back with the other hand.

Inhale deeply.

While exhaling, bend forward, keeping the spine straight.

Bring the forehead to the floor or as close as is comfortable.

Relax the whole body in the final position, breathing slowly and deeply. Be aware of the pressure of the heels on the abdomen.

Stay in the final position for as long as is comfortable.

Do not strain the back, ankles, knees or thighs by forcing the body into the posture or staying in it for too long.

Slowly return to the starting position.

Repeat the pose with the legs crossed the other way around.

Breathing: Inhale slowly and deeply in the starting position. Exhale while bending forward.

Breathe deeply and slowly in the final position.

Inhale while returning to the starting pose.

Duration: Remain in the final position for one or two minutes if comfortable.

Awareness: Physical–on the back, abdomen or breathing. Spiritual–on manipura chakra.

Sequence: Ideally preceded or followed by a backward bending asana such as matsyasana (with the legs stretched out), ushtrasana or bhujangasana.

Contra-indications: People with serious eye, back or heart conditions, or with high blood pressure, and those in the early post-operative or post-delivery period should not attempt this asana.

Benefits: This is an excellent asana for massaging the abdominal organs, removing constipation and indigestion. It stretches the back, freeing the spinal nerves which emerge from the spaces between the vertebrae, thus contributing to good general health. Yogamudrasana is used to awaken manipura chakra.

Variation: (for beginners)

This variation follows the same method as the basic technique except that instead of remaining in the final position, the body is raised and lowered a number of times.

It is particularly useful for those who are stiff and cannot touch the floor with their foreheads. Synchronize the movement with the breath.

MATSYASANA

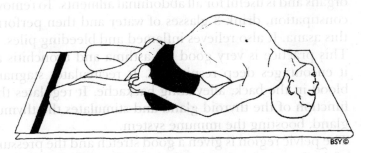

BSY©

Matsyasana (fish pose)

Sit in padmasana and relax the whole body.

Carefully bend backward, supporting the body with the arms and elbows. Lift the chest slightly, take the head back and lower the crown of the head to the floor.

Hold the big toes and rest the elbows on the floor.

Adjust the position of the head so that the maximum arch of the back is attained.

185

Relax the arms and the whole body, allowing the head, buttocks and legs to support the weight of the body.

Close the eyes and breathe slowly and deeply.

Return to the starting position, reversing the order of movements.

Repeat the asana, with the legs crossed the other way.

Breathing: Breathe deeply and slowly in the final position.

Duration: The final position may be held for up to 5 minutes, although 1 to 3 minutes is sufficient for general health.

Awareness: Physical – on the abdomen, chest, neck and head or breath.

Spiritual – on manipura or anahata chakra.

Sequence: Halasana or sarvangasana are the ideal counterposes as they stretch the neck in the opposite direction, releasing any muscular tension.

Contra-indications: People who suffer from heart disease, peptic ulcers, hernia, back conditions or any serious illness should not practise this asana. Pregnant women should also not attempt it.

Benefits: This asana stretches the intestines and abdominal organs and is useful for all abdominal ailments. To remove constipation, drink 3 glasses of water and then perform this asana. It also relieves inflamed and bleeding piles.

This practice is very good for asthma and bronchitis as it encourages deep respiration. It recirculates stagnant blood in the back, alleviating backache. It regulates the function of the thyroid gland and stimulates the thymus gland, boosting the immune system.

The pelvic region is given a good stretch and the pressure of the feet on the thighs greatly reduces blood circulation in the legs, diverting it to the pelvic organs. Youthfulness and vitality are increased.

Practice note: It is important that the body is slowly lowered into and raised from the final position by using the elbows as a support. The movement should be performed with control and care as it is very easy to injure the spine.

Note: *The way of folding the legs in matsyasana resembles the tail of a fish, while the rest of the body represents its body and head.*

Variation 1: This variation follows the basic technique except for the position of the hands.

Interlock the fingers of both hands. Place the hands behind the head and rest the back of the head in the open palms.

Variation 2: (for beginners)

Sit with the legs stretched forward.

Fold one leg, placing the foot on the opposite thigh as in ardha padmasana, the half lotus pose.

Keep the other leg straight in front of the body.

Slowly bend backward, using the elbows for support, and lower the crown of the head to the floor.

Hold the foot of the bent leg with both hands.

Accentuate the arch of the back as much as possible without straining.

Relax the whole body and close the eyes.

Remain in the final position for a comfortable length of time and then return to the starting position.

Repeat the same pose with the other leg folded.

As an alternative, rest the back of the head on the floor instead of the top of the head.

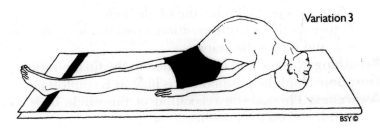

Variation 3

BSY©

Variation 3: (for beginners)

Stretch both legs straight in front of the body.

Lean backward, using the arms for support, and rest the top of the head on the floor. Arch the back and place both palms on the thighs or let them rest on the floor. As an alternative, this can be done from the lying position. Return to the starting position after some time in the final position.

187

GUPTA PADMASANA

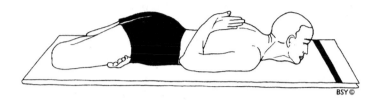

BSY©

Gupta Padmasana (hidden lotus pose)
Assume padmasana.
Place the hands on the floor in front of the knees. Leaning on the arms, raise the buttocks and stand on the knees.
Slowly lower the front side of the body to the floor in the prone position.
Rest the chin on the floor.
Place the palms together behind the back.
The fingers may point downward, or upward in hamsa mudra. If possible, touch the back of the head with the middle fingers.
Close the eyes and relax the whole body.
Return to the starting position, cross the legs the other way and repeat the asana.
Breathing: Normal and unrestrained in the final position.
Duration: Hold the position for as long as is comfortable.
Awareness: Physical–on relaxation of the whole body and mind, and on the breath.
Spiritual–on anahata chakra.
Benefits: This asana helps to correct postural defects of the spine and so is useful in achieving a productive meditation posture. It may be used as a relaxation pose as it induces peace, stability and emotional balance.
Variation: For complete relaxation, the hands may rest on the floor beside the body with the palms upward. Also the head can be turned to one side, resting one cheek on the floor. After some time, gently turn the head to the other side for an equal length of time.

188

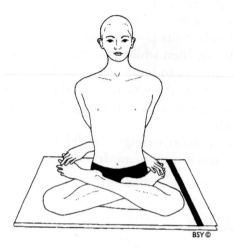

BSY©

Baddha Padmasana (locked lotus pose)

Sit in padmasana.

Take the arms behind the back and cross them.

Exhale, leaning forward slightly, and reach for the right big toe with the right hand and the left big toe with the left hand.

If it is difficult to grasp the toes, stretch the shoulders back so that the shoulder blades are brought nearer to each other. Hold the big toe of the foot which is uppermost first.

Remain in the final position for as long as is comfortable. Return to padmasana, cross the legs the other way around and repeat the practice.

Breathing: Deep and slow in the final position.

Awareness: Physical – on the abdomen or breathing process. Spiritual – on anahata chakra.

Contra-indications: People with serious eye, back or heart conditions, or with high blood pressure, hernia or hydrocele should not practise this asana or its variation, also those in the early post-operative or post-delivery period.

Benefits: It alleviates pain in the shoulders, arms and back. It encourages normal growth in children with poorly developed chests. Spiritually, it is used in the process of awakening kundalini.

Sequence: An excellent preliminary for meditation practices.

Variation: Sit in baddha padmasana.

Inhale deeply then while exhaling bend forward without straining and try to touch the forehead to the floor.

Remain in the final position while comfortable with normal breathing. Inhale while returning to the upright position. Gently release.

Benefits: The variation massages the abdominal organs, stretches the back, and is used to awaken manipura chakra.

LOLASANA

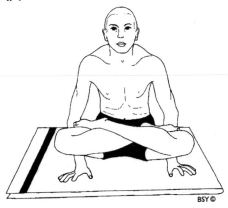

BSY©

Lolasana (swinging pose)

Sit in padmasana.

Place the palms on the floor beside the thighs.

Inhale deeply.

Raise the whole body from the floor, balancing only on the hands.

Swing the body backward and forward between the arms.

Lower the buttocks and legs to the ground.

Rest in the sitting position.

Repeat the pose with the legs crossed the other way.

Practise 3 to 5 rounds.

Breathing: Inhale before lifting the body off the floor.
Retain the breath inside while raising and swinging backward and forward.
Exhale on returning to the floor.

Awareness: Physical – on the strength of the arms, contraction of the perineal floor, the sensation of movement and energy coordinated with the breath, and the balance.
Spiritual – on anahata chakra.

Contra-indications: This is a strenuous asana, not suitable for people with heart conditions, high blood pressure, prolapse, hernia or back pain.

Benefits: The arms, wrists, shoulders and abdominal muscles are strengthened and the chest is opened. It generates control and balance.

KUKKUTASANA

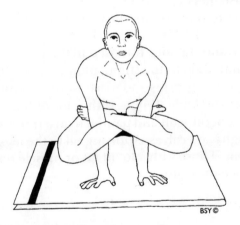

BSY©

Kukkutasana (cockerel pose)

Sit in padmasana.
Insert the hands between the calves and thighs, near the knees.
Gradually push the arms through the legs up to the elbows. Place the palms of the hands firmly on the floor with the fingers pointing forward.

191

Keeping the head straight and the eyes fixed on a point in front, raise the body from the floor, balancing only on the hands.

Hold the back straight.

Remain in the final position for as long as is comfortable. Return to the floor and slowly release the arms, hands and legs.

Change the leg position and repeat the pose.

Breathing: Take a deep breath in and raise the body.
Breathe normally in the final position.
Exhale while lowering.

Awareness: Physical – on the contraction of the perineum and the strength in the arms and shoulders, and on the breath in the nostrils while maintaining balance.
Spiritual – on mooladhara chakra.

Contra-indications: This is a strenuous asana, not suitable for people with heart conditions, high blood pressure, prolapse, hernia or back pain.

Benefits: This posture strengthens the arm and shoulder muscles, and stretches the chest. It develops a sense of balance and stability. It is used in the process of kundalini awakening due to the stimulation of mooladhara chakra.

Practice note: The arms and wrists must be strong enough to support the body. People with a lot of hair on their legs may find it difficult and painful to insert the arms between the thighs and calves. Applying oil to the legs will ease the problem. Those with a lot of fat or muscle on the legs will also have difficulty.

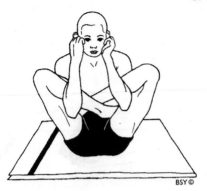

BSY©

Garbhasana (womb pose)

Sit in padmasana. Insert an arm between the thigh and calf of each leg and bend the elbows under the calves.

Fold the arms upward and raise the legs. Hold the ears, balancing the whole body on the coccyx.

The eyes may be open or closed.

Maintain the final position for as long as is comfortable.

Let go of the ears, lower the legs and slowly release the arms from the legs.

Cross the legs the other way around and repeat the pose.

This asana may also be performed lying on the back.

Breathing: Exhale while bringing the hands to the ears.

Breathe normally in the final position.

In the final position the breath will be shallow because the stomach and lungs are compressed.

Awareness: Physical – on the compression of the abdomen, on maintaining balance, and on the breath.

Spiritual – on manipura chakra.

Benefits: This asana has a regulating effect on the adrenal glands and calms an excited mind. It helps emotional stability generally, giving a sense of security, while those who experience uncontrollable anger may practise this pose regularly. It massages and tones the abdominal organs, stimulates the digestive fire and increases the appetite. It also develops the sense of balance.

TOLANGULASANA

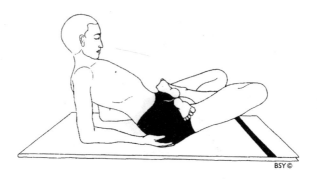

BSY©

Tolangulasana (weighing scale pose)

Sit in padmasana.

Slowly and carefully lower the back to a 45 degrees angle with the floor, using the hands and elbows to assist the movement. Place the palms of the hands underneath the buttocks. Raise the trunk and legs so that the whole body is supported only on the buttocks and forearms.

Perform jalandhara bandha. Advanced practitioners may also practise moola bandha.

Remain in the final position for a comfortable period of time without straining. Slowly lower the body to the floor. Repeat up to 5 times.

Breathing: Inhale in the raised position and retain the breath while doing jalandhara bandha. Do not retain the breath for longer than is comfortable.

Release jalandhara bandha and exhale while returning to the starting position.

Awareness: Physical—on the sense of balance and tranquillity and on retention of the breath.

Spiritual—on vishuddhi chakra.

Benefits: This asana tones the abdominal organs and lower abdominal muscles, and removes excess weight. It strengthens the back, and especially the thigh muscles. It induces a state of relaxation and equanimity.

Backward Bending Asanas

Backward bending asanas are postures which turn the body out to face the world. They are stimulating and extroverting. Because they expand the chest and encourage inhalation, they are associated with the attitude of embracing life. They are also dynamic postures which move counter to gravity and, therefore, require strength and energy to perform.

On a physical level, the backward bending asanas stretch the abdominal muscles, and tone and strengthen the muscles controlling the spine. The spinal nerves, which emerge from between the adjoining vertebrae, are decompressed. This has beneficial repercussions throughout the body since these nerves give energy to all the other nerves, organs and muscles in the body.

The spinal column is a 'stacked pile' of vertebrae and discs. Groups of muscles extend all along it, covering and supporting it from all sides. Maintenance of the spine in a straight and aligned position, despite all movement, depends totally on the balanced, supportive contraction and tone of the muscles. The muscles themselves are controlled unconsciously through posture.

Subconscious tensions and 'hang-ups' are often reflected in the tonic activity of the back muscles, resulting in too hard or too lax zones instead of homogeneous consistency. Research has shown that ninety percent of backache has its origin in muscular imbalance. If these imbalances are prolonged, then the 'stack pile' of the vertebral column is disaligned, the ligaments are

195

strained and symptoms of spondylitis, slipped disc, sciatica and osteoarthritis begin to manifest.

The practice of a balanced regime of backward and forward bending asanas can correct postural defects and neuro-muscular imbalances of the vertebral column. As with all asanas, it is important to perform these practices with proper control and synchronization of the breath so that the whole group of muscles is uniformly contracted.

Impure blood has a tendency to accumulate in the back region where circulation tends to be sluggish due to continuous maintenance of an upright position. These asanas help to circulate, purify and enrich the blood in this region. Backward bending asanas create a negative pressure in the abdomen and pelvis, helping neuro-circulatory toning of all the related organs. They also massage the abdomen and pelvic organs by stretching the muscles in this area, especially the rectus abdomini.

People with excessive lower back curve (lumbar lordosis) should not practise the asanas in this section, apart from saral bhujangasana, ardha shalabasana and gomukhasana. Generally, during pregnancy, asanas where the stomach is weight-bearing are not recommended. Of the asanas in this section, kandharasana practised gently will give the benefits of backward bends. In general, the specific contra-indications for each practice should also be carefully observed.

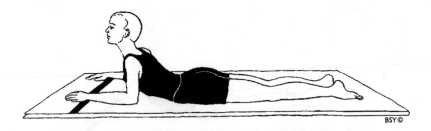

Saral Bhujangasana (easy cobra pose)

Lie flat on the stomach with the forehead resting on the floor, the legs straight, feet together, and the soles of the feet uppermost.

Bend the arms and place the forearms on the floor with the palms downward on each side of the head. The fingertips point forward, but are in line with the crown of the head. The forearms and elbows are close to the body.

Relax the whole body.

Raise the head, shoulders and chest by bringing the upper arms to the vertical position.

The elbows, forearms and hands will remain on the floor. Relax in the position for a comfortable length of time and then slowly lower the body.

This is one round.

Breathing: Inhale while raising the head, shoulders and chest. Exhale while lowering to the floor.
Breathe normally in the final position.

Duration: Hold the position for 3 to 4 minutes as a static pose or practise up to 5 rounds as a dynamic pose.

Awareness: Physical–on the sensation in the arms and shoulders, on relaxing the back, and on the breath.
Spiritual–on swadhisthana chakra.

Sequence: A good preparatory pose for bhujangasana. Follow with a forward bending asana.

Benefits: This asana strengthens the arms and shoulders and is especially good for stiff backs.

Note: *This posture is also known as sphinx asana.*

BHUJANGASANA

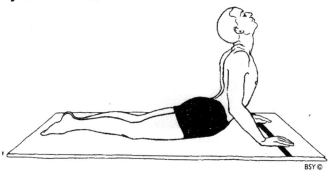

BSY©

Bhujangasana (cobra pose)

Lie flat on the stomach with the legs straight, feet together and the soles of the feet uppermost.

Place the palms of the hands flat on the floor, below and slightly to the side of the shoulders, with the fingers together and pointing forward.

Position the arms so that the elbows point backward and are close to the sides of the body.

Rest the forehead on the floor and close the eyes.

Relax the whole body, especially the lower back.

Slowly raise the head.

Gently tilt the head backward, so that the chin points forward and the back of the neck is compressed, then raise the neck and then the shoulders.

Straighten the elbows, using the back muscles first, then the arm muscles to raise the trunk further and arch the back.

In the final position, the pubic bone remains in contact with the floor and the navel is raised a maximum of 3 cm. If the navel is raised too high, the bend tends to be in the knees and not in the back.

The arms may or may not be straight; this will depend on the flexibility of the back.

Hold the final position.

To return to the starting position, slowly release the upper back by bending the arms, lower the navel, chest, shoulders and finally the forehead to the floor.

Relax the lower back muscles.

This is one round.

Breathing: Inhale while raising the torso.
Breathe normally in the final position or retain the breath if the pose is held for a short time.
Exhale while lowering the torso.

Duration: Practise up to 5 rounds, gradually increasing the length of time in the final position.

Awareness: Physical – on the smooth, systematic arching movement of the back, the stretching of the abdomen, and on synchronizing the breath with the movement.
Spiritual – on swadhisthana chakra.

Sequence: This asana gives maximum benefits if preceded or followed by a forward bending asana. It may also be performed in conjunction with shalabhasana and dhanurasana for effective general health of the back and spine.

Contra-indications: People suffering from peptic ulcer, hernia, intestinal tuberculosis or hyperthyroidism should not practise this asana without the guidance of a competent teacher.

Benefits: This asana improves and deepens breathing. It can help to remove backache and keep the spine supple and healthy. It tones the ovaries and uterus, and helps in menstrual and some other gynaecological disorders. It stimulates the appetite, alleviates constipation and is beneficial for all the abdominal organs, especially the liver and kidneys.

Note: *This is position 7 in surya namaskara and position 8 in chandra namaskara.*

TIRYAKA BHUJANGASANA

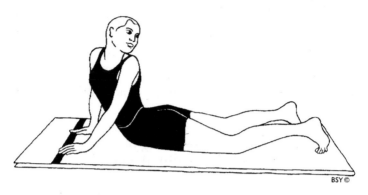

Tiryaka Bhujangasana (twisting cobra pose)

Lie flat on the stomach with the legs separated about half a metre. The toes should be tucked under and the heels raised so that the foot rests on the ball of the foot.

Place the palms of the hands flat on the floor, below and slightly to the side of the shoulders.

The fingers should be together and pointing forward.

The arms should be positioned so that the elbows point backward and are close to the sides of the body.

Rest the forehead on the floor and close the eyes.

Relax the whole body, especially the lower back

Slowly raise the head, neck and shoulders.

Straightening the elbows, raise the trunk as high as comfortable. Use the back muscles more than the arm muscles.

The head should be facing forward, instead of bending backward as in bhujangasana.

Twist the head and upper portion of the trunk, and look over the left shoulder.

Gaze at the heel of the right foot.

In the final position, the arms remain straight or slightly bent as the shoulders and trunk are twisted.

Relax the back and keep the navel close to the floor.

Stay in the final position for a few seconds.

Face forward again and repeat the twist on the other side

200

without lowering the trunk.

Return to the centre and lower the body to the floor.

This is one round. Practise 3 to 5 rounds.

Breathing: Inhale while raising the torso.

Exhale while twisting to the side, inhale to centre, exhale to the other side and again inhale to centre.

Exhale while lowering the torso to the floor.

Awareness: Physical – on the stretch of the muscles of the back and intestines, and the diagonal stretch of the abdomen. Spiritual – on swadhisthana chakra.

Benefits: As for bhujangasana, with increased influence on the arms and the intestines.

Note: *This asana is performed as part of the shankhaprakshalana series.*

SARPASANA

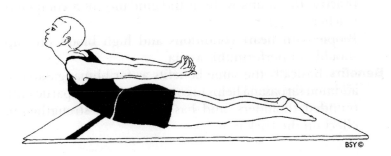

BSY©

Sarpasana (snake pose)

Lie flat on the stomach with the legs straight and the feet together.

Interlock the fingers and place the hands on top of the buttocks. Place the chin on the floor.

This is the starting position.

Using the lower back muscles, raise the chest as far as possible from the floor.

Push the hands further back and raise the arms as high as is comfortable. Imagine the arms are being pulled from behind.

Raise the body as high as possible without straining.

Squeeze the shoulder blades together and look forward.

Hold for as long as is comfortable.

Slowly return to the starting position and relax the whole body. Release the hands and relax the arms by the sides of the body. Turn the head to one side.

This is one round. Practise up to 5 rounds.

Breathing: Inhale deeply and slowly in the starting position prior to raising.

Retain while raising and in the final position.

Exhale while lowering.

Awareness: Physical – on the uniform contraction of the spinal muscles and arms.

Spiritual – on anahata chakra.

Sequence: A good preparatory pose for bhujangasana.

Contra-indications: People suffering from peptic ulcer, hernia, intestinal tuberculosis or hyperthyroidism should not practise this asana without the guidance of a competent teacher.

People with heart conditions and high blood pressure should not perform this asana.

Benefits: Basically the same benefits as for bhujangasana; in addition sarpasana helps to correct the posture, particularly rounded shoulders, and has a profound strengthening effect on the back muscles.

ARDHA SHALABHASANA

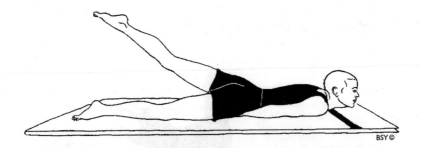

BSY©

Ardha Shalabhasana (half locust pose)
> Lie flat on the stomach with the hands under the thighs, palms downwards or hands clenched.
> Keep both the legs straight throughout the practice.
> Place the chin on the floor, slightly stretched forward, to give the best possible stretch to the neck muscles and nerves.
> Using the back muscles, raise the left leg as high as possible, keeping the other leg straight, relaxed and in contact with the floor.
> Retain the position for as long as is possible without strain.
> Do not tilt or twist the pelvis.
> Lower the leg to the floor.
> Repeat the same movement with the right leg.
> This is one round.

Breathing: Inhale in the starting position.
> Retain the breath inside while raising the leg and in the final position.
> Exhale while lowering the leg to the starting position.

Duration: Up to 5 rounds when performed dynamically. Up to 3 rounds when performed statically.

Awareness: Physical–on the lower back, abdomen and heart, and on synchronizing the breath with the movement. Spiritual–on swadhisthana chakra.

Benefits: Ardha shalabhasana is an excellent asana for the back and pelvic organs. It can release tension in the pelvic area.

203

Practice note: The left leg should be raised first so that pressure is applied on the right side of the abdomen to massage the ascending colon of the large intestine, following the direction of intestinal peristalsis.

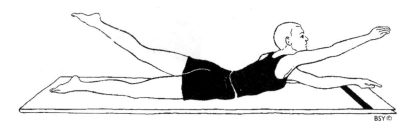

Variation: Lie on the stomach with the legs and feet together and the forehead touching the floor.

Stretch both arms above the head in advasana. Place the chin on the floor.

Keep the arms and legs straight throughout the practice. Simultaneously, raise the left leg, the head and right arm as high as possible.

The left leg should be stretched backwards and the right arm stretched forward as they are raised.

Retain the position for as long as possible without straining. Lower the leg, head and arm to the starting position.

Relax in advasana, allowing the respiration to return to normal.

Repeat the same movement with the right leg and left arm.

This is one round. Practise up to 5 rounds.

Breathing: Inhale while raising the leg, arm and head.

Retain while holding the position.

Exhale while lowering the leg, arm and head to the starting position.

Awareness: Physical – on synchronizing the breath with the movement and on the diagonal stretch through the body from the tips of the toes of the raised leg to the fingertips of the opposite hand.

Spiritual – on swadhisthana chakra.

Benefits: This variation is beneficial for beginners with weak and stiff backs as it helps to tone the back muscles and stimulate the nerves, particularly in the lower back, while simultaneously giving a strong diagonal stretch to the body. It develops concentration through awareness of coordination of movement with breath.

SHALABHASANA

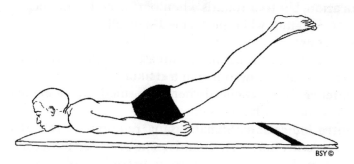

BSY ©

Shalabhasana (locust pose)

Lie flat on the stomach with the legs and feet together and the soles of the feet uppermost.

The arms may be placed either under the body or by the sides, with the palms downward or the hands clenched.

Stretch the chin slightly forward and rest it on the floor throughout the practice.

Close the eyes and relax the body.

This is the starting position.

Slowly raise the legs as high as possible without straining, keeping them straight and together.

The elevation of the legs is produced by applying pressure with the arms against the floor and contracting the lower back muscles.

Hold the final position for as long as is comfortable without strain.

Slowly lower the legs to the floor.

This is one round.

Return to the starting position and relax the body with the head turned to one side.

Allow the respiration and heartbeat to return to normal.

Breathing: Inhale deeply in the starting position.
Retain the breath inside while raising the legs and holding the position. Exhale while lowering the legs.
Beginners may find it helpful to inhale while raising the legs.
Advanced practitioners may exhale after returning to the starting position.

Duration: Up to 5 rounds when performed dynamically. Up to 3 rounds when performed statically.

Awareness: Physical – on the lower back, abdomen and heart, and on synchronizing the breath with the movement.
Spiritual – on swadhisthana chakra.

Sequence: Most beneficial when performed after bhujangasana and before dhanurasana.

Contra-indications: Shalabhasana requires a great deal of physical effort, so it should not be practised by people with a weak heart, coronary thrombosis or high blood pressure. Those suffering from peptic ulcer, hernia, intestinal tuberculosis and other such conditions are also advised not to practise this asana.

Benefits: Shalabhasana strengthens the lower back and pelvic organs, and provides relief from backache, mild sciatica and slipped disc as long as the condition is not serious. It tones and balances the functioning of the liver, stomach, bowels and other abdominal organs, and stimulates the appetite. It tightens the muscles of the buttocks and causes the body to do vajroli mudra spontaneously.

Variation: Lie on the stomach with the legs and feet together and the forehead touching the floor.
Stretch both arms above the head in advasana. Place the chin on the floor.
Keep the arms and legs straight throughout the practice. Simultaneously raise both legs, the head and both arms as high as is comfortable.

Retain the position, balancing on the abdominal muscles for as long as possible without straining.
Lower the legs, head and arms to the starting position.
Relax in advasana, allowing the respiration to return to normal.
This is one round.

SARAL DHANURASANA

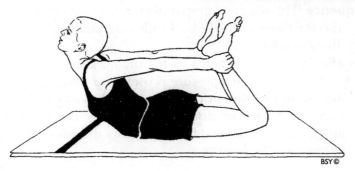

BSY©

Saral Dhanurasana (easy bow pose)

Lie flat on the stomach with the legs and feet together, and the arms and hands beside the body.
Bend the knees and bring the heels close to the buttocks.
Grasp the ankles with the hands.
Keep the knees and thighs firmly on the floor and the arms straight throughout the practice.
Place the chin on the floor.
This is the starting position.
Tense the legs and push the feet backwards while raising the head and chest as high as possible from the floor without straining.
Use the backward movement of the legs to assist the raising of the body, allowing the back muscles to remain passive.
In the final position the head is tilted back.
Hold the final position for as long as is comfortable.
Slowly lower the chest and head to the ground by releasing the legs.

207

Relax in the prone position until the respiration returns to normal.

This is one round. Practise up to 5 rounds.

Breathing: Inhale deeply in the starting position.
Retain the breath inside while raising the body.
Breathe deeply and slowly in the final position.
Exhale while returning to the starting position.

Awareness: Physical – on the abdominal or back regions or on deep breathing in the final position.
Spiritual – on vishuddhi chakra.

Sequence: This is a good preparatory asana for beginners and also for those with stiff backs who are unable to perform dhanurasana.

Benefits: The same benefits as for dhanurasana, but at decreased levels. This posture is useful for lower back pain due to slipped disc or cervical spondylitis when it can be performed without discomfort. It tones the heart and lungs, and is beneficial for respiratory disorders. It helps to improve the posture.

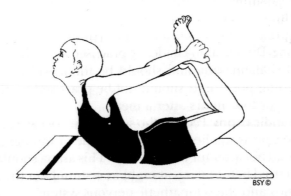

BSY©

Dhanurasana (bow pose)

Lie flat on the stomach with the legs and feet together, and the arms and hands beside the body.

Bend the knees and bring the heels close to the buttocks.

Clasp the hands around the ankles.

Place the chin on the floor.

This is the starting position.

Tense the leg muscles and push the feet away from the body. Arch the back, lifting the thighs, chest and head together. Keep the arms straight.

In the final position the head is tilted back and the abdomen supports the entire body on the floor. The only muscular contraction is in the legs; the back and arms remain relaxed.

Hold the final position for as long as is comfortable and then, slowly relaxing the leg muscles, lower the legs, chest and head to the starting position.

Release the pose and relax in the prone position until the respiration returns to normal.

This is one round. Practise 3 or up to 5 rounds.

Breathing: Inhale deeply in the starting position.

Retain the breath while raising the body.

Retain the breath inside in the final position or practise slow, deep breathing so that the body rocks gently in unison with the breath.

Exhale while returning to the prone position.

Awareness: Physical–on the abdominal region, the back, or the rhythmic expansion and contraction of the abdomen to the slow, deep breathing.

Spiritual–on manipura or ajna chakra.

Sequence: Dhanurasana is ideally practised after bhujangasana and shalabhasana and should be followed by a forward bending posture. It should not be practised until at least three or four hours after a meal.

Contra-indications: People who suffer from a weak heart, high blood pressure, hernia, colitis, peptic or duodenal ulcers should not attempt this practice. This asana should not be practised before sleep at night as it stimulates the adrenal glands and the sympathetic nervous system.

Benefits: The entire alimentary canal is reconditioned by this asana. The liver, abdominal organs and muscles are massaged. The pancreas and adrenal glands are toned, balancing their secretions. The kidneys are massaged and excess weight is reduced around the abdominal area.

This leads to improved functioning of the digestive, excretory and reproductive organs and helps to remove gastrointestinal disorders, dyspepsia, chronic constipation and sluggishness of the liver.

It is useful for the management of diabetes and menstrual disorders. It improves blood circulation generally. The spinal column is realigned and the ligaments, muscles and nerves are activated, removing stiffness. It helps to correct hunching of the upper back. It strengthens leg muscles, especially the thighs.

Dhanurasana is useful for freeing nervous energy in the cervical and thoracic area, generally improving respiration.

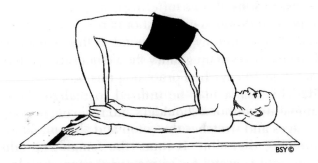

BSY©

Kandharasana (shoulder pose)

Lie flat on the back.

Bend the knees, placing the soles of the feet flat on the floor with the heels touching the buttocks.

The feet and knees may be hip width apart.

Grasp the ankles with the hands.

This is the starting position.

Raise the buttocks and arch the back upward.

Raise the chest and navel as high as possible without straining, pushing the chest up towards the chin and head, but without moving the position of the feet or shoulders.

Keep the feet flat on the floor.

In the final position, the body is supported by the head, neck, shoulders, arms and feet.

Hold the pose for as long as is comfortable and then lower the body to the starting position.

Release the ankles and relax with the legs outstretched.

Practise 5 to 10 rounds.

Breathing: Inhale deeply in the starting position.

Retain the breath inside while raising and holding the final position.

Alternatively, breathe slowly and deeply in the final position. Exhale while lowering to the starting position.

Awareness: Physical–on the movement, the abdominal region, thyroid gland or accentuation of flexion of the back.

Spiritual–on vishuddhi or anahata chakra.

Sequence: Perform before or after a forward bending asana. It is a good preparatory pose for chakrasana.

Contra-indications: People suffering from peptic or duodenal ulcers, or abdominal hernia should not practise kandharasana. It is generally recommended that women in the advanced stages of pregnancy should not raise the buttocks more than 15 cm when practising this pose.

Benefits: This asana may be utilized to realign the spine, eliminating rounded shoulders and relieving backache. It massages and stretches the colon and abdominal organs, improving digestion. It tones the female reproductive organs and is useful for women who have a tendency to miscarry, for the management of menstrual disorders, prolapse, asthma, and various bronchial and thyroid conditions.

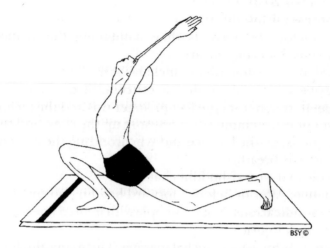

Ardha Chandrasana (half-moon pose)

Practise ashwa sanchalanasana.

In the final position maintain the balance and raise the hands, bringing the palms together in front of the chest in prayer position.

Keeping the palms together, raise the arms up over the head.

Arch the head and upper trunk as far back as comfortable without straining.

There should be a gentle curve from the tips of the fingers to the toes of the right leg, resembling a crescent moon.

Balance in the final posture.

To release, lower the hands back to prayer position then smoothly to the floor, and look forward, returning to ashwa sanchalanasana.

Releasing ashwa sanchalanasa and return to its starting position.

This is one round. Continue with the forward and backward lunges on this side.

Before practising an equal number of rounds on the other side, relax in vajrasana (as for ashwa sanchalanasana). Practise 5 to 10 rounds.

Breathing: Exhale while moving slowly forward into ashwa sanchalanasana.

Inhale raising the arms into ardha chandrasana.

Hold for a few seconds while maintaining the balance.

Exhale lowering the arms.

Inhale releasing ashwa sanchalanasana.

Awareness: Physical – on the smooth controlled movement, the deep stretch from the feet to finger tips and the feeling of spaciousness induced by opening up the chest and throat regions; on the balance and synchronizing the movement with the breath.

Spiritual – on vishuddhi chakra.

Sequence: After or before a forward bending posture.

Contra-indications: Not for people with injured knees, ankles or back injuries.

Benefits: As for ashwa sanchalanasana. This asana also limbers and strengthens the entire skeletal structure. It gives a good stretch to the neck, shoulders, back and chest, releasing feelings of congestion. It improves the sense of balance.

Note: *The addition of this key posture changes surya namskara to chandra namaskara.*

214

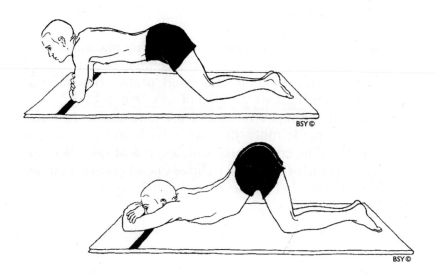

BSY©

Utthan Pristhasana (lizard pose)

Lie on the stomach with the arms crossed under the chest, the hands holding the upper arms.

Separate the legs slightly and keep the feet flat.

Raise the head so that the face looks forward.

This is the starting position.

The elbows should not move during the practice.

Raise the trunk and buttocks so that the body is supported by the knees and elbows, as in the first diagram.

Stretch the torso back, placing the chin and chest on, or as close as possible to, the floor behind the forearms.

Return to the raised position and then to the starting position.

This is one round.

Breathing: Inhale while raising the trunk, exhale into the stretch. Breathe normally while holding the position. Inhale coming up on to the knees and elbows. Exhale while lowering the body back to the ground.

Duration: Up to 10 rounds if practising dynamically, less if holding the stretch for a comfortable length of time.

Awareness: Physical – on the stretch in the upper arms, shoulders, chest and back, especially the region between the shoulder blades; on synchronizing the movement with the breath.

Spiritual – on swadhisthana, manipura or anahata chakra.

Sequence: Perform after a forward bending asana such as paschimottanasana. It is a good preparation for the ashtanga namaskara position of surya namaskara.

Benefits: This asana exercises and strengthens the chest and diaphragm. It tones the entire back and gives many benefits of inverted asanas with less risk of side effects. It is excellent for relieving tightness between the shoulder blades. When held for some time, it helps to relieve constipation and piles.

SETU ASANA

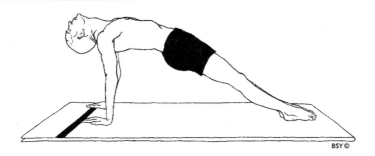

BSY©

Setu Asana (bridge pose)

Sit with the legs stretched forward.

Place the palms on the floor on either side of the body, about 30 cm behind the buttocks.

The elbows should be straight, the fingers pointing back and the trunk slightly reclined.

This is the starting position.

Raise the buttocks and lift the body upward.

Let the head hang back and down.

216

Try to place the soles of the feet flat on the ground.
Keep the arms and legs straight.
Hold the final position for as long as is comfortable.
Lower the buttocks to the floor.
This is one round. Practise up to 5 times.

Breathing: Inhale in the starting position.
Retain the breath inside while raising the body and holding the final position.
Exhale while lowering to the starting position.

Awareness: Physical – on the wrists, arms, back and abdomen.
Spiritual – on manipura chakra.

Sequence: As a preliminary practice to chakrasana.

Contra-indications: This asana should not be practised by those with high blood pressure, heart disease, cervical spondylosis, hernia, stomach ulcers or weak wrists.

Benefits: This asana has similar benefits to chakrasana. It is generally strengthening for shoulders, thighs and wrists, and also tones the lumbar region of the spine and the Achilles' tendons.

GOMUKHASANA

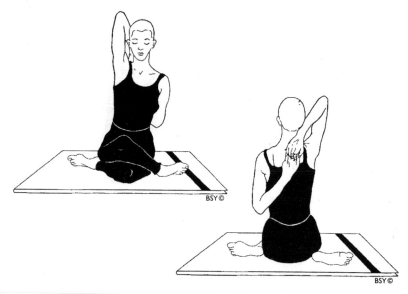

Gomukhasana (cow's face pose)

Sit in dhyana veerasana so that the right knee is directly above the left knee.

Stretch the left arm to the side and then fold it behind the back.

Stretch the right arm up above the head, then fold it over the right shoulder.

The back of the left hand should lie in contact with the spine while the palm of the right hand rests against the spine.

Try to clasp the fingers of both hands behind the back.

Bring the raised elbow behind the head so that the head presses against the inside of the raised arm.

The spine should be erect and the head back. Close the eyes.

Stay in this position for up to 2 minutes.

Unclasp the hands, straighten the legs and repeat with the left knee uppermost and the left arm over the left shoulder.

Breathing: Normal in the final position.
Awareness: Physical–on respiration.
   Spiritual–on ajna or anahata chakra.
Benefits: Gomukhasana is an excellent asana for inducing relaxation. If practised for 10 minutes or more, it will alleviate tiredness, tension and anxiety. It relieves backache, sciatica, rheumatism and general stiffness in the shoulders and neck, and improves posture by increasing energy, awareness, and generally opening the chest area. It alleviates cramp in the legs and makes the leg muscles supple.

Forward Bending Asanas

Generally speaking, forward bending is a passive process in which gravity is utilized to stretch the muscle groups being focused upon. While backward bends move the body away from the confines of gravity, forward bending asanas use gravity to help release tension and pain. It is a process of introversion, counteracting the extroversion and dynamic opening up of bending backwards. Forward bending, associated with chest compression and exhalation, induces relaxation.

Many people lead sedentary lifestyles with little or no exercise and, as a result, the body becomes stiff and unable to bend forward. City living encourages mental tension and physical rigidity, both of which are counteracted by forward bending asanas. At another level, forward bending is associated with bowing and humility. An inability to bend forward may indicate a stiff, proud or stubborn personality. Difficulty bending forward is also associated with fear. Human beings face forward to see the world, but some people live in constant fear of attack from behind and the backs of their bodies unconsciously freeze. Forward bending asanas release this rigidity.

Forward bending asanas loosen up the back, maintaining good health and increasing vitality. These practices move the spine into the position known as the primary curve, the shape it takes in the womb. During a forward bending asana each of the vertebra is separated, stimulating the nerves, improving circulation around the spine and nourishing the spinal cord. This has a positive impact on the organs of the body generally and on the brain specifically. This group of asanas is also very important for making the back muscles supple and strong, compressing and massaging the abdominal organs, including the liver, kidneys, pancreas and intestines, and stretching the leg muscles and tendons.

Most forward bending asanas described in this book start by bending from the hips and not the waist. Bending from the hips gives greater flexibility of movement and creates a stronger pressure against the abdomen. Care must be taken not to force the back to bend further forward than present flexibility will allow; rather, the muscles should be relaxed, allowing gravity and exhalation to move the body. With regular practice, even the most rigid back will develop increased flexibility.

It is not advisable to practise all the forward bending asanas one after the other. Start with the preliminary practices and gradually build up to the more advanced ones as the back becomes more flexible. A balanced program of forward and then backward bending asanas should be carefully maintained. People with any kind of back condition and those suffering from backache should consult a doctor before practising these asanas. In general, also carefully observe the specific contra-indications for each practice.

Right-handed people will find these asanas are easily learned with the right side leading. They should then be practised with the left side leading as a counterbalance.

When practising forward bending asanas from a sitting position, particularly those in which the legs are separated, it is helpful to sit with the perineum on the floor, rather than sitting on the coccyx. The correct position is obtained by sitting with the legs slightly separated and placing the hands on the floor, on either side of the hips, with the fingertips pointing forward. Then, using the arms and hands as supports, lift the buttocks slightly from the floor and, while lowering them, tilt the pelvis forward.

SAITHALYASANA

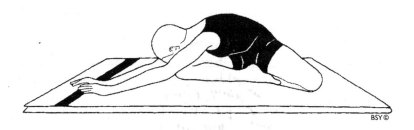

Saithalyasana (animal relaxation pose)
Sit on the floor with the legs outstretched.
Carefully bend the right knee and place the sole of the
foot against the inside of the left thigh.
Bend the left knee and place the left heel to the outside
of the left buttock.
Turn the torso to the right and rest the hands on the right
knee.
Raise the arms above the head, keeping them straight and
shoulder width apart.
Bend forward over the right knee, bringing the forehead
to the floor. Relax in the position.
To return to the starting position, raise the arms and
trunk in one straight line, then lower the hands to the
right knee.
Practise 5 times on the right, then 5 times on the left side.
Breathing: Inhale while raising the arms.
Exhale while bending forward.
Breathe normally in the final position.
Inhale while returning to the upright position.
Exhale while lowering the arms.
Awareness: Physical–on synchronization of the movement
with the breath and relaxation of the back.
Spiritual–on manipura chakra.
Sequence: This is a preparatory practice for meditation poses
and may precede any backward bending asana such as
bhujangasana, saral dhanurasana or dhanurasana which

particularly stretch the neck and pelvic region in the opposite direction.

Contra-indications: People who have lower back conditions should only bend forward as far as is comfortable.

Benefits: This asana stretches the back, pelvic region, insides of the thighs and opens up the hip joints. It balances the nervous system. It also massages the abdominal organs by gently compressing each side alternately against the thighs.

PASCHIMOTTANASANA

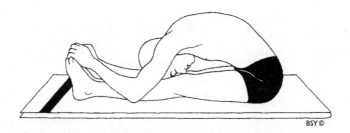

BSY©

Paschimottanasana (back stretching pose)

Sit on the floor with the legs outstretched, feet together and hands on the knees.

This is the starting position.

Relax the whole body.

Slowly bend forward from the hips, sliding the hands down the legs. Try to grasp the big toes with the fingers and thumbs. If this is impossible, hold the heels, ankles or any part of the legs that can be reached comfortably. Move slowly without forcing or jerking.

Hold the position for a few seconds. Relax the back and leg muscles, allowing them to gently stretch.

Keeping the legs straight and utilizing the arm muscles, not the back muscles, begin to bend the elbows and gently bring the trunk down towards the legs, maintaining a firm grip on the toes, feet or legs.

223

Try to touch the knees with the forehead. Do not strain.
This is the final position.
Hold the position for as long as is comfortable and relax.
Slowly return to the starting position.
This is one round.

Breathing: Inhale in the starting position.
Exhale slowly while bending forward.
Inhale in the static position.
Exhale while bringing the trunk further towards the legs with the arms.
Breathe slowly and deeply in the final position or retain the breath out if holding for a short duration.
Inhale while returning to the starting position.

Duration: Beginners should perform up to 5 rounds, staying in the final position for only a short length of time. Adepts may maintain the final position for up to 5 minutes.

Awareness: Physical – on the abdomen, relaxation of the back and leg muscles, or the slow breathing process.
Spiritual – on swadhisthana chakra.

Sequence: This asana should precede or follow backward bending asanas such as setu asana, chakrasana, bhujang-asana or matsyasana.

Contra-indications: People who suffer from slipped disc, sciatica or hernia should not practise paschimottanasana.

Benefits: This asana stretches the hamstring muscles and increases flexibility in the hip joints. It tones and massages the entire abdominal and pelvic region, including the liver, pancreas, spleen, uro-genital system, kidneys and adrenal glands. It helps to remove excess weight in this area and stimulates circulation to the nerves and muscles of the spine.

Practice note: Paschimottanasana can also be commenced by inhaling and raising the arms in the starting position, and then exhaling into the forward bend, instead of sliding the hands down the legs.

GATYATMAK PASCHIMOTTANASANA

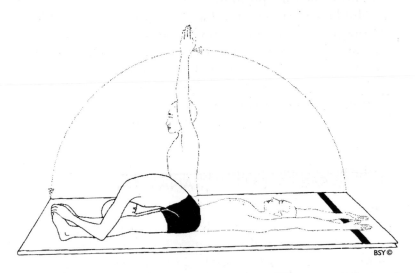

Gatyatmak Paschimottanasana (dynamic back stretch pose)
Lie flat on the back with the feet together. Raise the arms over the head and bring them to the floor with the palms facing up. This is the starting position.
Relax the whole body.
Raise the trunk to the sitting position with the arms straight above the head and the spine straight. Bend forward into paschimottanasana in a smooth movement.
Hold the final position for a short time.
Return to the sitting position with the arms straight above the head.
Lean backwards and return to the starting position.
This is one round. Practise up to 10 rounds.

Breathing: Breathe normally in the starting position.
Inhale while coming into the sitting position.
Exhale while bending forward into paschimottanasana.
Inhale while sitting up.
Exhale while returning to the starting position.

Awareness: Physical – on synchronizing the movement with the breath.
Spiritual – on swadhisthana chakra.

225

Contra-indications: As for paschimottanasana. In addition, this is a strenuous practice, not suitable for people with heart conditions, high blood pressure or any back problem.

Benefits: The benefits are the same as for paschimottanasana although at a reduced level. This is a dynamic practice which speeds up the circulation and metabolic processes. In addition, it renders the whole body more flexible, stimulating physical and pranic energy.

PADA PRASAR PASCHIMOTTANASANA

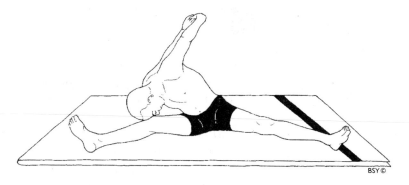

Pada Prasar Paschimottanasana (legs spread back stretch pose)

Sit with the legs spread apart as wide as possible.
Interlock the fingers behind the back.
This is the starting position.
Turn the trunk to the right.
Raise the arms up behind the back and bend forward over the right leg. Keep the arms straight.
Bring the nose towards the knee without bending the leg, but do not strain to make contact.
Hold the position for as long as is comfortable.
Raise the trunk and lower the arms.
Turn to the left and repeat the movement on this side.
Return to the centre.

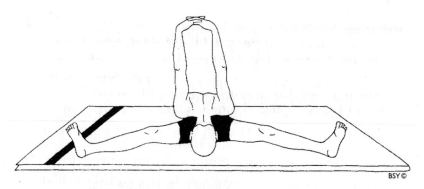

Bend forward and bring the forehead towards the floor directly in front of the body while raising the arms as high as possible without straining.

Hold the position for as long as is comfortable.

Return to the upright position, lowering the arms.

This completes one round. Practise 3 to 5 rounds.

Breathing: Inhale in the starting position.

Exhale while bending forward.

Breathe slowly and deeply in the final position or retain the breath out if the position is held for only a short time.

Inhale while returning to the starting position.

Awareness: Physical – on the stretch in the legs, back, shoulders and arms, on finding the beneficial amount of stretch without strain, and on synchronizing the movement with the breath.

Spiritual – on mooladhara or swadhisthana chakra.

Sequence: This asana should precede or follow backward bending asanas such as tiryaka bhujangasana, chakrasana or matsyasana.

Contra-indications: As for paschimottanasana. This practice should not be attempted until paschimottanasana has been mastered.

Benefits: As well as providing essentially the same benefits as paschimottanasana, this asana gives an extended stretch to the inside of the legs and the muscles under and between the shoulder blades. The chest is opened more than in paschimottanasana and the effect of the asana is distributed throughout both the upper and lower parts of the body.

Variation: Assume the same starting position as above, but with the hands in front of the body on the floor.

Slowly bend forward and grasp the big toes with the fingers. If this can be done without strain, place the forehead on the floor directly in front of the body.

Gradually bring the chest, abdomen and pelvic region to the floor. Raise the head so that the throat and chin are also on the floor.

This is the final position.

Hold the position for as long as is comfortable.

Release the hands and return to the starting position.

JANU SIRSHASANA

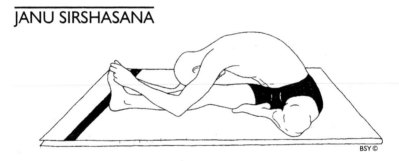

Janu Sirshasana (head to knee pose)

Sit with the legs outstretched and the feet together.

Bend the left leg, placing the heel of the foot against the perineum and the sole of the foot against the inside of the right thigh. Keep the left knee on the floor.

Place the hands on top of the right knee, keeping the spine straight and the back muscles relaxed.

This is the starting position.

Slowly bend forward, sliding the hands down the right leg, and grasp the right foot. If possible, hold the big toe with the index finger, middle finger and thumb of the left hand and the outside edge of the foot with the right hand.

Try to touch the knee with the forehead.

This is the final position.

Keep the back relaxed and do not strain.

Hold the position for as long as is comfortable.

Return to the starting position and rest the hands on the knees.

Change sides and repeat with the right leg bent and the left leg straight.

Practise up to 5 times with each leg.

Breathing: Inhale in the starting position.

Exhale while bending forward.

Retain the breath outside if holding the final position for a short time.

Breathe normally if holding the pose for a longer time.

Inhale while returning to the starting position.

Other details: As for paschimottanasana.

Benefits: This practice gives basically the same benefits as paschimottanasana as well as loosening up the legs in preparation for meditation asanas.

Practice note: Sometimes known as ardha paschimottanasana. It may be practised before paschimottanasana as a preparatory asana.

ARDHA PADMA PASCHIMOTTANASANA

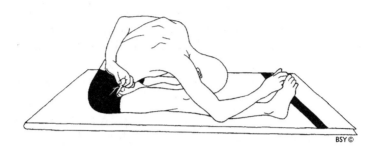

Ardha Padma Paschimottanasana (half lotus back stretching pose)

Sit with both legs outstretched.

Bend the left leg and place the left foot as high as possible on the right thigh, turning the sole of the foot up.

Press the heel firmly into the abdomen.

Bend forward slightly, fold the left arm behind the back and try to grasp the toes of the left foot with the left hand.

Sit upright again.

Relax the whole body, especially the back muscles.

Lean forward and grasp the toes of the right foot with the right hand.

Utilizing the arms, not the back muscles, slowly pull the trunk forward so that the forehead is near to or resting on the straight knee.

This is the final position.

Hold the pose for as long as is comfortable.

Release the hands and slowly sit up.

Repeat the technique with the other leg.

Practise up to 3 rounds, gradually extending the duration.

Breathing: Inhale in the upright position.

Exhale bending forward into the final position.

Breathe slowly and deeply in the final position or retain the breath outside if holding the pose for a short time.

Inhale while returning to the upright position.

Other details: As for paschimottanasana.

Benefits: Although the benefits of this asana are almost identical to janu sirshasana and paschimottanasana, it has one distinct characteristic: the foot of the bent leg applies an intense massage to the abdominal organs. Each leg is bent in turn, which helps to stimulate intestinal peristalsis and alleviate constipation. This asana also prepares the legs and hips for prolonged sitting in meditation asanas.

HASTA PADA ANGUSHTHASANA

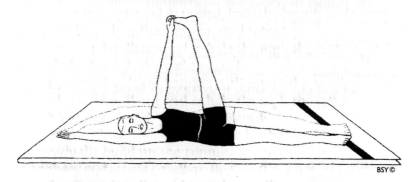

BSY©

Hasta Pada Angushthasana (finger to toe stretch)
Lie on the right side with the arms stretched over the head, so that the whole body is balanced in one straight line along the floor. The palm of the left hand should rest on top of the palm of the right hand.
The left foot should rest on top of the right foot.
This is the starting position.
Keep the arms and legs straight throughout the practice.
Raise the left leg and arm to their full extent and, keeping them straight, take hold of the big toe without bending the knee. If this is impossible, take hold of a suitable point on the leg to give support while gently stretching the hip.
This is the final position.
Hold the final position for a short duration.
Lower the arm and leg to the starting position.

231

Practise a maximum of 10 times on this side.

Lie in shavasana to relax with normal breathing.

Roll over to the other side and repeat.

Breathing: Inhale while raising the limbs.

Exhale while lowering.

Awareness: Physical – on the stretch in the hip and raised leg while holding the pose, on the balance, or on synchronizing the movement with the breath,

Spiritual – on mooladhara or swadhisthana chakra.

Contra-indications: Those suffering from sciatica should not practise this asana.

Benefits: This practice makes the hip joints flexible. It helps the proper development and shaping of the pelvis in young girls. It reduces excess weight on the hips and thighs and develops a sense of balance and coordination, making the posture and gait more steady and graceful.

Practice note: Make sure that the whole body stays in a straight line, without allowing it to curve or bend at the buttocks.

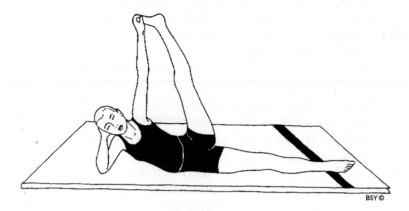

BSY©

Meru Akarshanasana (spinal bending pose)
Lie on the right side with the left leg on top of the right leg.
Bend the right arm, placing the elbow on the floor.
Raise the torso and head, supporting them on the right elbow.
Rest the head in the right palm. The forearm and upper arm should be nearly vertical.
Place the left arm on the left thigh.
This is the starting position.
Raise the left leg as high as possible without straining, and slide the left hand to the foot and grasp the big toe. If this is too difficult, hold the leg as close to the foot as possible.
Keep the legs straight. This is the final position.
Lower the raised leg and arm to the starting position.
Practise a maximum of 10 times. Relax in shavasana.
Repeat on the other side.
Breathing: Inhale while raising the arm and leg.
Retain the breath in while holding the final position.
Exhale while lowering.
Awareness: Physical – on synchronizing the movement with the breath, on the stretch in the hip and raised leg while holding the pose.
Spiritual – on swadhisthana chakra.

Contra-indications: People suffering from slipped disc, sciatica or cervical spondylitis should not practise this asana.

Benefits: This asana relaxes the hamstring, inner thigh and abdominal muscles and stretches the muscles of the sides of the body, rendering them stronger and more flexible. It reduces weight on the hips and thighs and develops a sense of balance and coordination, making the posture and gait more steady and graceful.

Variation: Instead of raising the torso, bend the right elbow and rest the head on the inside of the right arm. The rest of the practice is the same as above.

PADAHASTASANA

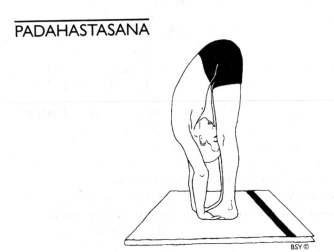

BSY ©

Padahastasana (hand to foot pose)

Stand with the spine erect, feet together and hands beside the body. Relax the body.

This is the starting position.

Distribute the weight of the body evenly on both feet. Slowly bend forward, first bending the head, taking the chin towards the chest, then bending the upper trunk, relaxing the shoulders forward and letting the arms go limp. Bend the mid-trunk and finally the lower trunk. While bending forward, imagine that the body has no bones or muscles. Do not strain or force the body.

Place the fingers underneath the toes or bring the palms to the floor beside the feet. If this is not possible, bring the fingertips as near to the floor as possible.

Relax the back of the neck. The body is bent forward with the knees straight and the forehead close to or touching the knees.

Hold the position, relaxing the whole back.

Slowly return to the starting position in the reverse order. This completes one round.

Relax in the upright position before continuing the next round.

Breathing: Inhale in the starting position.

Exhale while bending forward.

Breathe slowly and deeply in the final position.

Inhale while returning to the starting position.

Duration: Practise up to 5 rounds, gradually increasing the time that the posture is held and decreasing the number of rounds, or practise one round for 3 to 5 minutes.

Awareness: Physical–on the movement, relaxation of the back muscles or the breath.

Spiritual–on swadhisthana chakra.

Sequence: This asana may be practised before or after backward bending asanas and may be used as a preliminary to other forward bending poses to encourage maximum flexibility.

Contra-indications: This asana should not be practised by people suffering from serious back complaints, sciatica, heart disease, high blood pressure or abdominal hernia. Cautions for inverted postures apply.

Benefits: This asana massages and tones the digestive organs, alleviates flatulence, constipation and indigestion. Spinal nerves are stimulated and toned. Inverting the trunk can increase vitality, improve metabolism and concentration and help with nasal and throat diseases.

The dynamic form of padahastasana also helps to remove excess weight.

Variation: (dynamic forward bending)

Stand upright with the feet together, arms beside the body and the palms of the hands facing backward. The fingers should be together and straight.

Raise the arms above the head, keeping them straight and shoulder width apart.

Lean backward slightly to stretch the whole body.

Bend forward from the hips, keeping the knees straight, and bring the hands towards the floor. If possible without straining, place the hands on either side of the feet with the tips of the fingers in line with the toes.

Bring the forehead towards the knees.

Do not strain the hamstring muscles by using excessive force.

Hold the final position for one or two seconds.

Raise the body to the upright position, keeping the arms straight above the head.

Lower the arms to the sides.

Breathing: Inhale raising the arms, and exhale bending forward, inhale coming back to the upright position, exhale lowering the arms to the sides.

Duration: 5 to 10 rounds to begin with. Advanced practitioners may increase this number up to 30.

Practice note: Beginners should try to bring the fingertips to the floor beside the toes. If this is not possible, they can grasp the ankles or calves.

Note: *This variation is used in surya namaskara and chandra namaskara as positions 2 and 3.*

BSY©

236

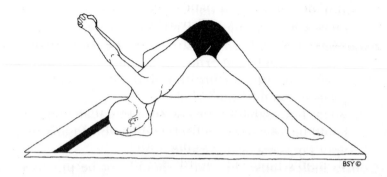

Sirsha Angustha Yogasana (head to toe pose)

Stand upright with the feet about two shoulder widths apart.

Interlock the fingers behind the back with the palms up. Keep the arms straight.

This is the starting position.

Twist the trunk to the right and turn the right foot slightly out to the side.

Bend forward at the waist, stretching the arms up as high as possible.

Bring the head down to the inside of the right foot.

Bend the right knee slightly to assume this position.

As the head comes closer to the foot, relax the shoulders, keep the arms straight and allow them to fall forward.

Hold the position for as long as is comfortable.

To avoid overbalancing when raising the body, first raise the head, straightening the neck and spine and lower the arms on to the back. Straighten the leg a little, but keep the knee bent and only straighten it once the torso is upright, then re-centre the body.

Repeat on the other side.

This completes one round.

Practise a maximum of 5 rounds.

Breathing: Inhale while in the starting position and while twisting.

237

Exhale while bending.

Retain the breath out while holding the position or breathe normally breathing if holding the stretch for some time.

Inhale while raising the trunk and recentring the body.

Awareness: Physical – on the stretch in the leg muscles and spine, shoulders and arms, on keeping the balance, and on synchronizing the breath with the movement.

Spiritual – on manipura chakra.

Sequence: This asana may be preceded by padahastasana and should be followed by a backward bending asana such as supta vajrasana or matsyasana.

Contra-indications: This asana should not be practised by people suffering from heart disease, high blood pressure, back conditions such as slipped disc or sciatica. Cautions for inverted postures apply.

Benefits: This asana stretches the hamstring, the thigh muscles, the area between the shoulder blades, and provides a lateral stretch to the body. It stimulates the nervous system and the appetite, and helps to remove abdominal complaints. It reduces excess weight around the waist.

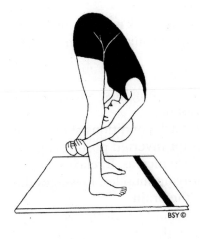 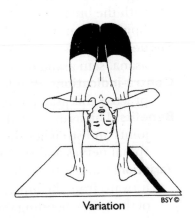

Variation

Utthita Janu Sirshasana (standing head between knees pose)
Stand with the feet about shoulder width apart, arms beside
the body. This is the starting position.
Raise the arms in front of the body, level with the chest.
Bend forward from the hips and take the arms around
the outside of the legs. Either grasp one wrist or clasp the
hands behind the calves.
Bring the head towards the knees by slightly bending the
elbows and using the strength of the arm muscles to achieve
this. The legs should remain straight. Do not strain.
In the final position the trunk rests against the thighs and
the wrists or elbows are held behind the lower legs.
Hold the final position for as long as is comfortable.
Release the hands and slowly raise the body to the upright
position with the arms stretched out in front of the chest.
Lower the arms to the starting position.
Practise up to 5 rounds.

Breathing: Inhale while raising the arms in front of the chest.
Exhale fully before bending.
Retain the breath outside while bending forward and
holding the final position.

Inhale while returning to the upright position.
Exhale while lowering the arms.

Awareness: Physical – on relaxing the back muscles and keeping the legs straight, and on synchronizing the movement with the breath.

Spiritual – on swadhisthana chakra.

Sequence: Follow by a backward bending pose such as sarpasana, setu asana or dhanurasana.

Contra-indications: People with back conditions should not practise this asana. Cautions for inverted postures apply.

Benefits: This asana stimulates the pancreas. It relaxes the hip joints and stretches the hamstring muscles, massages the spinal nerves and revitalizes the brain.

Variation: Stand with the feet about shoulder width apart. Bend forward from the hips and wrap the arms around the back of the knees, bending the legs slightly. The arms should be horizontal with the elbows pointing out to the sides.

Keeping the legs bent, try to bring the hands forward in between the legs and firmly interlock the fingers behind the back of the neck. Relax the back muscles.

Slowly straighten the legs without letting the fingers slip from behind the neck. Do not strain. The action of straightening the legs will apply a strong leverage on the neck and a firm compression of the abdomen.

In the final position the head will face backward.

Hold the pose for a short duration.

Release the position by bending the knees and unclasping the hands. Slowly return to the upright position.

Breathing: Exhale before bending forward.

Inhale after interlocking the fingers behind the neck.

Exhale while straightening the legs.

Retain the breath out or breathe normally in the final position. Inhale while returning to the upright posture.

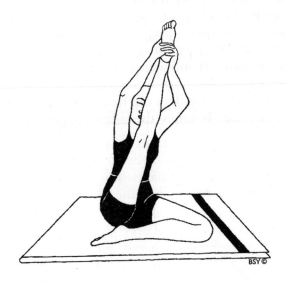

Eka Padottanasana (one leg raised to head pose)
Sit with the legs outstretched.
Bend the right knee and place the foot flat on the floor in front of the right buttock.
Fold the left leg, keeping the knee on the ground, and place the heel under the perineum.
Interlock the fingers under the sole of the right foot.
This is the starting position.
Raise the right foot and straighten the knee. Keep the spine straight.
Bring the knee to the nose.
Hold the pose for as long as is comfortable.
Bend the knee and lower the foot to the floor.
Practise a maximum of 5 times.
Repeat on the other side.
Breathing: Inhale in the starting position.
Retain the breath in while raising and lowering the leg.
Retain the breath in the final position or breathe normally if held for an extended duration.
Exhale in the starting position.

241

Awareness: Physical – on relaxation of the muscles of the straight leg, particularly the hamstrings.

Spiritual – on manipura chakra.

Sequence: This asana is a preparatory practice for meditative and forward bending asanas.

Contra-indications: People with back complaints or a displaced coccyx should not practise this asana.

Benefits: This asana renders the hamstring muscles and hip joints flexible. It tones the adrenals and reproductive system.

Spinal Twisting Asanas

This is an important series of asanas for spinal health. Every asana program should include at least one practice from this group, preferably following the forward and backward bending postures. The twist imposed on the spine and the whole trunk exercises the muscles, makes the spinal column more flexible and stimulates the spinal nerves. It also has a strong influence on the abdominal muscles, alternately stretching and compressing them as the body twists from one direction to the other. Beginners must be careful not to twist the trunk more than flexibility will allow. During pregnancy, meru wakrasana is the only asana recommended from this group. In general, also carefully observe the specific contra-indications for each practice.

Most of the spinal twist asanas enhance the pranic flow in the samana region, around the navel. This nourishes organs such as the pancreas, kidneys, stomach, small intestines, liver and gall bladder, relieves associated disorders and rejuvenates the tissues generally. The samana region is also related to manipura chakra, a plexus of major nadis or pranic channels, supplying the whole body. These asanas therefore have a strong effect on total health and vitality.

On the emotional and psychic levels, controlled twisting and untwisting represents a means of managing the knots and problems we encounter. These asanas give insight and inspire a systematic approach to untying the tangled knots of life.

243

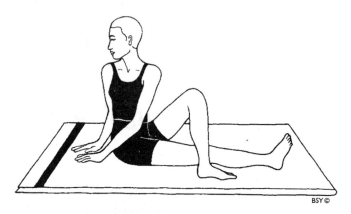

BSY©

Meru Wakrasana (spinal twist)

Sit with the legs outstretched.

Turn the trunk slightly to the right and place the right hand behind the body, close to the left buttock, with the fingers pointing backward.

Place the left hand behind and slightly to the side of the right buttock, as close as possible to the right hand.

Bend the left knee and place the foot outside the right knee. Twist the head and trunk as far to the right as is comfortable, using the arms as levers, while keeping the spine upright and straight.

The buttocks should remain on the floor. The right elbow may bend a little.

Hold the final position, relaxing the back. Look over the right shoulder as far as possible without straining.

Re-centre the trunk and relax for a few seconds.

Practise up to 5 times and then repeat on the other side.

Breathing: Inhale deeply, exhale while twisting.

Retain the breath outside, or breathe normally if holding the pose.

Inhale while recentring.

Awareness: Physical – on the twist and relaxation of the spine, and on breath awareness in the final position.

Spiritual – on manipura chakra.

Sequence: Meru wakrasana is a preparatory asana for ardha matsyendrasana and may be practised after forward and backward bending asanas and before inverted asanas.

Benefits: Meru wakrasana stretches the spine, loosening the vertebrae and toning the nerves. It alleviates backache, neck pain, lumbago and mild forms of sciatica. It is a good asana for beginners, preparing the back for the more difficult spinal twists.

BHU NAMANASANA

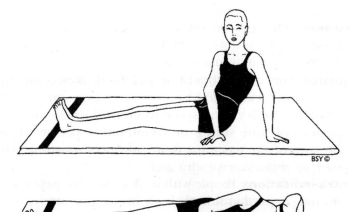

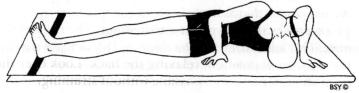

Bhu Namanasana (spinal twist prostration pose)

Sit with the spine erect and the legs outstretched.

Place the hands to the side of the right hip.

Move the right hand back slightly further behind the body with the fingers pointing backward.

Twist the trunk 90 degrees to the right, using the arms and shoulders as levers. Slowly bend the torso and bring the forehead to the floor, close to the hand placed behind

the body. The spine should be as straight as possible.
Try to keep both buttocks on the floor.
Hold the final position for a short time.
Slowly raise and return to the starting position.
Repeat the movement on the other side. This completes one round.
Practise up to 5 rounds.

Breathing: Inhale while facing forward.
Retain the breath in while twisting.
Exhale while bending.
Retain the breath out in the final position or breathe normally if holding the asana for some time.
Inhale while raising the trunk.
Exhale while recentring the body.

Awareness: Physical–on relaxation of the back and on the breath.
Spiritual–on manipura chakra.

Sequence: This asana should be practised after completing a series of forward and backward bending asanas. It also stretches the legs and spine when performed after long periods of time sitting in a meditation posture. It is a preparatory practice for more advanced twisting asanas such as ardha matsyendrasana.

Contra-indications: People with back problems, peptic ulcer, hernia, hyperthyroidism, high blood pressure or heart problems should not practise this asana.

Benefits: This asana stretches the spine and lower back, making the muscles supple and stimulating the nerves.

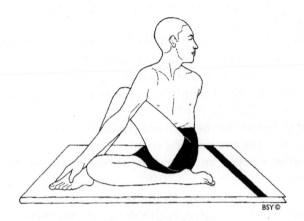

BSY©

Ardha Matsyendrasana (half spinal twist)

Sit with the legs stretched out in front of the body.

Bend the right leg and place the right foot flat on the floor on the outside of the left knee.

The toes of the right foot should face forward.

Bend the left leg and bring the foot around to the right buttock. The outside edge of the foot should be in contact with the floor.

Pass the left arm through the space between the chest and the right knee, and place it against the outside of the right leg.

Hold the right foot or ankle with the left hand so that the right knee is close to the left armpit.

Sit up as straight as possible.

Raise the right arm in front of the body and gaze at the fingertips.

Slowly twist to the right, simultaneously moving the arm, trunk and head.

Use the left arm as a lever against the right leg to twist the trunk as far as possible without using the back muscles.

Follow the tips of the fingers of the right hand with the gaze and look over the right shoulder.

Do not strain the back.

247

Bend the right elbow and place the arm around the back of the waist.

The back of the right hand should wrap around the left side of the waist.

Alternatively, it can be placed as high as possible between the shoulder blades with the fingers pointing up. This arm position enforces the straightness of the spine.

Reverse the movements to come out of the posture and repeat on the other side.

Breathing: Inhale in the forward position.

Exhale while twisting the trunk.

Breathe deeply and slowly without strain in the final position.

Inhale while returning to the starting position.

Duration: Practise once on each side, gradually increasing the holding time to 1 or 2 minutes on each side of the body or up to 30 breaths.

Awareness: Physical – on keeping the spine straight, and on the movement of the abdomen created by the breath in the final position.

Spiritual – on ajna chakra.

Sequence: This asana should be performed after completing a series of forward and backward bending asanas.

Contra-indications: Pregnant women should avoid this practice. People suffering from peptic ulcer, hernia or hyperthyroidism should only practise this pose under the guidance of a competent teacher.

People with sciatica or slipped disc should not practise it.

Benefits: This asana simultaneously stretches the muscles on one side of the back and abdomen while contracting the muscles on the other side.

It tones the nerves of the spine, makes the back muscles supple, relieves lumbago and muscular spasms, and reduces the tendency of adjoining vertebrae to develop inflammatory problems and calcium deposits. It massages the abdominal organs, alleviating digestive ailments. It regulates the secretions of the adrenal gland, liver and pancreas, and is beneficial for the kidneys.

Variation: For beginners and those with stiff bodies or bulky thighs, instead of bending one leg and placing its foot by the side of the buttock, that leg can remain straight. Also, instead of one hand holding the ankle, wrap the arm around the thigh, hugging the knee to the chest.

PARIVRITTI JANU SIRSHASANA

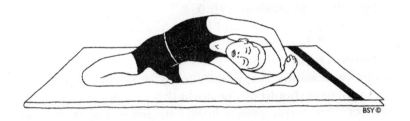

Parivritti Janu Sirshasana (spiralled head to knee pose)
Sit with the legs about a metre apart.
Bend the left knee and place the heel against the perineum.
Bend forward, inclining the body to the right to hold the right foot with the right hand.
The fingers should be in contact with the arch of the foot and the thumb should be on top.
Place the elbow on the floor on the inside of the straight leg.
Move the right shoulder down towards the right leg.
Bring the left arm over the head and grasp the right foot with the left hand.
Contracting the arms, slowly pull the right shoulder towards the right foot.
Ease the head under the left arm, relax the back and twist the trunk as much as possible so that the chest is open and facing forward.
Hold the pose for a comfortable length of time.
Release the hands, raising the left arm over the head,

249

and slowly return to the upright position.
Repeat the movement on the other side.

Breathing: Breathe normally while positioning the legs.
Exhale while inclining the trunk and placing the arms and hands into position, then inhale.
Exhale while pulling the body sideways.
Breathe normally while holding the final position.
Inhale while returning to the upright position.

Duration: Practise once on each side. Discontinue the pose if any discomfort is experienced.

Awareness: Physical – on the twist and stretch of the body.
Spiritual – on manipura chakra.

Sequence: This asana should be practised after forward and backward bending asanas. It is a twisting asana with a forward bend.

Contra-indications: Pregnant women or people with back complaints should not perform this practice.

Benefits: This asana gives a lateral stretch to the body, and also stretches the hamstrings and behind the shoulders. It gives a beneficial compression of the abdominal muscles and organs on one side of the body and simultaneously stretches them on the other side. It prepares the body for long hours of sitting in meditation asanas.

Inverted Asanas

Inverted asanas reverse the action of gravity on the body; instead of everything being pulled towards the feet, the orientation shifts towards the head. Similarly, on the emotional and psychic levels, inverted asanas change the normal patterns, throwing a new light on old patterns of behaviour and being. Generally, these practices are refreshing and revitalizing. They improve health, reduce anxiety and stress, and increase self-confidence. They also increase mental power, concentration and the capacity to sustain large workloads without strain.

Inverted asanas encourage blood to flow to the brain, nourishing the neurones and flushing out toxins. Blood and lymph, accumulated in the lower limbs, pelvis and abdomen, are drained back to the heart, then circulated to the lungs, purified and re-circulated to all parts of the body. This process nourishes the cells of the whole human organism. The enriched blood flow also allows the pituitary gland to operate more efficiently, tuning the entire endocrine system. This has a positive effect on the metabolic processes and even on ways of thinking.

While the body is in an inverted asana, the breath becomes slow and deep, maximizing the exchange of carbon dioxide and oxygen, and generally encouraging correct respiration. In addition, the abdominal organs: the liver, spleen, stomach, kidneys and pancreas, receive a powerful massage, helping them to perform their functions more efficiently.

Traditionally, inverted asanas are used to sublimate and transform sexual energy into spiritual energy. The aim of

251

the practices, in this context, is to stimulate the chakras, open sushumna nadi and raise the kundalini to bring about psychic awakening. While it is unlikely that kundalini will be raised through practice of these asanas alone, inverted postures undoubtedly improve the quality of meditation and concentration, refining the consciousness and enabling it to enter unexplored levels of the mind.

This important group of asanas must be performed correctly and with the utmost care. It is emphasized that these are powerful practices and that the following observances should be strictly adhered to.

Time of practice: Do not practise inverted asanas until at least three hours after taking food. Do not perform inverted asanas immediately after vigorous exercise.

Equipment: Always practise these asanas on a folded blanket or yoga mat thick enough to protect the vertebrae of the neck and back of the head. Never practise on a soft mattress, spring bed or cushions.

Duration: Beginners should only remain in the final positions for a few seconds. Once an asana can be maintained without experiencing the slightest difficulty, the duration may be increased gradually until it can be held for the recommended time.

Rest: Always follow inverted poses with shavasana. Rest until the breath and heartbeat are completely normal, then practise the recommended counterpose.

Precautions: Do not practise near furniture or anything that might impede a free fall to the floor. During a backward or forward fall, aim to break the fall with the feet. While falling, the body should be completely relaxed, never tense. If any discomfort occurs, discontinue the practice.

Cautions for inverted asanas: People recovering from operations, or going through pregnancy, people with inflammatory conditions or who are presently infirm, and the elderly, should carefully note the contra-indications for individual asanas, and those cautions and contra-indications given below. They apply to all inverted asanas, not just the ones in this section.

Inverted asanas include:

1. Semi-inverted positions where the trunk and head are horizontal, but the feet are raised above the head, e.g. poorwa halasana. Generally, they are not so challenging, but more care is needed if they are also strenuous practices, e.g. padotthanasana when performed with both legs raised.
2. Semi-inverted positions where the head is below the trunk, where the contra-indications must be fully observed, e.g. pada hastasana, and more so if the asanas are also strenuous, e.g. sirshapada bhumi sparshasana.
3. Fully inverted positions such as sarvangasana or sirshasana, which are also strenuous, e.g. vrischikasana.

Contra-indications: People suffering from heart conditions, high blood pressure or back conditions, especially slipped disc, should not practise these asanas. Those with illnesses that make the blood impure should not perform inverted asanas until the blood is purified. People with arteriosclerosis, glaucoma, an active ear infection or any disease of the brain should refrain from inverted postures. Those with cervical problems should not practise postures where the neck is bearing weight. Women should not practise inverted postures during pregnancy or menstruation.

Practice note: Assume the postures slowly and gently. Inverted asanas with their counterposes are usually placed at the end of an asana program. Never combine mayurasana with inverted asanas in one practice session.

BHUMI PADA MASTAKASANA

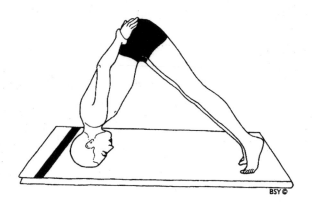

Bhumi Pada Mastakasana (half headstand)

Assume marjari-asana.

Turn the toes under.

Place the crown of the head on the floor between the hands.

Straighten the knees and raise the buttocks, balancing on the head and feet.

Bring the heels together and separate the toes.

Raise the arms and clasp the hands or take hold of one wrist behind the back.

Come up on to the toes as high as possible.

Hold the final pose for as long as is comfortable.

Lower the arms and place the hands beside the head. Slowly return to marjari-asana and then lower into shashankasana for a few moments.

This is one round.

After completing the practice, lie in shavasana before continuing with the counterpose.

Breathing: Normal breathing.

Duration: Practise up to 3 rounds, gradually extending the period in the asana.

Awareness: Physical – on the sensation at the crown of the head, in the neck and spine, on the balance and breath.

Spiritual – on sahasrara chakra.

Sequence: This asana should be followed by tadasana.

Contra-indications: People with high blood pressure, heart conditions, inflammation of the ear, weak eye capillaries, severe near-sightedness, problems in the pituitary or thyroid glands, arteriosclerosis, cerebral or other thrombosis, severe asthma, tuberculosis, cold or sinusitis, excessively impure blood, slipped disc, weak spine or vertigo should not practise this asana.

Benefits: This asana helps in cases of low blood pressure. It balances the nervous system, strengthens the neck muscles and brings a rich supply of blood to the brain. As a preliminary pose to sirshasana, it accustoms the brain to the increased influx of blood and the crown to supporting the weight of the body.

MOORDHASANA

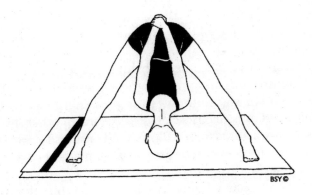

Moordhasana (crown-based pose)

Stand erect with the feet about a metre apart.

Bend forward from the hips and place the hands in front of the feet. The weight of the body should be evenly distributed and supported by the limbs.

Stage I: Place the crown of the head on the floor between the hands.

Raise the arms and take hold of one wrist behind the back.

255

Stage 2: Raise the heels and balance on the head and toes. This is the final position.

Hold the position for as long as is comfortable.

Replace the hands and soles of the feet on the floor and then return to the upright position.

Relax in the standing position until the body regains its equilibrium.

Breathing: Inhale in the standing position.

Exhale while bending forward.

Breathe normally while holding the position.

Inhale while returning to the standing position.

Duration: Practise up to 3 rounds. When first practising this asana hold the pose for a few seconds only, then gradually, over a period of a few weeks, extend the time to one minute.

Awareness: Physical – on the sensation at the crown of the head, in the neck and spine, on the balance, and on the breath.

Spiritual – on sahásrara chakra.

Sequence: At the end of the asana program, before sirshasana and followed by tadasana as the recommended counterpose.

Contra-indications: People with high blood pressure, heart conditions, inflammation of the ear, weak eye capillaries, severe near-sightedness, problems in the pituitary or thyroid glands, arteriosclerosis, cerebral or other thrombosis, severe asthma, tuberculosis, cold or sinusitis, excessively impure blood, slipped disc, weak spine or vertigo should not practise this asana.

Benefits: This asana helps in cases of low blood pressure. It balances the nervous system, strengthens the neck muscles and brings a rich supply of blood to the brain. As a preliminary pose to sirshasana, it accustoms the brain to the increased influx of blood and the crown to supporting the weight of the body.

VIPAREETA KARANI ASANA

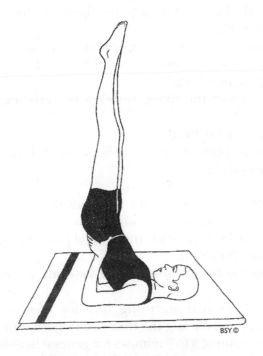

BSY ©

Vipareeta Karani Asana (inverted pose)

Lie flat on the back with the legs and feet together in a straight line. Place the hands and arms close to the body with the palms facing down.

Relax the whole body.

Raise both legs, keeping them straight and together.

Move the legs over the body towards the head.

Push down on the arms and hands, raising the buttocks.

Roll the spine from the floor, taking the legs further over the head.

Turn the palms up, bend the elbows and let the top of the hips rest on the base of the palms near the wrists. The hands cup the hips and support the weight of the body.

Raise the legs to the vertical position and relax the feet.

In the final position, the weight of the body rests on the shoulders, neck and elbows, the trunk is at a 45 degree

257

angle to the floor and the legs are vertical. Note that the chin does not press firmly against the chest.

Close the eyes and relax in the final pose for as long as is comfortable.

To return to the starting position, lower the legs over the head, then place the arms and hands close to the body, palms facing down.

Slowly lower the spine, vertebra by vertebra, along the floor.

Do not lift the head.

When the buttocks reach the floor, lower the legs, keeping them straight.

Relax the body in shavasana.

Breathing: Inhale while in the lying position.

Retain the breath inside while assuming the final pose.

Once the body is steady in the final pose, practise normal or ujjayi breathing.

Retain the breath inside while lowering the body to the floor.

Duration: When first practising, hold for a few seconds only, gradually increasing the time over a period of months to an optimum of 3 to 5 minutes for general health purposes. This practice should be performed only once during the asana program.

Other details: As for sarvangasana.

Practice note: This asana can be a preparatory practice for sarvangasana. It is highly recommended as it gives similar benefits to sarvangasana with less pressure on the neck. To begin with, it may be necessary to bend the knees when raising and lowering the legs.

Note: *This posture provides the basis for vipareeta karani mudra.*

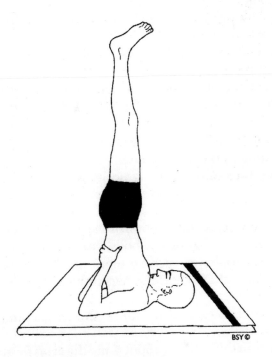

BSY©

Sarvangasana (shoulder stand pose)

Lie on the back on a folded blanket.

Check that the head and spine are aligned and that the legs are straight with the feet together.

Place the hands beside the body with the palms facing down.

Relax the entire body and mind.

Contract the abdominal muscles and, with the support of the arms, slowly raise the legs to the vertical position, keeping them straight.

When the legs are vertical, press the arms and hands down on the floor.

Slowly and smoothly roll the buttocks and spine off the floor, raising the trunk to a vertical position.

Turn the palms of the hands upward, bend the elbows and place the hands behind the ribcage, slightly away from the

259

spine, to support the back. The elbows should be about shoulder width apart.

Gently push the chest forward so that it presses firmly against the chin.

In the final position, the legs are vertical, together and in a straight line with the trunk. The body is supported by the shoulders, nape of the neck and back of the head. The arms provide stability, the chest rests against the chin and the feet are relaxed.

Close the eyes. Relax the whole body in the final pose for as long as is comfortable.

To return to the starting position, bring the legs forward until the feet are above and behind the back of the head. Keep the legs straight.

Slowly release the position of the hands and place the arms on the floor beside the body with the palms down.

Gradually lower each vertebra to the floor, followed by the buttocks, so that the legs resume their initial vertical position.

Lower the legs to the floor slowly, keeping the knees straight.

Perform this action without using the arms for support. The whole movement should combine balance with control so that the body contacts the floor slowly and gently.

Relax in shavasana until the respiration and heartbeat return to normal.

Breathing: Inhale in the starting position.

Retain the breath inside while assuming the final pose.

Practise slow, deep abdominal breathing in the final pose.

Retain the breath inside while lowering the body to the floor.

Duration: When first practising, hold the final position for a few seconds only, gradually increasing the time over a period of weeks to an optimum of 3 to 5 minutes for general health. This practice should be performed only once during the asana program.

Awareness: Physical – on the various sensations of the body adjusting to its inversion, on control of the movement, on

260

the neck or thyroid gland, and on the breath.
Spiritual – on vishuddhi chakra.

Sequence: Sarvangasana is ideally practised immediately before halasana. After halasana, either matsyasana, ushtrasana or supta vajrasana should be practised as a counterpose for half the combined duration of sarvangasana and halasana.

Contra-indications: This asana should not be practised by people suffering from enlarged thyroid, liver or spleen, cervical spondylitis, slipped disc, high blood pressure or other heart ailments, weak blood vessels in the eyes, thrombosis or impure blood. It should be avoided during menstruation and advanced stages of pregnancy.

Benefits: By pressing the chest against the chin, this asana stimulates the thyroid gland. It generally balances the circulatory, respiratory, digestive, reproductive, nervous and endocrine systems. It also tranquillizes the mind, relieves mental and emotional stress, and helps clear psychological disturbances, boosting the immune system. Its influence on the parathyroid glands ensures normal development and regeneration of the bones.

Abdominal breathing is induced, improving the exchange of air in the body, relieving stress and massaging the abdominal organs. Sarvangasana releases the normal gravitational pressure from the anal muscles, relieving haemorrhoids. It tones the legs, abdomen and reproductive organs, draining stagnant blood and fluid, and increasing circulation to these areas.

Flexibility of the neck vertebrae is improved and the nerves passing through the neck to the brain are toned. Circulation is increased in this area generally, revitalizing the ears, eyes and tonsils.

Variation I: Assume sarvangasana.

Exhale and lower one leg forward over the body until it is horizontal to the floor. The other leg should be vertical. Hold the pose for a few seconds.

Inhale, return the leg to the vertical position and resume sarvangasana. Repeat on the other side.

261

Variation 2: Assume sarvangasana.

Exhale, bend the hips forward, and lower both the straight legs over the head until they are parallel to the floor.
Hold for a few seconds.
Inhale and raise the legs to the vertical position.

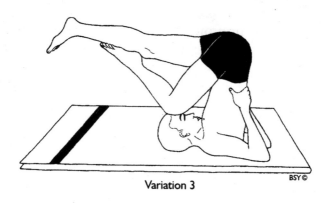

Variation 3

Variation 3: Assume sarvangasana.

Inhale and bend the right knee. Place the right foot on the left knee.
Exhale, bend the hips forward and place the right knee on the forehead. The left leg should be horizontal to the floor.
Retain the breath inside while holding this position.
Return to sarvangasana.
Repeat on the other side.

262

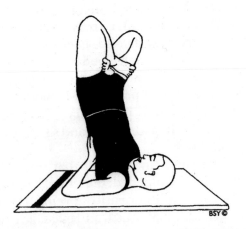

Padma Sarvangasana (shoulder stand lotus pose)

Assume sarvangasana.

Fold the legs into padmasana in the final pose.

Variation: Sit with the spine straight and the legs stretched out in front of the body.

Perform padmasana. Lean back and, carefully using the support of the elbows, lie flat on the back. Relax fully.

Raise the folded legs to the vertical position and assume sarvangasana.

Hold the final pose for as long as is comfortable.

Return to the starting position in the reverse order.

Breathing: Breathe normally while relaxing, then inhale deeply and retain the breath while raising the legs and coming into sarvangasana.

Practise normal breathing in the final pose, then inhale and retain the breath while releasing back to the floor.

Duration: When first practising, hold the final position for a few seconds only, gradually increasing the time over a period of weeks to about 3 minutes. This practice should be performed only once during the asana program.

Awareness: Physical–on the legs, spine and neck, on control of the movement, and on the breath.

Spiritual–on vishuddhi chakra.

263

Sequence: Matsyasana, ushtrasana or supta vajrasana should be practised as a counterpose.

Contra-indications: This asana is for a strong and healthy body only. Those who suffer from sciatica or weak or injured knees, enlarged thyroid, liver or spleen, cervical spondylitis, slipped disc, high blood pressure or other heart ailments, weak blood vessels in the eyes, thrombosis or impure blood should not practise it. It should be avoided during menstruation and pregnancy. This asana should not be attempted until padmasana and sarvangasana have both been mastered.

Benefits: As for sarvangasana, except that free drainage of blood from the legs is impeded; therefore, it is not effective in the treatment of piles or varicose veins. However, this asana gives an additional stretch and massage to the pelvic region and internal organs. It strengthens and coordinates the leg muscles and improves the sense of balance.

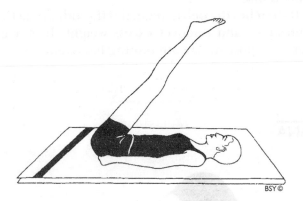

Poorwa Halasana (preliminary plough pose)

Lie on the back with the legs and feet together.

Place the arms close to the body, either with the palms of the hands facing down or with the hands made into fists and placed under the buttocks.

This is the starting position.

Raise both the legs to the vertical position.

The buttocks should rest on the floor or on the fists.

Bring the feet towards the head, making a 45 degrees angle between the legs and torso.

Separate the legs as far as is comfortable and then bring them together again.

Slowly lower the legs to the floor, keeping them straight.

This is one round. Practise 5 to 10 rounds.

Breathing: Inhale in the starting position.

Retain the breath inside while raising, separating, bringing together and lowering the legs.

Exhale after returning to the starting position.

Awareness: Physical–on the controlled movement with the breath or on the thyroid gland.

Spiritual–on manipura or vishuddhi chakra.

Sequence: This pose should be followed by a backward bending counterpose such as bhujangasana or shalabhasana.

Contra-indications: This asana should not be practised by those who are old or infirm, suffering from hernia, sciatica or slipped disc.

Benefits: It stretches the pelvis, regulates the kidneys, activates the intestines and removes excess weight. It is a good preparatory pose before attempting halasana.

HALASANA

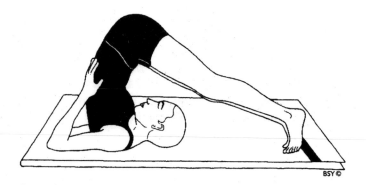

Halasana (plough pose)

Lie flat on the back with the legs and feet together. Place the arms beside the body with the palms facing down. Relax the whole body.

Raise both legs to the vertical position, keeping them straight and together, using only the abdominal muscles. Press down on the arms and lift the buttocks, rolling the back away from the floor. Lower the legs over the head. Bring the toes towards the floor behind the head without straining, but do not force the toes to touch the floor.

Turn the palms up, bend the elbows and place the hands behind the ribcage to support the back, as in sarvangasana. Relax and hold the final pose for as long as is comfortable. Return to the starting position by lowering the arms with the palms facing down, then gradually lower each vertebra of the spine to the floor, followed by the buttocks, so that the legs resume their initial vertical position.

Using the abdominal muscles, lower the legs to the starting position, keeping the knees straight.

Breathing: Inhale while in the lying position.

Retain the breath inside while assuming the final pose.

Breathe slowly and deeply in the final pose.

Retain the breath inside while returning to the starting position.

Duration: Beginners should hold the pose for 15 seconds, gradually adding a few seconds per week until it can be held for one minute.

Adepts may hold the final pose up to 10 minutes or longer.

Awareness: Physical – on the abdomen, relaxation of the back muscles and neck, the respiration, or the thyroid.

Spiritual – on manipura or vishuddhi chakra.

Sequence: If possible, perform this asana immediately after sarvangasana. To move from sarvangasana to halasana, bring the feet slightly over the head for balance, slowly remove the arms from their position behind the back and place them on the floor in the starting position, palms facing down. Relax the body and slowly lower the legs over the head, keeping them straight and together, until the toes touch the floor. Release as described above.

Follow halasana with either matsyasana, ushtrasana or supta vajrasana as a counterpose, practised for half the combined duration of sarvangasana and halasana. Halasana is a good preparatory practice for paschimottanasana.

Contra-indications: This asana should not be practised by those who suffer from hernia, slipped disc, sciatica, high blood pressure or any serious back problem, especially arthritis of the neck.

Benefits: The movement of the diaphragm which takes place during the practice of halasana massages all the internal organs, activates the digestion, relieving constipation and dyspepsia, revitalizes the spleen and the suprarenal glands, promotes the production of insulin by the pancreas and improves liver and kidney function. It strengthens the abdominal muscles, relieves spasms in the back muscles, tones the spinal nerves and increases blood circulation to the whole area. It regulates the activities of the thyroid gland, which balances the body's metabolic rate. It also improves the immune system.

Variation I: In the final pose, walk the feet away from the head until the body is completely stretched and a tight chin lock is performed. Breathe normally for as long as is comfortable in the final pose.

Benefits: This variation stretches the shoulders and the upper back, including the neck, giving more flexibility to the upper spine.

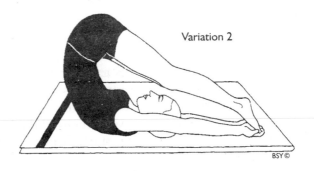

Variation 2

BSY©

Variation 2: In the final pose, begin to walk the toes towards the back of the head, keeping the legs straight and together. Take hold of the toes, keeping the arms straight. Breathe normally for as long as is comfortable in the final pose.

Benefits: This variation stretches the shoulders and increases flexibility in the lumbo-sacral region of the spine.

Sequence: After practising these variations, return to halasana and then to the starting position.

268

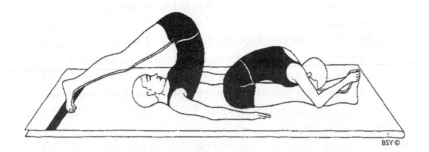

Druta Halasana (dynamic plough pose)
Lie flat on the back with the legs and feet together.
Place the arms close to the body with the palms facing
down. Relax the whole body.
Press down on the arms. Rapidly roll the legs over the head,
keeping the legs straight, and touch the floor behind the
head with the toes.
Hold the position for 1 or 2 seconds.
Roll the body rapidly back to the starting position.
Immediately sit up and bend the body forward into
paschimottanasana. Keep the legs straight and bring the
knees towards the forehead, hold the toes, feet or lower
legs. The practice should be performed with an even
flowing movement.
Resume the seated position. This completes one round.
Practise up to 10 rounds.
Breathing: Inhale and exhale deeply in the lying position
before starting. Inhaling roll backwards into halasana.
Exhale coming forward into paschimottanasana.
Awareness: Physical – on the stretch in the back and compression of the abdomen, and on the flow of the movement
with the breath.
Spiritual – on manipura chakra.
Sequence: This practice should be followed by a backward
bending counterpose such as matsyasana or supta vajrasana
to release the compression in the neck and abdomen.

Contra-indications: Druta halasana should not be practised by people with hernia, sciatica or other back or neck ailments, or by those with high blood pressure or heart ailments.

Benefits: This practice has the benefits of both halasana and paschimottanasana. It strengthens the back and abdominal muscles, activates intestinal peristalsis, improving digestion and removing constipation. It facilitates the breakdown of fats by exercising the liver and gall bladder, and stretches the pelvic region.

Practice note: The body should be completely stretched out in the lying position before moving into either halasana or paschimottanasana. This aspect can easily be overlooked as the momentum gathers. Be careful not to strain the muscles of the back or legs. Do not hit the back of the head on the floor.

ARDHA PADMA HALASANA

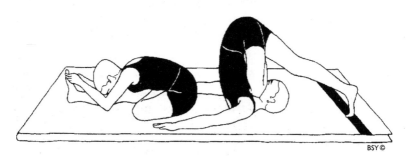

BSY©

Ardha Padma Halasana (half lotus plough pose)
Sit with the legs outstretched and the feet together.
Bend the left leg and place the foot on top of the right thigh in the half lotus position. Place the arms close to the body with the palms facing down.
Press down with the hands and roll backward.
Move the straight leg over the head and touch the ground with the toes.

Roll back to the upright position and, without breaking the movement or straining, bend forward from the hips, bringing the head towards the knee and holding the toes of the outstretched leg.

Resume the upright position.

Repeat with the right leg folded in ardha padmasana.

Practise up to 5 times with each leg folded.

Contra-indications: As for druta halasana. In addition, people with knee problems should refrain from this practice.

Other details: As for druta halasana.

STAMBHAN ASANA

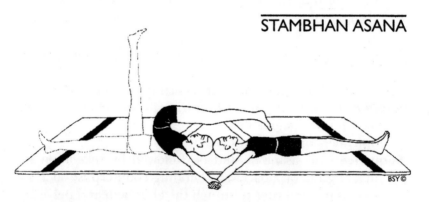

Stambhan Asana (posture of retention)

This asana requires the participation of two people of similar height and build.

Lie on the back with the crown of the head touching that of the other person.

The arms should rest beside the body with the legs and feet together.

The two bodies should be in a single, straight line.

Stretch the arms out to the sides at shoulder level and take hold of each other's hands.

Tense the arms and keep them flat on the floor with the elbows straight throughout the practice.

The tops of the heads must press against each other.

This is the starting position.

271

Partner one should raise the legs, keeping them together, until they are perpendicular to the floor.

Hold this position for a few seconds.

Lower the legs to the floor.

Again the same partner should raise both legs and buttocks from the floor and lower the legs into a horizontal position over the partner so the toes are above the partner's navel.

Hold the position for a few seconds, then slowly lower the legs and buttocks to the floor, resuming the starting position.

Partner two then performs the practice in the same way.

Each partner should practise up to 5 times.

Breathing: Inhale and exhale deeply while in the starting position.

Retain the breath outside while raising, holding and lowering the legs.

Inhale while returning to the starting position.

Awareness: Physical – on synchronizing the movement and the breath with the partner.

Spiritual – on manipura chakra.

Sequence: This asana should be followed by relaxation in makarasana or a backward bending counterpose such as setu asana, in order to stretch the abdomen and pelvis in the opposite direction.

Other details: As for druta halasana.

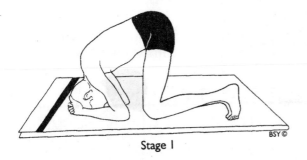

Stage I

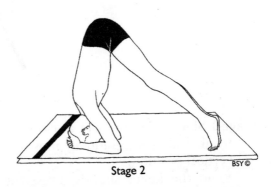

Stage 2

Sirshasana (headstand pose)
Stage I: Sit in vajrasana.

Close the eyes and relax the whole body.

After a few minutes, open the eyes, bend forward and place the forearms on a folded blanket with the fingers interlocked and the elbows in front of the knees.

The distance between the elbows should be equal to the distance from each elbow to the interlocked fingers, forming an equilateral triangle.

Place the crown of the head on the blanket between the interlocked fingers. Wrap the hands around the head to make a firm support so that it cannot roll backward when pressure is applied.

Stage 2: Lift the knees and buttocks off the floor and straighten the legs.

273

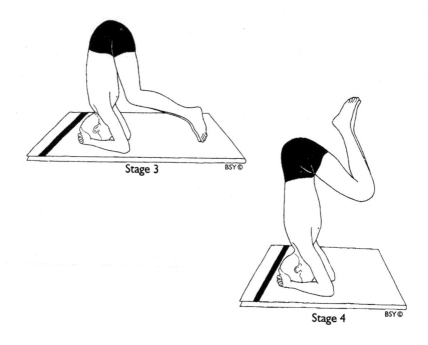

Stage 3   BSY©

Stage 4   BSY©

Stage 3: Slowly walk the feet as close as possible towards the trunk and head, gradually moving the back towards the vertical position.

Bend the knees slightly, press the thighs against the abdomen and lower chest.

Transfer the body weight slowly from the toes on to the head and arms, maintaining a steady balance.

Raise one foot off the floor about 20 cm, carefully balance, then raise the other foot and balance on the head and arms.

Stage 4: Bending the knees, gradually raise the lower legs in a controlled movement. Adjust the trunk slightly to counter-balance the weight of the legs.

Fold the legs back so the heels move towards the buttocks. To accomplish this movement contract the muscles of the lower back. The knees are now pointing down with the legs together.

Maintain the position for a few seconds, being aware of complete balance before proceeding.

274

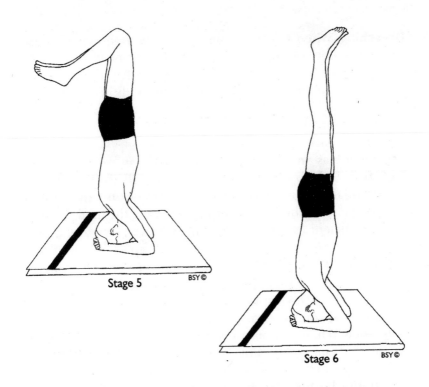

Stage 5   BSY©

Stage 6   BSY©

Stage 5: Raise the knees to the vertical position. Keeping the heels near the buttocks, slowly straighten the hips so that the thighs move up and away from the torso.
Raise the knees until they point directly upward and the thighs are in line with the trunk.
Balance the body.

Stage 6: Slowly straighten the knees and raise the lower legs. The whole body should be in one straight line with the feet relaxed.
This is the final position.
Close the eyes and balance the whole body, relaxing in the final position for as long as is comfortable.

Stage 7: Return to the starting position.
Slowly bend the knees and lower the body with control, in the reverse order, until the toes touch the floor. Remain with the head on the ground in the kneeling position for a short time, then slowly return to the upright position.

Breathing: When first learning sirshasana, one may practise normal breathing while coming into the posture.

Otherwise, inhale at the end of stage 1, and retain the breath inside while raising the body into the final position.

Breathe normally in the final position.

The breath should become increasingly subtle in this posture as one becomes accustomed to it.

Duration: Start by holding the pose for 10 to 30 seconds, gradually adding a few seconds each week until the desired period is reached. 3 to 5 minutes spent in the final position is sufficient for general health. However, sirshasana may be practised by adepts for periods of up to 30 minutes.

Awareness: Physical – when first practising, on maintaining the balance. For adepts, on the brain, on the centre of the head or on the respiration.

Spiritual – on sahasrara chakra.

Sequence: When first learning, practise sirshasana at the end of the asana program; more experienced practitioners may perform it either at the beginning or the end. It should be followed by tadasana, as a counterpose, and then shavasana.

Contra-indications: Sirshasana should not be practised by people with neck problems, headache or migraine, high blood pressure, heart disease, thrombosis, arteriosclerosis, chronic catarrh, chronic constipation, kidney problems, impure blood, severe near-sightedness, weak blood vessels in the eye, conjunctivitis, chronic glaucoma, inflammation of the ears or any form of blood haemorrhage in the head. It should not be practised during pregnancy or menstruation.

Benefits: This asana is very powerful for awakening sahasrara chakra and therefore it is considered the greatest of all asanas.

Sirshasana revitalizes the entire body and mind. It relieves anxiety and other psychological disturbances which form the root cause of many disorders such as asthma, hay fever, diabetes and menopausal imbalance.

It also helps to rectify many forms of nervous and glandular disorders, especially those related to the reproductive system.

This asana reverses the effect of gravity on the body. Strain on the back is thus alleviated and the reversed flow of blood in the legs and visceral regions aids tissue regeneration. The weight of the abdominal organs on the diaphragm encourages deep exhalation so that larger amounts of carbon dioxide are removed from the lungs.

Practice note: In the final position, most of the weight of the body is sustained by the top of the head, the arms being used to maintain balance only. Beginners, however, may use the arms for support until the neck is strong enough to bear the full weight of the body, and a reasonable sense of balance has been developed.

If the practitioner should fall during the practice, the body should be kept as relaxed as possible. If the fall is forward, try to fold the knees into the chest so that the impact on the floor is sustained by the feet. If falling backwards, arch the back again so that the feet sustain the impact.

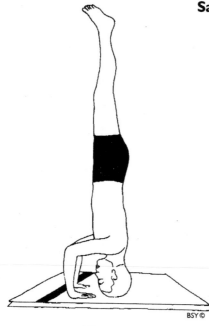

Salamba Sirshasana (supported headstand pose)

Assume marjari-asana.

Place the crown of the head on the blanket between the hands.

Move the hands back towards each side of the knees and adjust the position so that the hands form the corners of an equilateral triangle with the head. The forearms should be vertical and the elbows bent.

Lift the knees from the floor, straightening the legs and raising the buttocks.

Walk the feet forward until the thighs are near the chest and the back is almost vertical.

Slowly raise one foot off the floor, balance and then raise the other foot.

Utilising the arms for support, raise the legs and straighten the knees so that the body is fully erect (see stages 4, 5, and 6 of sirshasana).

Keep the spine and legs in a single vertical line.

This is the final position.

Hold the pose for as long as is comfortable.

Return to the starting position. Slowly refold the legs and lower the body with control, in the reverse order, until the toes touch the ground.

Remain in the kneeling position with the head on the floor for a short time.

Slowly return to the upright position.

Breathing: Retain the breath inside while assuming the final position. Breathe normally in the final position.
Retain the breath inside while lowering the body.

Other details: As for sirshasana.

Variation: (preparatory practice)
Assume the same base position as for salamba sirshasana.
Straighten both legs and walk the feet forward until the thighs are near the chest.
Raise the right foot, place the right knee on the right upper arm and balance. Raise the left foot and place the left knee on the left upper arm.
Hold the position for a few seconds, being aware of balance.

NIRALAMBA SIRSHASANA

Niralamba Sirshasana (unsupported headstand pose)

Stage I: Assume marjari-asana.
Place the crown of the head on the blanket between the hands.
Straighten the arms in front of the chest and place the hands flat on the floor about shoulder width apart.
Straighten the legs, allowing the weight of the body to be supported by the hands, feet and head.

Stage 2: Progressively walk the feet towards the head, keeping the legs straight, until the trunk is vertical.
Applying pressure on the hands, slowly bend the legs and raise the feet off the floor, bringing the knees to the chest.

Stage 3: Slowly raise the knees until they point upward.
Maintain balance in this position for a few moments.
Gradually straighten the knees until the feet point upwards in a relaxed position.
In the final pose the whole body is vertical and, ideally, all the weight of the body is supported by the head.
The hands should only provide balance.
Hold the final pose for as long as is comfortable.

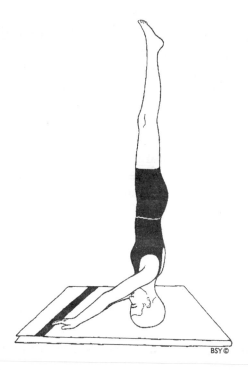

Stage 4: Return to the starting position.

Lower the body in the reverse order until the feet touch the floor.

Place the hands beside the head and bend the knees to the floor.

Relax with the head on the floor for a short time.

Duration: This asana is not as stable as sirshasana in the final position and is therefore unsuitable to be held for long periods of time.

Other details: As for sirshasana.

Practice note: Adepts may assume the vertical position directly without bending the knees first.

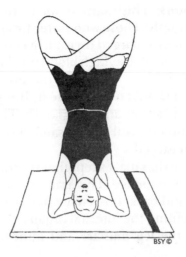

Oordhwa Padmasana (headstand lotus pose)

Perform sirshasana.

When balance has been established, slowly fold the legs into padmasana.

Remain in the final pose for as long as is comfortable.

Straighten the legs and balance again in sirshasana.

Return to the starting position as described for sirshasana.

Breathing: Inhale deeply and retain the breath while raising the legs and coming into sirshasana.

Practise normal breathing while balancing in sirshasana, folding the legs into padmasana, in the final pose and while releasing the legs from padmasana and resuming sirshasana. Inhale and retain the breath while releasing back to the floor.

Duration: When first practising, hold the final position for a few seconds only, gradually increasing the time over a period of weeks to about 3 minutes. This practice should be performed only once during the asana program.

Awareness: Physical – on alignment of the legs, back and neck, on the openness of the chest, and on the breath.

Spiritual – on sahasrara or anahata chakra.

Sequence: Tadasana and then shavasana should be practised as counterposes.

Contra-indications: This asana is for a strong, supple and healthy body only. Those who suffer from sciatica or weak or injured knees, enlarged thyroid, liver or spleen, cervical spondylitis, slipped disc, high blood pressure or other heart ailments, weak blood vessels in the eyes, thrombosis or impure blood should not practise it. It should be avoided during menstruation and pregnancy. This asana should not be attempted until padmasana and sirshasana have both been mastered.

Benefits: As for sirshasana, except that free drainage of blood from the legs is impeded. This asana induces full expansion of the chest and back. It stretches and massages the pelvic region, benefiting the internal organs. It strengthens and coordinates the leg muscles and improves the sense of balance.

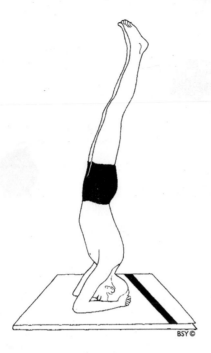

BSY©

Kapali Asana (forehead supported pose)

Perform sirshasana.

Maintain perfect balance for a short time, then slowly shift the angle of the head on to the forehead.

This is the point of balance.

In the final position, the spine and legs lean back a little to maintain balance.

Hold the final position for as long as is comfortable.

Return to sirshasana before lowering the body.

Variation I: Assume kapali asana.

Bend the right knee and place the sole of the right foot on the front of the left thigh.

The right knee should point forward.

Bend the left knee so that the foot points towards the floor behind the body.

Hold the final pose for as long as is comfortable.

Return to kapali asana and repeat with the opposite leg.

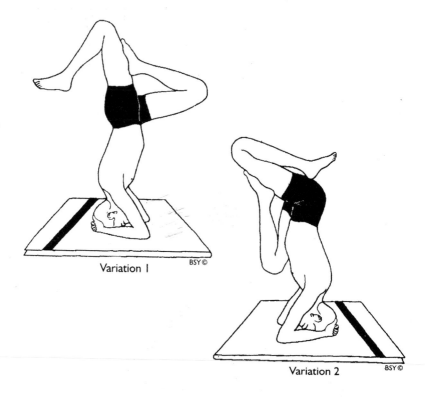

Variation I

Variation 2

Variation 2: Assume kapali asana.

> Bend the right knee and touch the right buttock with the heel.
>
> Tilt the hips forward, bend the left leg and bring the left knee to the chest.
>
> The sole of the left foot rests against the right thigh.
>
> In the final pose the right knee points forward and the left knee points downward.
>
> Hold the final pose for as long as is comfortable.
>
> Repeat the practice with the opposite leg.

Other details: As for sirshasana, with increased strain on the neck.

Balancing Asanas

Balancing asanas develop the functions of the cerebellum, the brain centre that controls how the body works in motion. Most people are uncoordinated in their movements, so their bodies constantly have to compensate for their lack of balance in order to avoid falling or knocking things over. This expends maximum effort and energy for minimum results, creating considerable additional strain. Such people will benefit from this series. However, people with diseases of the cerebellum should not attempt it. Balancing asanas improve muscle coordination and posture, inducing physical and nervous balance, and stilling unconscious movement. This conserves energy and achieves grace and fluidity of motion.

The focus required to perform these asanas with steadiness develops concentration and balance at the emotional, mental and psychic levels, removing stress and anxiety. For relief of excessive tension these practices should be held for as long as comfortable. To steady the mind, practise concentration on one point, at eye or navel level, on the ground, or as indicated in the individual asana – this allows the body to maintain seemingly difficult positions for long periods of time.

Balancing asanas may be difficult to perform at first. However, the body is very adaptable and progress will quickly be made with a few weeks of regular practice. Carefully observe the contra-indications given for individual practices.

285

EKA PADA PRANAMASANA

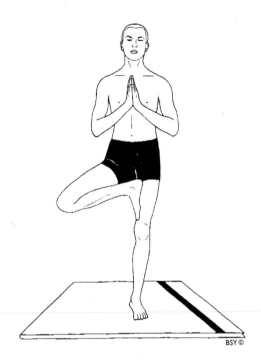

BSY©

Eka Pada Pranamasana (one-legged prayer pose)

Stand upright with the feet together and the arms at the sides. Focus the gaze on a fixed point in front of the body. Bend the right leg, grasp the ankle and place the sole of the foot on the inside of the left thigh. The heel should be close to the perineum and the right knee should point out to the side.

When the body is balanced, place the hands in prayer position in front of the chest for the final position.

Release the hands and then the foot.

Relax completely in the starting position, and change sides.

Breathing: Breathe normally throughout the practice.

Duration: Practise up to 3 rounds on each leg, holding the final position for up to 2 minutes.

Awareness: Physical – on a fixed point at eye level.
  Spiritual – on ajna or anahata chakra.
Benefits: This asana develops nervous balance. It also strengthens the leg, ankle and foot muscles.
Variation: Assume the final position of eka pada pranamasana. Keeping the gaze focused at eye level, inhale and raise the arms above the head, palms together. Hold the position with the breath inside and, on exhalation, lower the hands back in front of the chest. Repeat on the other side.

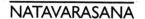

NATAVARASANA

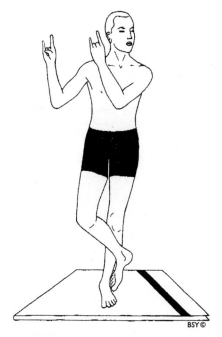

BSY©

Natavarasana (Lord Krishna's pose)

Stand with the feet together and focus on a fixed point. Bring the right leg a little forward and place the right foot to the outside of the left calf with the toes above the floor and the sole of the foot almost vertical.

287

Rest the side of the right calf against the left shin.

Raise both hands to the right as if playing a flute. The right palm should face forward and the left palm backward. The index and little fingers of the hands are straight and the middle fingers are curled into the base of the thumb.

Turn the head slightly to the left and focus the eyes at a fixed point.

Hold the final position for as long as is comfortable.

To release, bring the head to the centre, lower the arms to the sides and the raised foot to the floor.

Repeat the stance on the other side.

Breathing: Breathe normally throughout the practice.

Duration: Practise up to 3 rounds on each leg, holding the final position for up to 2 minutes.

Awareness: Physical – on maintaining balance while focusing on a fixed point.

Spiritual – on ajna chakra.

Sequence: This asana may be practised as a preparatory pose for meditation.

Benefits: Natavarasana helps develop nervous balance and concentration.

GARUDASANA

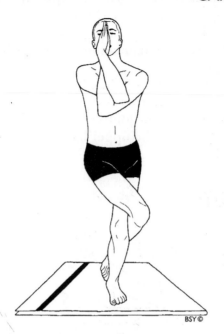

Garudasana (eagle pose)

Assume the standing position and focus the gaze on a fixed spot.

Bend the right leg and twist it around the left leg. The right thigh should be in front of the left thigh and the top of the right foot should rest on the calf of the left leg.

Bend the elbows and bring them in front of the chest.

Twist the forearms around each other with the left elbow remaining below.

Place the palms together to resemble an eagle's beak.

Balance in this position for some time, then slowly bend the left knee and lower the body, keeping the back straight, until the elbows come down to the knees and the tip of the right big toe touches the floor.

Keep the eyes focused on the fixed point.

Hold the final position for as long as is comfortable, then raise the body, and release the legs and arms.

Relax with the eyes closed.

289

Repeat with the legs and arms the opposite way around.
Practise up to 3 rounds on each side.

Breathing: Breathe normally throughout the practice.

Awareness: Physical – on maintaining balance while lowering and raising the body.

Spiritual – on mooladhara chakra.

Benefits: Garudasana improves concentration, strengthens the muscles and loosens the joints of the shoulders, arms and legs, and is good for the upper back.

TANDAVASANA

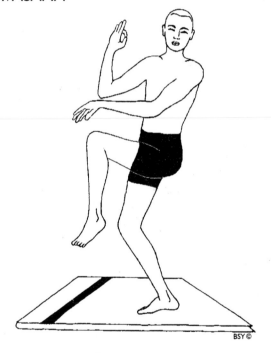

Tandavasana (Lord Shiva's dance)

Stand upright with the feet slightly apart.

Bend and raise the left knee so the thigh is horizontal, the foot pointing away from the body and slightly to the right of the right leg. Bend the right knee slightly.

Place the left arm across the body in line with the left thigh, with the palm and fingers facing down.
Bend the right elbow so that the right palm faces forward and the forearm is vertical.
The right elbow should be just behind the left wrist.
Practise jnana mudra with the right hand and gaze toward the horizon.
This is the final position.

Breathing: Breathe normally throughout the practice.

Duration: Up to 3 times on each side, holding each time for as long as possible without strain.

Awareness: Physical – on maintaining balance while focusing on jnana mudra.
Spiritual – on ajna chakra.

Benefits: This asana balances the nervous system, develops control of the body and mental concentration, and makes the legs supple.

SARAL NATARAJASANA

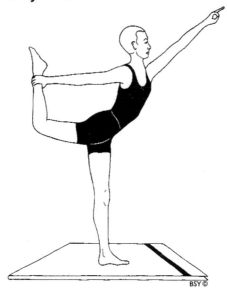

Saral Natarajasana (preparatory Lord Shiva's pose)

Stand with the feet together and focus on a fixed point.
Bend the right knee and grasp the ankle with the right
hand behind the body.

Keep both knees together and maintain the balance.

Slowly raise and stretch the right leg backward, as high
as comfortable.

Make sure the right hip does not twist and the leg is raised
directly behind the body.

Reach upward and forward with the left arm, bringing the
tip of the index finger and thumb of the left hand together
to form jnana mudra. Focus the gaze on the left hand.
This is the final position.

Hold the position for as long as is comfortable.

Lower the left arm to the side. Lower the right leg, bringing
the knees together. Release the right ankle and lower the
foot to the floor. Lower the right arm to the side. Relax,
then repeat with the left leg.

Other details: As for natarajasana.

NATARAJASANA

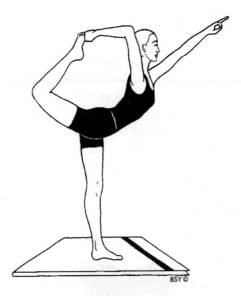

Natarajasana (Lord Shiva's pose)

Stand with the feet together and gaze at a fixed point.
Bend the right knee and grasp the right big toe.
As the right leg is raised, swivel the shoulder, so that the elbow of the arm holding the big toe points upward. This position of the hand and arm will allow the foot to be raised nearer to the back of the head.
Make sure the right hip does not twist and the leg is raised directly behind the body.
Reach upward and forward with the left arm, bringing the tip of the index finger and thumb of the left hand together to form jnana mudra.
Focus the gaze on the left hand.
This is the final position.
Hold the position for as long as comfortable.
Lower the left arm to the side. Lower the right leg, releasing the right foot to the floor and the right arm to the side.
Relax, then repeat on the other side.
Practise up to 3 times on each side.
Breathing: Breathe normally throughout the practice.

Contra-indications: People who suffer from a weak heart, high blood pressure, back problems, hernia, colitis, peptic or duodenal ulcers, or vertigo should not practise this asana.

Benefits: This asana strengthens the back, shoulders, arms, hips and legs. It helps develop a sense of balance and coordination and improves concentration.

Variation: Advanced practitioners with flexible bodies may be able to touch the back of the head with the toes or to hold the toes with both hands.

EKA PADASANA

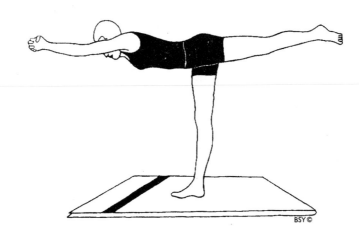

Eka Padasana (one foot pose)

Stand relaxed, with the feet together.

Raise the arms directly above the head and interlock the fingers with the palms together.

Bend forward slowly from the hips, keeping the trunk, head and arms in a straight line and transferring the weight on to the right leg.

Simultaneously raise the left leg straight back, keeping it in line with the trunk.

The body should pivot from the right hip joint.

In the final position the left leg, trunk, head and arms are all in one straight, horizontal line. The right leg is straight and vertical.

Focus the gaze on the hands.

Hold the final position for as long as is comfortable and then, keeping the arms, back and leg aligned, return to the upright position.

Slowly lower the arms and return to the starting position.

Repeat the movement, raising the right leg back.

Breathing: Inhale while raising the arms.

Exhale while bending to assume the final position.

Breathe normally in the final position.

Inhale while returning to the upright position.

Exhale while lowering the arms.

Duration: Up to 3 times on each side, holding for as long as is comfortable each time.

Awareness: Physical–on maintaining the alignment of limbs and spine, and on maintaining balance.

Spiritual–on swadhisthana or manipura chakra.

Sequence: This asana should be preceded or followed by a backward bending asana such as makarasana. This posture may be used as a preliminary practice to bakasana.

Contra-indications: People with lower back problems, heart problems or high blood pressure should not do this asana.

Benefits: This asana strengthens the arms, wrists, back, hips and leg muscles. It helps to develop muscular coordination, nervous balance and concentration.

BAKASANA

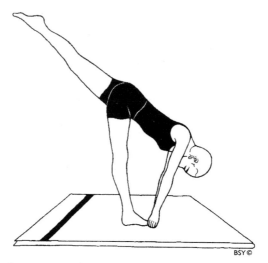

Bakasana (crane pose)

Relax in the standing position with the feet together.

Raise the arms in front of the body over the head.

Bend forward from the hips, transferring the weight to the right foot, and touch the toes of the right foot with both hands. Simultaneously, slowly stretch the left leg behind, raising it as high as is comfortable and bring the forehead towards the right knee.

Keep both legs straight.

To release, lower the leg and return to the upright position, keeping the arms straight as they are raised above the head. Then lower the arms and relax in the standing position.

Repeat the practice on the other side.

Breathing: Inhale while raising the arms.

Exhale while bending forward.

Breathe normally in the final position.

Inhale while returning to the upright position.

Exhale while lowering the arms.

Duration: Up to 3 times on each side, holding for as long as is comfortable each time.

Awareness: Physical–on maintaining balance.
Spiritual–on swadhisthana or manipura chakra.
Contra-indications: People with back or heart problems, high
blood pressure or vertigo should not practise this asana.
Cautions for inverted asanas apply.
Benefits: Strengthens the back, hip and leg muscles, improves
blood circulation and gives a beneficial compression to
the abdominal organs. It aids concentration, balance and
nervous coordination.

UTTHITA HASTA PADANGUSTHASANA

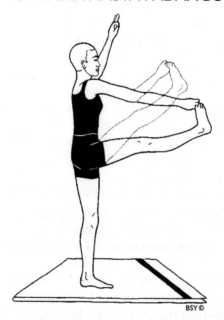

Utthita Hasta Padangusthasana (raised hand to big toe pose)

Stand upright with the feet together and relax the whole
body.
Focus the gaze on a fixed point.
Bend the right knee, bringing the thigh as close as possible
to the chest.

Place the right arm around the outside of the bent leg and take hold of the big toe.

Straighten the right leg in front of the body, then slowly pull it up closer to the body.

Do not strain the leg muscles.

Raise the left arm to the side for balance and perform chin or jnana mudra with that hand.

Hold the final position for as long as is comfortable.

Bend the knee, release the toe and slowly lower the foot to the floor.

Relax the arms.

Repeat on the other side.

Breathing: Inhale after grasping the big toe.

Exhale while straightening the raised leg, then inhale.

Exhale while pulling the leg higher.

Breathe deeply in the final position.

Exhale while lowering the leg.

Duration: Hold the final position for up to 60 seconds. Those people who are unable to maintain the pose may repeat up to 5 times with each leg.

Awareness: Physical – on the stretch along the back of the leg, on the hips, and on maintaining balance by focusing on the chosen fixed point.

Spiritual – on mooladhara or swadhisthana chakra.

Contra-indications: This asana should not be practised by people with sciatica or hip complaints.

Benefits: Improves concentration and coordinates muscular and nervous balance. The hips and leg muscles are strengthened and toned, and the hamstrings are stretched, helping the knee and ankle joints.

Variation I: Repeat the basic form, but hold the raised straight leg with both hands.

Clasp the fingers together and place them behind the heel.

Using the arms as levers, gently pull the leg as near as possible to the head without straining.

Advanced practitioners may be able to touch their chin to the raised leg.

Variation 2: Stand upright with the feet together and focus on a fixed point.

Bend the right knee and raise the thigh towards the chest. Place the right arm along the inside of the right leg and hold the big toe with the hand.

Turn the knee out to the right and slowly straighten the leg to the side.

Raise the left arm to the side to assist with balance and adopt jnana mudra.

Raise the leg higher and bring it closer to the body.

Hold the final position for as long as is comfortable.

Bend the right knee and bring the leg back to the centre.

Release the upright arm, then the toe, and lower the leg to the floor.

Repeat on the other side.

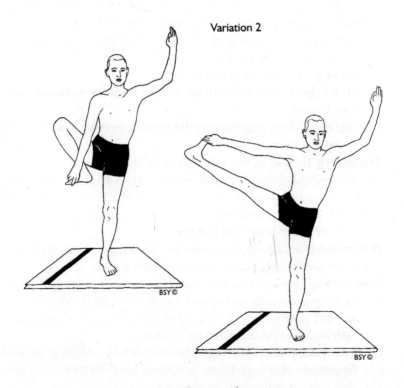

Variation 2

MERUDANDASANA

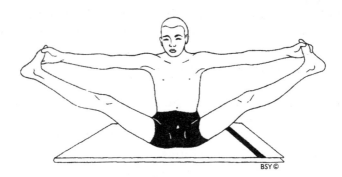

BSY ©

Merudandasana (spinal column pose)
Sit with the legs outstretched.
Bend the knees and place the feet flat on the floor in front
of the buttocks, about half a metre apart. Holding the big
toes, slowly lean backward, balancing on the coccyx.
Straighten the legs and arms, raising them upward.
Steady the body, keeping the spine straight, then separate
the legs as wide as possible. Do not strain.
Hold the final position, keeping the gaze focused on a
fixed point.
Bring the legs together at the centre, bend the knees and
lower the feet to the floor.
Breathing: Inhale in the sitting position.
Retain the breath inside while stretching the legs and
holding the final position. If holding the pose for some
time, breathe normally.
Exhale after lowering the feet.
Duration: Practise up to 5 rounds, holding the breath in the
final position for as long as is comfortable.
Awareness: Physical – on the stretch in the arms, legs and groin,
and on maintaining balance on the coccyx by focusing on
a fixed point.
Spiritual – on swadhisthana chakra.
Contra-indications: Merudandasana should not be practised
by people with high blood pressure, heart ailments, slipped
disc, sacral infections or sciatica.

Benefits: This asana tones the abdominal organs, especially the liver, and strengthens the abdominal muscles. It helps to stimulate intestinal peristalsis, alleviating constipation. It tones the sympathetic and parasympathetic nervous systems, strengthens the muscles of the back and helps to realign the spine. It helps to remove tiredness from the legs, giving a feeling of lightness and balance, and is good for the knees.

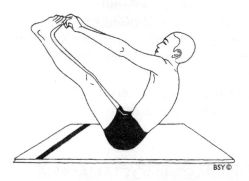

Variation 1: Utthita Hasta Merudandasana (raised hand and spine pose)

The instructions are the same as for merudandasana except that instead of separating the legs in the final position, bring them together.

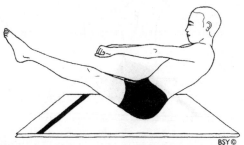

Variation 2: Mukta Hasta Merudandasana (rocking horse)

Sit with the legs outstretched and the feet together.
Bend the knees and bring them to the chest, keeping the feet flat on the floor.
Bend the arms and place the fists outside the knees.

301

Focus the gaze on a fixed point.

Lean backwards, simultaneously straightening and raising the arms and legs.

Keep the fists above the knees and the spine straight.

The whole body should be balanced on the buttocks.

Raise the legs as high as possible.

Maintain the final position for a short time and then return to the starting position in the reverse order.

Relax and repeat several times.

Breathing: Inhale while leaning backwards and raising the legs. Exhale while placing the feet back on the floor and bringing the knees to the chest. Breathe normally if holding the position.

Contra-indications: As for merudandasana, but this variation is also a strenuous practice.

NIRALAMBA PASCHIMOTTANASANA

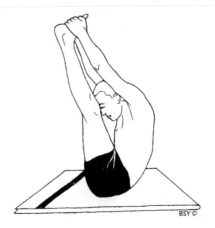

Niralamba Paschimottanasana (unsupported back stretching pose)

Sit with the legs outstretched and the feet together.

Bend the knees and bring them to the chest, keeping the feet flat on the floor. Place the arms outside the legs and grasp the soles of the feet.

Relax the whole body and focus on a fixed point.
Lean backwards slightly on to the coccyx, lifting the feet off the floor.
Slowly raise the feet and straighten the knees.
Balance on the buttocks.
Pulling the arms back, draw the knees towards the head.
Relax the back as much as possible in the final position. Do not strain.
Hold the position for as long as is comfortable.
Keeping the balance, slowly bend the knees and lower the feet to the floor.
Stretch the legs forward.
Relax the whole body.

Breathing: Inhale in the sitting position.
Retain the breath in while raising and lowering the legs and while balancing, or breathe deeply and slowly if holding the pose for an extended period.
Exhale after lowering the feet.

Duration: Practise up to 3 rounds, or hold once for up to 3 minutes.

Awareness: Physical – on the stretch in the limbs, on relaxing the back muscles, and on maintaining balance by focusing on a fixed point.
Spiritual – on swadhisthana chakra.

Sequence: This practice may be followed by bhujangasana or makarasana.

Contra-indications: People suffering from slipped disc, sciatica, sacral infections, high blood pressure or heart disease should not practise this asana.

Benefits: This practice has similar benefits to paschimottanasana. In addition, it helps to improve the sense of balance.

ARDHA PADMA PADOTTANASANA

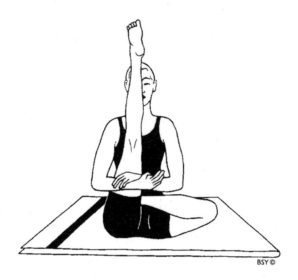

Ardha Padma Padottanasana (half lotus leg stretch pose)
Sit with the legs outstretched.
Bend the left knee and place the left foot on top of the right thigh in the half lotus position.
Bend the right knee and place the foot flat on the floor.
Fold the forearms under the right thigh.
Focus the gaze on a fixed point in front.
Lean backward on to the coccyx. Slowly raise the right leg and straighten the knee.
Balance on the back of the buttocks, bring the raised leg closer to the body, using the clasped arms to support it.
Hold the final position for as long as is comfortable.
Bend the right knee, lower the foot to the floor and stretch the leg forward. Practise up to 5 times on each side.
Repeat on the other side.
Breathing: Inhale while seated.
Retain the breath in while assuming and holding the final position, or breathe normally if holding for extended periods.
Exhale after lowering the foot to the floor.

Awareness: Physical—on maintaining balance while focused
on a fixed point.
Spiritual—on swadhisthana chakra.
Benefits: This asana helps improves the sense of balance and
activates intestinal peristalsis, alleviating constipation.

ARDHA BADDHA PADMOTTANASANA

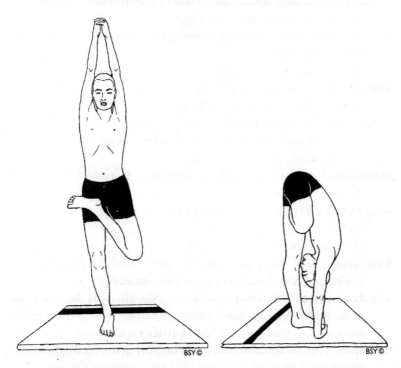

Ardha Baddha Padmottanasana (half lotus forward bending)
Stand with the feet together.
Focus the gaze on a fixed point.
While balancing on the left leg, bend the right knee and
place the foot as high as possible on the left thigh, in the
half lotus position.
Raise the arms above the head and interlock the fingers,
palms down. The elbows should be straight.

Relax and steady the whole body.

This is the starting position.

Slowly bend forward, keeping the arms straight. Bring the interlocked fingers down to the left foot or place the palms of the hands flat on the floor. Bring the forehead to the left knee.

Hold the final position for as long as is comfortable.

Slowly raise the torso and arms to the starting position with the hands above the head. Lower the arms beside the body and release the right leg.

Close the eyes and relax in the standing position with both feet on the floor.

Repeat on the other side.

Breathing: Inhale in the starting position.

Exhale while bending forward.

Breathe normally in the final position.

Inhale while returning to the starting position.

Exhale while lowering the arms.

Duration: Practise one round, holding the pose for up to 2 minutes on each side.

Awareness: Physical – on maintaining balance or on the breath.

Spiritual – on swadhisthana chakra.

Sequence: This asana should be preceded or followed by bhujangasana, chakrasana or dhanurasana.

Contra-indications: People with sciatica, slipped disc, hernia, weak legs or high blood pressure should not practise this asana. Cautions for inverted postures apply.

Benefits: This asana stimulates digestion, removes constipation, improves blood circulation and strengthens the legs.

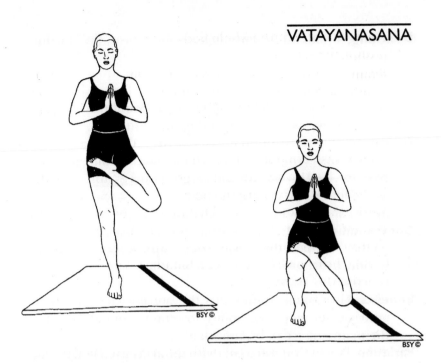

BSY©

BSY©

Vatayanasana (flying horse pose)

Stand with the feet together.

Focus the gaze on a fixed point.

Shift the weight of the body to the right leg.

Bend the left knee and place the foot on the right thigh in the half lotus position.

Hold the left ankle until the body is steady, then place the palms of the hands together in front of the chest.

Slowly bend the right knee and lower the body, maintaining balance, until the left knee rests on the floor.

Hold the final position for a short while, resting with the weight evenly balanced on the right foot and left knee.

Transfer the weight back on to the right leg and slowly raise the body, straightening the right knee, and returning to the starting position.

Release the left leg and lower it to the floor. Relax in the standing position with the eyes closed.

Repeat to the opposite side.

Practise up to 3 times on each side.

Breathing: Inhale while standing on one foot in the starting position.
Retain the breath while lowering the body.
Breath normally in the final position.
Inhale and retain the breath while raising the body.
Exhale when once more standing upright.

Awareness: Physical – on maintaining the balance, especially while transferring the weight in the different stages of the practice, and on the upward surge of energy and strength in the legs while raising the body.
Spiritual – on swadhisthana chakra.

Contra-indications: This is a strenuous practice. People with sciatica, slipped disc, weak back, hips, knees or ankles, hernia, heart problems or high blood pressure should not practise this asana.

Benefits: This asana strengthens the leg muscles and knee joints. It develops the ability to retain seminal fluid for the maintenance of brahmacharya.

Variation: Practise vatayanasana with the arms stretched downward at a 45 degrees angle from the body or stretched sideways like the wings of a bird.

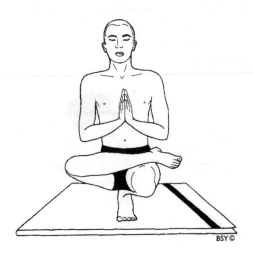

BSY©

Pada Angushthasana (tiptoe pose)

Squat, with the gaze focused on a fixed point.

Raise the heels and balance on the tiptoes.

Allow the knees to come forward slightly so that the thighs are horizontal.

Adjust the heel of the left foot so that it presses against the perineum.

Transfer the weight on to the left foot and place the right foot on top of the left thigh, turning the sole upward.

Balance the whole body and then place the palms together in front of the chest.

Stay in this final position for as long as is comfortable.

Replace the right foot on the floor.

Relax for a short time and repeat on the other side.

Practise 2 to 3 times on each side.

Breathing: Breathe normally throughout the practice.

Awareness: Physical – on the pressure of the heel while maintaining balance.

Spiritual – on mooladhara chakra.

Contra-indications: People with sciatica, slipped disc, ankle or knee problems should not practise this asana.

Benefits: This asana helps to maintain brahmacharya and regulates the reproductive system. It strengthens the toes and ankles. Concentration is improved.

BAKA DHYANASANA

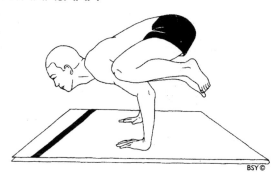

Baka Dhyanasana (patient crane pose)

Squat on the floor with the feet apart.

Balance on the toes and place the hands flat on the floor directly in front of the feet, with the fingers pointing forward. The elbows should be slightly bent.

Lean forward and adjust the knees so that the inside of the knees touch the outside of the upper arms as near as possible to the armpits.

Lean forward further, transferring the body weight on to the arms and lifting the feet off the floor.

Balance on the hands with the knees resting firmly on the upper arms. Bring the feet together.

Focus the gaze at the nosetip.

Hold the final position for as long as is comfortable.

Slowly lower the feet to the floor and relax.

Breathing: Retain the breath inside in the final position if holding the pose for a short period.

Breathe normally if holding for longer periods.

Duration: Practise holding the pose once for 2 or 3 minutes or practise raising and lowering the feet several times.

Awareness: Physical – on maintaining balance.

Spiritual – on the nosetip as in nasikagra drishti.

Sequence: Relax in advasana following this asana.

Contra-indications: People with high blood pressure, heart disease or cerebral thrombosis should not attempt this practice.

Benefits: This asana balances the nervous system. It strengthens the arms and wrists and develops the sense of physical balance.

Practice note: This asana requires more coordination than muscular strength.

EKA PADA BAKA DHYANASANA

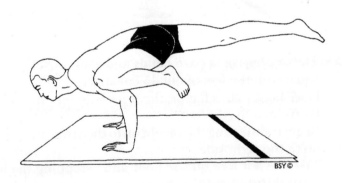

Eka Pada Baka Dhyanasana (one-legged crane pose)

Assume the final position of baka dhyanasana.

Focus the gaze at the nosetip.

Maintaining the balance, transfer more weight on to the left arm and slowly stretch the right leg back until it is straight.

Hold this position for as long as possible without straining.

Return the right knee to rest on the upper right arm.

Lower the feet to the floor and relax.

Practise again, stretching the left leg back.

Breathing: Retain the breath inside in the final position if holding the pose for a short time.

Breathe normally if holding for longer periods.

Other details: As for baka dhyanasana.

DWI HASTA BHUJASANA

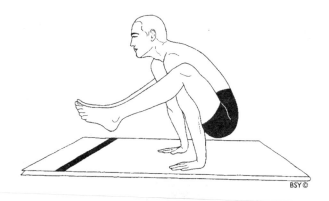

Dwi Hasta Bhujasana (two hands and arms pose)

Squat with the feet about 45 cm apart.

Place both palms flat on the floor between the feet.

Focus on a fixed point.

Begin transferring the weight on to the arms, and especially on to the right side.

Take the left foot off the floor and, wrapping the left leg around the outside of the left arm, rest the thigh on the upper arm.

Maintain the balance.

Transfer the weight of the body more equally on to both arms and, raising the right foot, slowly rest the right leg on the outside of the right arm above the elbow.

In the final position the whole body is supported by the arms and hands.

Hold the position for as long as is comfortable.

Slowly reverse the order of movements and resume the starting position. Relax for a short time.

Repeat leading with the right foot.

Practise once or twice on each side.

Breathing: Breathe normally throughout the practice.

Awareness: Physical – on carefully transferring the weight to avoid overbalancing, and on the strength in the arms and shoulders.

Spiritual – on vishuddhi chakra.

Sequence: Relax in advasana or jyestikasana after the practice.

Contra-indications: People with sciatica, slipped disc, weak back, hernia, heart problems or high blood pressure should not practise this asana.

Benefits: This asana develops the arm muscles and increases flexibility in the shoulder joints and lower back. It massages and tones the abdomen and visceral organs, stimulating the pancreas.

EKA HASTA BHUJASANA

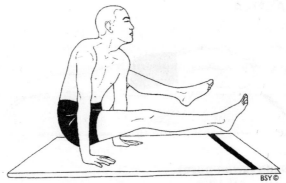

Eka Hasta Bhujasana (single hand and arm pose)

Sit on the floor with both legs outstretched.

Bend the left leg and place the inner knee as high as possible on the outside of the left upper arm.

Squeeze so that there is a grip between the leg and the arm capable of bearing some weight.

Place both palms flat on the floor with the right palm on the outside of the right leg.

313

Focus on a fixed point.

Raise the whole body off the ground, keeping the right leg straight and parallel to the floor between the arms.

Hold the final position for a comfortable length of time.

Lower the body to the floor and completely relax in the seated position.

Repeat the practice with the left leg held straight.

Breathing: Inhale while seated on the floor.

Retain the breath inside while raising and balancing the body. Exhale while returning to the floor.

Benefits: This asana strengthens the arm muscles and increases flexibility in the shoulders, hips and lower back. It strengthens the abdominal organs and tones the perineum as the muscles contract. Thus it helps with the preservation of sexual energy for spiritual purposes.

Other details: As for dwi hasta bhujasana.

HAMSASANA

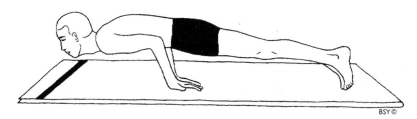

BSY©

Hamsasana (swan pose)

Kneel on the floor with the feet together and the knees apart.

Place the palms flat on the floor with the fingers pointing towards the feet. Bring the wrists and forearms together so that they touch.

Lean forward so that the abdomen rests on top of the elbows and the chest rests on the upper arms.

Maintain the balance and slowly stretch the legs backward until they are straight.

314

Keep the feet together and place the tips of the toes on the floor.

Raise the head slightly and focus the gaze on a fixed point in front at eye level.

In the final position, all the weight of the body should rest on the hands and the tips of the toes.

Hold the position for as long as is comfortable.

Do not strain.

Lower the knees to the floor and sit up in vajrasana.

Relax the whole body.

Breathing: Exhale completely before moving into the first position.

Hold the breath out if holding the final position for a short time, or breathe deeply and slowly if holding the pose for an extended period.

Hold the breath out when lowering the body.

Inhale after returning to the sitting position.

Duration: Adepts may hold the final position for up to 3 minutes. Beginners should hold the pose for a few seconds, gradually increasing the duration over a period of weeks.

Practise up to 3 rounds.

Awareness: Physical – on the abdomen, the sense of balance and on the breath.

Spiritual – on manipura chakra.

Sequence: This pose is a preparation for mayurasana and may be performed as an alternative by people who do not have the muscular strength required for that practice. It should not precede inverted asanas.

Contra-indications: People suffering from peptic or duodenal ulcers, hyperacidity, hernia or high blood pressure should not practise this asana. Pregnant women are strictly advised not to attempt this asana.

Benefits: Hamsasana massages and stimulates the abdominal organs and muscles, and is beneficial for a healthy digestive system.

315

SANTOLANASANA

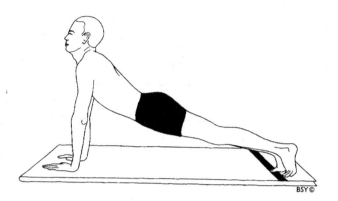

Santolanasana (balancing pose)

Come into the starting position of marjari-asana.

Grasp the ground with the toes.

Straighten the knees, move the shoulders forward and drop the buttocks until the body is straight. The arms should be vertical.

Focus the gaze on a fixed point in front.

Hold the final position for a short duration.

Lower the knees to the floor.

Relax in marjari-asana or shashankasana.

Practise up to 5 times.

Breathing: Breathe normally throughout the practice.

Awareness: Physical – on the strength in the arms, legs and back, and on maintaining balance.

Spiritual – on manipura chakra.

Benefits: This asana improves nervous balance and develops a sense of inner equilibrium and harmony. It strengthens the muscles of the thighs, arms, shoulders and spine.

Variation I: Assume the final position of santolanasana.

Slowly raise the left arm, keeping the body straight, and roll on to the right side so that the chest faces forward.

The outer side of the right foot must be firmly on the floor with the left foot resting on top of it.

Rest the upper arm and hand along the trunk and thigh.

316

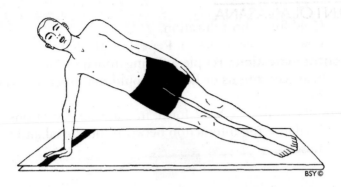

Balance in this position, keeping the body straight.
Roll back to the initial position and repeat the movement
to the left side.
Practise up to 5 times on each side.

Breathing: Breathe normally in the base position.
Retain the breath inside when practising the variations.

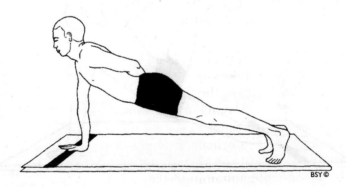

Variation 2: Assume the final position of santolanasana.
Focus the eyes on a point in front of the body.
Raise the left arm and place it behind the back so that the
forearm rests across the small of the back.
Lower the arm and repeat on the other side.

Variation 3: Assume the final position of santolanasana.
Focus the eyes on a point in front of the body.
Either keep both hands on the floor or assume the raised
arm position of variation 2.
Raise the right leg, stretching it back and up.

317

Hold for a short duration.
Lower the leg and arm. Repeat on the left side.

Contra-indications: People suffering from high blood pressure, heart conditions or hernia should not practise variations 2 or 3.

Benefits: As for the basic form; in addition, variations 2 and 3 balance the interaction between the dorsal and ventral muscles.

VASHISHTHASANA

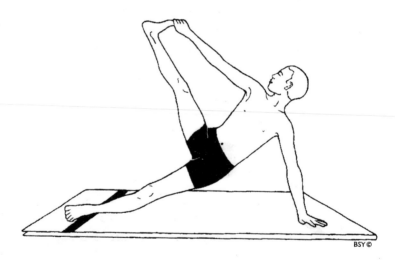

Vashishthasana (Sage Vashishtha's pose)

Assume the final position of santolanasana variation 1.
Balance in this position, keeping the body straight.
Bend the right knee and take hold of the big toe.
Straighten the knee and raise the leg to the vertical position.
Turn the head and focus the gaze on the right big toe.
Balance the body, keeping the legs and arms straight.
Hold the final position for a short duration. Do not strain.
Bend the right knee and release the toe. Lower the leg and return to santolanasana.

Lower the knees to the floor and relax in marjari-asana or shashankasana.

Repeat the practice on the other side.

Practice up to 3 times on each side.

Breathing: Breathe normally while in santolanasana.

Retain the breath inside while assuming the final position. Continue to retain the breath inside in the final position and while lowering the leg if holding the pose for a short period. Breathe normally if holding for longer periods. Exhale while moving back into santolanasana.

Awareness: Physical – on maintaining balance and relaxing the leg muscles.

Spiritual – on manipura chakra.

Contra-indications: This asana should not be practised by people with hernia, high blood pressure, heart ailments, back conditions, vertigo or weakness of the limbs.

Benefits: This asana improves nervous balance. It also makes the leg muscles supple, strengthens the arms and tones the lower back.

Asana

Advanced Group

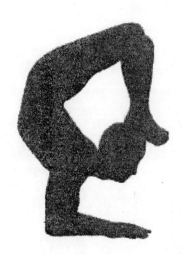

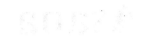

Advanced Asanas

The advanced asana group should not be attempted unless the body is very flexible. The asanas in the beginners and intermediate groups must be mastered before trying to perform any of these postures. While practising the advanced asanas, it is essential to avoid overstraining the body in any way. These practices require the limbs and joints to move into unusual positions to which they are not habituated. Any strain may damage them. Gently coaxing the body to perform advanced asanas over a period of time is far better than trying to achieve quick results through force. The asanas are usually described with the right side leading, but this should be alternated.

Generally speaking, these asanas are designed to further improve the health of a person who is already very healthy. They are not designed for therapeutic purposes. They are not recommended during pregnancy. Carefully observe the contra-indications given for the individual asanas, and the asanas recommended as preparatory.

These asanas strongly affect the energy of the body. The chakras and associated physical, mental, emotional and psychic dimensions of the personality are stimulated and harmonized, contributing to positive transformations in one's character.

POORNA BHUJANGASANA

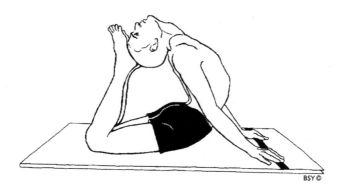

BSY ©

Poorna Bhujangasana (full cobra pose)

Assume bhujangasana.

Holding the position, breathe in and out normally a few times.

Bend the knees and raise the feet.

Stretch the head, neck and shoulders back a little further and try to touch the back of the head with the toes or with the soles of the feet.

This is the final position.

Hold the final position for as long as is comfortable.

To return to the starting position, lower the feet.

Relax in bhujangasana for a few moments.

Release the pose and relax with the arms by the side of the body and the head turned to one side.

This is one round.

After completing each round, allow the respiration and heartbeat to return to normal.

Breathing: Inhale while assuming bhujangasana.

Exhale while raising the toes to touch the head.

Breathe normally in the final position.

Exhale while returning to bhujangasana and while returning to the prone position.

Duration: Up to 3 rounds, gradually extending the duration in the pose.

Awareness: Physical – on relaxing the spine and on the stretch in the abdominal and chest areas.

Spiritual – on swadhisthana chakra.

Sequence: This asana gives maximum benefits if preceded or followed by a forward bending asana.

Practice note: This variation is only suitable for adepts or children over the age of 12 with very supple backs.

Contra-indications: People suffering from peptic ulcer, hernia, intestinal tuberculosis or hyperthyroidism should not practise this asana without the guidance of a competent teacher. Those with any back condition, cervical spondylitis, high blood pressure or heart condition should not practise this asana.

Benefits: This asana keeps the spine supple and healthy. It tones the ovaries and uterus, and is beneficial for all the abdominal organs, especially the liver and kidneys.

On a pranic level, this asana has a strong effect on all the organs related to swadhisthana, manipura, anahata and vishuddhi chakras.

KOORMASANA

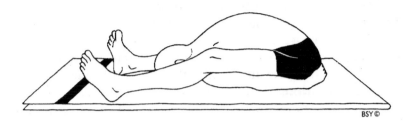

BSY©

Koormasana (tortoise pose)

Sit on the ground with the legs outstretched.

Separate the feet as wide apart as is comfortable.

Bend the knees slightly, keeping the heels in contact with the floor.

Lean forward from the hips and place the hands under the knees, palms facing either up or down.

Lean further forward and slowly slide the arms under the legs.

The knees may be bent more if necessary.

Slide the arms sideways and backward until the elbows lie near the back of the buttocks.

Do not tense the back muscles.

Slowly push the heels forward and straighten the legs as far as possible. The body will simultaneously bend further forward as leverage is applied on the hands and legs.

Gradually, keeping the awareness on breath and relaxation, move the body forward until the forehead or chin touches the floor between the legs.

Do not force or strain in any way.

Fold the arms around the back and interlock the fingers of both hands under the buttocks.

This is the final position.

Relax the whole body, close the eyes and breathe slowly and deeply.

Stay in the final position for as long as is comfortable.

Return to the starting position.

Perform a counterpose and then relax in shavasana.

Breathing: Exhale while bending forward.

Breathe normally in the final position.

Duration: Hold the pose for up to 3 minutes.

For spiritual purposes, it may be held for longer periods.

Awareness: Physical – on relaxing the spine, back muscles and abdomen, and on the breath in the final position.

Spiritual – on swadhisthana or manipura chakra.

Sequence: Follow or precede with a backward bending asana such as bhujangasana, matsyasana or supta vajrasana. Poorna dhanurasana is the perfect counterpose for koormasana.

Contra-indications: Those suffering from slipped disc, sciatica, hernia or chronic arthritis should not perform this asana. It should only be attempted if the spine is sufficiently flexible.

Benefits: Koormasana tones all the organs of the abdomen and is helpful in managing diabetes, flatulence and constipation. It increases circulation in the spine, soothing the nerves and relieving head and neck ache. It induces introversion, mental relaxation, composure and a sense of inner security and surrender. Passion, fear and anger subside, and the body and mind are refreshed through this practice.

Note: *This asana induces spontaneous* pratyahara, *sense withdrawal, which is symbolized by the tortoise. The* Bhagavad Gita *(2:58) states, "When one can withdraw the senses from association with other objects, as a tortoise withdraws its limbs from external danger, then one is firmly fixed on the path towards wisdom." Koorma means 'tortoise', and this posture looks like one too.*

POORNA SHALABHASANA

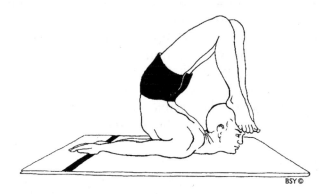

Poorna Shalabhasana (full locust pose)

Assume the final position of shalabhasana with the legs raised in the air as high as possible.

Tense the arm muscles.

Keep the arms and shoulders in firm contact with the floor to support the body.

Lift the legs with a jerk to the vertical position and balance on the shoulders, chin and arms.

Once the point of balance is obtained, gradually bend the knees and bring the toes down to touch the head.

This is the final position.

The final position may sometimes be more easily achieved by rhythmically swinging the legs up to progressively higher levels until the point of balance is reached.

Hold the final position for as long as is comfortable.

To return to the starting position, lift the feet from the head and find the point of balance. Then slowly lower the body to the starting position.

Turn the head to one side, or practise advasana, and allow the respiration and heartbeat to return to normal.

Breathing: Inhale while in the prone position.

Retain the breath inside while raising the body into the final position.

Breathe normally in the final position.

Retain the breath inside while lowering the body to the prone position.

Duration: Practise 1 or 2 rounds, slowly increasing the length of time in the final position.

Awareness: Physical – on the abdomen, relaxing the back and maintaining balance.

Spiritual – on vishuddhi chakra.

Sequence: This asana gives maximum benefits if preceded or followed by a forward bending asana.

Contra-indications: This advanced form of shalabhasana should only be performed by people who are physically fit and who have very supple backs. It should not be practised by people with a weak heart, coronary thrombosis or high blood pressure, cervical spondylitis or hyperthyriodism. Those suffering from peptic ulcer, hernia, intestinal tuberculosis and other such conditions are also advised not to practise this asana.

The cautions for strenuous inverted asanas apply.

Benefits: Poorna shalabhasana strengthens the back and pelvic organs. It tones and balances the functioning of the liver, stomach, bowels and other abdominal organs, and stimulates the appetite. It tightens the muscles of the buttocks and causes the body to do vajroli mudra spontaneously. Many of the benefits of inverted asanas also apply.

POORNA DHANURASANA

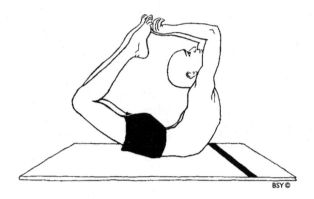

Poorna Dhanurasana (full bow pose)

Lie on the stomach and bend the knees.

Clasp the feet with the hands; the fingers should be in contact with the top of the foot with the thumb on the sole, or the fingers should clasp the big toe.

This is the starting position.

Raise the head, chest and thighs, pulling the feet as close to the head as possible. The elbows point upward.

In the final position the body resembles a fully stretched bow.

Hold the position for as long as is comfortable.

Slowly release the legs and return to the prone position.

This is one round, and is generally sufficient.

Relax until the respiration and heartbeat return to normal.

Breathing: Inhale deeply in the starting position.

Retain the breath inside while coming into the final position.

In the final position, retain the breath inside or practise slow, deep breathing.

Exhale while returning to the starting position.

Awareness: Physical–on the abdomen or back.

Spiritual–on manipura chakra.

Sequence: This asana gives maximum benefits if preceded or followed by a forward bending asana.

Contra-indications: This asana is for advanced practitioners and should only be practised if the back is very supple. People who suffer from a weak heart, high blood pressure, hernia, colitis, peptic or duodenal ulcers should not attempt this practice. It should not be practised before sleep at night as it stimulates the adrenal glands and the sympathetic nervous system.

Benefits: The entire alimentary canal is reconditioned by this asana. The abdominal organs and muscles are massaged. The liver, pancreas, kidneys and adrenal glands are toned, balancing their secretions. This leads to improved functioning of the digestive, excretory and reproductive organs. It improves blood circulation generally.

The spinal column is realigned and the ligaments, muscles and nerves are activated. It strengthens the shoulder, arm and leg muscles, especially the thighs.

It is useful for freeing nervous energy in the cervical and thoracic area, generally improving respiration.

DHANURAKARSHANASANA

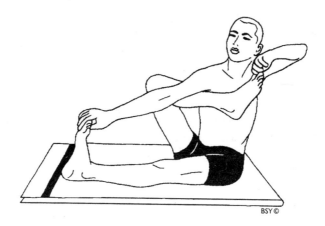

BSY©

Dhanurakarshanasana (archer's pose)
Sit in ardha padmasana with the right foot on top of the thigh and gaze steadily at a fixed point, as at a target.
This is the base position.
Grasp the right foot with the left hand and the left foot, or toe, with the right hand.
Keep the spine and head erect.
Raise the right foot towards the left ear.
This is the final position.
Hold for as long as is comfortable.
Rest the right foot back on the left thigh in ardha padmasana, release the left foot, and relax.
Repeat on the other side.
Practise up to 3 times on each side.
Breathing: Inhale while drawing the foot towards the ear. Retain the breath for a comfortable duration in the final position.
Exhale while returning the foot to the thigh.
Awareness: Physical – on the flexibility of the knee, foot and hip, and on maintaining the back and head straight and on focusing on the target while coordinating the movement with the breath.
Spiritual – on swadhisthana chakra.

Sequence: This asana may be performed at any stage during the asana program.

Contra-indications: Those suffering from slipped disc, sciatica or dislocation of the hip joints should not practise it.

Benefits: This is an excellent asana for loosening the hip joints and making the legs supple. It strengthens the arms and tones the abdominal organs. It helps to relieve tension in the back and neck, and is helpful for people with hydrocele.

Variation: Once this basic form can be performed effortlessly, the practice can be attempted with the heel of the right foot resting in the palm of the left hand.

Note: *The word* dhanu *means 'bow' and* akarshan *means 'drawing' or 'pulling back'. This pose is very graceful. It should be practised until it comes effortlessly and gives the appearance of a trained archer discharging arrows from a bow.*

PRISHTHASANA

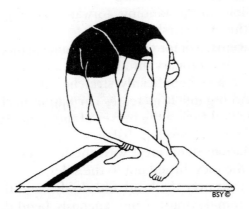

Prishthasana (back pose)

Stand erect with the feet about 30 cm apart and the toes turned out to the sides.

Bend the knees, bringing them as close to the floor as possible.

Simultaneously, bend the trunk backward from the waist.

333

Move the arms back and reach down to grasp the ankles. Bend the head back.

Without straining, lower the head and back nearer to the floor.

Hold the final position for as long as is comfortable.

Alternatively, the hands may be placed on the waist to support the backward movement of the spine, and then moved down the thighs and legs.

Breathing: Inhale while in the standing position.

Exhale while bending backwards and grasping the ankles.

Breathe normally in the final position.

Retain the breath inside while returning to the starting position.

Exhale in the standing position.

Duration: Practise a maximum of 3 times. Gradually extend the length of time in the posture.

Awareness: Physical – on relaxing the back and maintaining balance.

Spiritual – on manipura chakra.

Sequence: Follow with a standing, forward bending posture such as utthita janu sirshasana.

Contra-indications: Not for people with stomach ulcers, high blood pressure, coronary thrombosis or any back ailment.

Benefits: This asana beneficially stretches the abdominal muscles and organs. It increases circulation in the back, stimulating and toning the nerves of the spine. It strengthens the legs and develops balance.

Advanced variation: Stand erect with the feet about 30 cms apart and the toes turned out to the sides.

Raise the arms over the head and slowly bend the trunk backward from the waist. Simultaneously, bend the knees and bring them forward.

Move the arms to the sides and reach down to grasp the ankles.

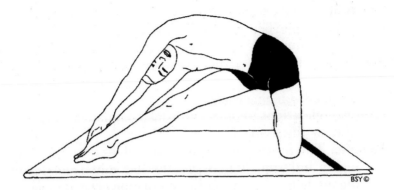

Parighasana (beam or cross-bar pose)

Kneel on the floor with the ankles together, toes flat on the floor and the trunk upright.

Mentally relax the whole body.

Stretch the right leg sideways to the right, keeping it in line with the trunk and the left knee.

Turn the right toes in slightly and rest the sole of the right foot on the ground.

Raise the arms sideways at shoulder level so that they form one straight line.

Move the trunk and right arm towards the extended leg.

Rest the right forearm and wrist on the right shin and ankle respectively, with the right palm facing upward.

The right ear will then rest on the right upper arm.

Move the left arm over the head and place the left palm on top of the right palm.

The left ear will now touch the left upper arm.

Make sure that the head and trunk face forward so the front of the body lies in one plane.

This is the final position.

Remain in this pose for as long as is comfortable, up to one minute.

Come back to the upright position.

Bend the right leg and kneel on the floor, keeping the ankles together in the starting position.

335

Repeat the pose on the other side for an equal length of time. Practise once on each side.

Breathing: Inhale while raising the arms horizontally.
Exhale while bending to the side.
Breathe normally in the final position.

Awareness: Physical – on the lateral stretch and on maintaining balance.
Spiritual – on ajna chakra.

Contra-indications: People with back complaints should not practise this asana.

Benefits: This posture gives a good lateral stretch to the pelvic region and trunk. It massages the abdominal muscles and organs, helping to prevent accumulation of fat and sagging skin around the abdomen.

Note: *In this posture, the body resembles the beam or bar, parigha, used to shut a gate.*

CHAKRASANA

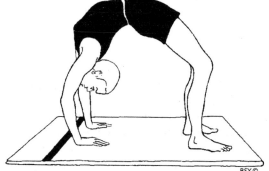

BSY©

Chakrasana (wheel pose)

Lie on the back with the knees bent and the heels touching the buttocks.

The feet and knees should be about 30 cm apart.

Place the palms on the floor beside the head with the fingers pointing towards the shoulders.

336

This is the starting position.

Slowly raise the body and arch the back, allowing the crown of the head to support the weight of the upper body.

Move the hands in further towards the body for more support if necessary.

Straighten the arms and legs as much as possible without straining and lift the head and trunk from the floor.

Arch the back as high as is comfortable in the final position.

Straighten the knees further by moving the trunk towards the head.

Let the head hang between the straight arms.

Lift the heels and balance on the balls of the feet and the hands for a few seconds, then lower the heels.

Hold the final position for as long as is comfortable.

Slowly lower the body so the head rests on the floor and then lower the rest of the body.

This is one round.

Breathing: Inhale in the starting position.

Retain the breath inside while raising the body.

Retain the breath inside or breathe normally in the final position. Exhale while lowering the body.

Duration: Hold for as long as is comfortable. Practise up to 3 rounds.

Awareness: Physical – on relaxing the spine in the final position and on the chest and abdomen.

Spiritual – on manipura chakra.

Sequence: Chakrasana should be practised only after mastery of preliminary and intermediate backward bending asanas. It may be followed with forward bending asanas such as halasana and sarvangasana which apply a tight forward lock on the neck.

Contra-indications: Chakrasana should not be practised by people with any illness, weak wrists, weak back, during pregnancy or when feeling generally tired. The cautions for inverted postures apply.

Benefits: Chakrasana strengthens the legs. It is beneficial to the nervous, digestive, respiratory, cardiovascular and glandular systems. It influences all the hormonal secretions and helps relieve various gynaecological disorders.

Practice note: Chakrasana should preferably be practised on a soft carpet, which will protect the head. It should not be practised on a blanket, which may slip.

This is an inverted asana in which the whole body and nervous system are being placed in an abnormal position. It may be difficult to raise the body because the nervous system is not ready. Do not strain. Practise easier postures as preparation, such as setu asana. If the sense of position in space, or proprioception, is lost, strength is also lost. Chakrasana develops this sense of position in space.

Variation I: (from the standing position)

Stand with the feet about 30 cm apart. Raise the arms straight up over the head about shoulder width apart.

Bend backward, bending first the knees, then the hips and finally the spine.

Bring the hands to the floor under the shoulders.

Variation 2: Poorna Chakrasana (full wheel pose)

Those people who are comfortable in chakrasana may extend the practice by carefully moving the hands towards the feet. In the final position, and only if the spine is extremely flexible, the hands grasp the feet, placing the elbows on the floor to form a complete wheel.

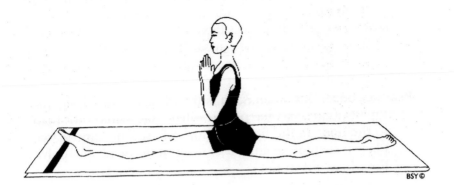

Hanumanasana (Hanuman's pose)

Kneel on the left knee and place the right foot about 30 cm in front of the left knee. Place the palms of the hands on the floor on either side of the right foot.

Gently and gradually slide the right foot forward. Simultaneously, support the weight of the body on the hands.

Straighten both legs, moving the right foot as far forward and the left as far backward as they will go without strain.

In the final position, the buttocks are lowered so that the pelvic floor and both legs rest on the ground in one straight line.

Close the eyes, relax the body and bring the palms together in front of the sternum.

Check that the back knee is straight.

Hold the position for as long as is comfortable.

Return to the starting position.

Repeat the asana with the opposite leg forward.

Breathing: Breathe normally throughout.

Duration: Once on each side.

Awareness: Physical–on the stretch of the hips, groin and leg muscles, and on the breath.

Spiritual–on mooladhara, ajna or anahata chakra.

Sequence: After completing this asana, sit with both of the legs extended forward for one or two minutes.

Contra-indications: People who suffer from conditions such as slipped disc, sciatica, hernia and dislocation of the hip joint are strictly advised not to attempt this asana.

Benefits: This pose improves flexibility and blood circulation in the legs and hips. It massages the abdominal organs, tones the reproductive system and makes the pelvic area supple.

Practice note: Hanumanasana is the ultimate test of leg and hip flexibility. Very few people will be able to lower the body to the floor in the final position. Those who cannot may place a cushion or folded blanket underneath the pelvic floor to avoid strain.

BRAHMACHARYASANA

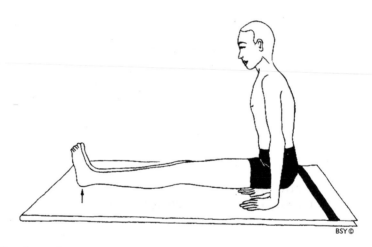

Brahmacharyasana (celibate's pose)

Sit with the legs together and outstretched in front of the body.

Place the palms of the hands on the floor on either side of the hips with the fingers pointing forward and the elbows straight.

Adjust the position of the hands, bringing them slightly forward, until the centre of gravity is found.

Push down with the arms, using the abdominal muscles to lift the buttocks, legs and feet from the floor.

In the final position only the palms of the hands remain on the floor. The whole body is supported and balanced on the hands alone.

The legs should be horizontal and straight; the spine may curve slightly.

Do not strain.

Hold the position for as long as is comfortable.

Slowly lower the buttocks and legs to the floor.

Relax for a few moments with the legs outstretched before performing the next round. Practise up to 3 rounds.

Breathing: Inhale while seated on the floor.
Retain inside while raising and balancing the body.
Exhale while returning to the floor.

Awareness: Physical–on the tension in the abdomen, hips, leg and arm muscles, or perineum.
Spiritual–on mooladhara or manipura chakra.

Sequence: Follow with shavasana or advasana.

Contra-indications: This asana should not be practised by people with high blood pressure or any heart ailment or hernia.

Benefits: This asana strengthens the abdominal organs and muscles, as well as the thighs and arms. The muscles of the perineum contract strongly while this asana is performed, automatically inducing vajroli mudra, ashwini mudra, and moola bandha. Consequently, it is an important asana for the conservation of sexual energy for spiritual purposes.

GRIVASANA

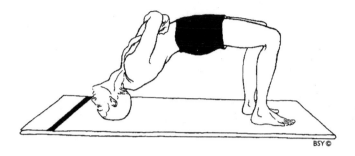

BSY ©

Grivasana (neck pose)
Lie flat on the back.
Bend the knees and bring the heels up to touch the buttocks.
The knees and feet should be slightly separated.
Place the palms on the ground on either side of the head, level with the temples.
Push down on the hands and feet and raise the trunk, placing the crown of the head on the floor.
Balance on the head and feet.
Raise the arms and cross them on the chest.
This is the final position.
Hold for as long as is comfortable.
Breathing: Inhale deeply in the starting position.
Retain the breath inside while raising.
In the final position, retain the breath or breathe normally.
Exhale while lowering the trunk.
Duration: Up to 3 rounds, gradually extending the final position.
Awareness: Physical – on the neck, thyroid gland or pelvic region, the crown of the head and the balance.
Spiritual – on vishuddhi or manipura chakra.
Sequence: Follow this asana with a forward bending pose such as paschimottanasana where the neck vertebrae are stretched.
Contra-indications: This is a strenuous posture. Only people in good, sound health should attempt it. People with neck conditions such as spondylitis, arthritis, slipped disc, high

blood pressure, coronary diseases, high myopia, serious eye problems, prolapse, hernia or acid stomach should not practise this asana. Cautions for inverted asanas apply.

Benefits: Grivasana strengthens the neck, back and thighs, and improves the sense of balance.

SIRSHAPADA BHUMI SPARSHASANA

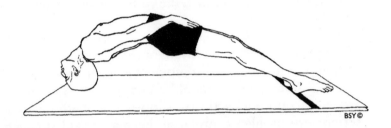

BSY©

Sirshapada Bhumi Sparshasana (head and foot touching the ground pose)

Lie in shavasana.

Relax the whole body.

Turn the palms of the hands to the floor.

Press down on the hands, elbows and lower arms, raising the head and shoulders. Place the top of the head on the floor.

Tense the body and, moving the body towards the head, raise the trunk off the ground as high as possible.

The arms and hands are kept on the ground to support the body until balance is obtained.

Try to straighten the legs.

Place the soles of the feet flat on the ground.

In the final position the palms of the hands are placed on the thighs. The entire body is supported by the head and feet only.

To release the final position, place the hands and arms on the floor for support and gently lower the body.

Relax and let the breathing return to normal.
This is one round.

Breathing: Inhale before raising the trunk and while holding the final position.
Exhale while lowering the body.

Duration: Hold for as long as is comfortable without strain. Practise up to 3 rounds.

Awareness: Physical–on the spine and back.
Spiritual–on manipura chakra.

Sequence: Follow with a forward bending practice such as paschimottanasana in which the vertebrae of the neck are stretched forward.

Contra-indications: Not to be practised by people with high blood pressure, heart conditions or any chronic condition, without the guidance of a competent teacher. Only people in good, sound health should attempt it. People having any neck condition, arthritis, slipped disc, high myopia, serious eye problems, prolapse, hernia or acid stomach should not practise this asana. Cautions for strenuous inverted asanas apply.

Benefits: This asana makes the back muscles strong and supple. It stimulates the spinal nerves and blood circulation, strengthens the thigh, neck and abdominal muscles and is an excellent pose for inducing relaxation.

POORNA MATSYENDRASANA

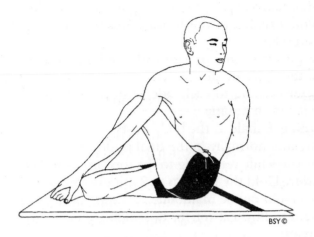

BSY©

Poorna Matsyendrasana (full spinal twist pose)

Sit on the floor with the legs stretched forward.

Relax the whole body.

Place the right foot on the left thigh as near to the waist as comfortable, as in ardha padmasana.

The right foot should press against the abdomen with the right knee remaining on the floor.

Bend the left knee and place the foot on the outside of the right knee with the sole on the floor.

Twist the body to the left, bringing the right armpit against the outside of the left knee and reach down to grasp the left ankle or toe with the right hand.

Try to keep the head and spine straight.

The right arm should eventually be straight and in line with the left calf.

Place the left arm behind the back and try to touch the right heel with the hand. Be careful not to strain the body in any way by either twisting the trunk more than its flexibility will allow or by placing the leg, in ardha padmasana, higher than it is able to go naturally.

Using the right arm as a lever, gently twist the trunk further to the left.

345

Finally, twist the head to the left.

This is the final position.

Maintain the pose for as long as is comfortable.

Slowly return to the forward position, release the limbs and relax.

Repeat the same process with the legs reversed and twist in the opposite direction.

After twisting to each side, stretch the legs forward and relax in shavasana.

Breathing: Exhale as the body twists.

Breathe normally in the final position.

Inhale while returning to the forward facing pose.

Duration: Hold the pose up to 2 minutes on each side.

It should not be maintained for long periods of time.

Awareness: Physical – on the twist of the spine or on the natural breath.

Spiritual – on ajna chakra.

Sequence: Only when padmasana and ardha matsyendrasana are mastered should this asana be attempted.

Contra-indications: People suffering from peptic ulcer, hernia or hyperthyroidism should not practise this pose.

People with sciatica or slipped disc should not practise it.

Benefits: This asana simultaneously stretches the muscles on one side of the back and abdomen while contracting the muscles on the other side.

It tones the nerves of the spine, makes the back muscles supple, relieves lumbago and muscular spasms, and reduces the tendency of adjoining vertebrae to develop inflammatory problems and calcium deposits. It massages the abdominal organs, alleviating digestive ailments. It regulates the secretions of the adrenal gland, liver and pancreas, and is beneficial for the kidneys.

Note: *This asana is dedicated to the great yogi Matsyendranath, who founded hatha vidya.*

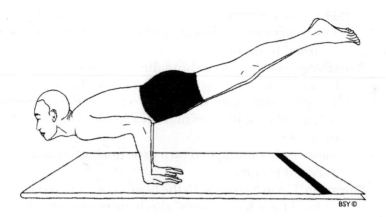

Mayurasana (peacock pose)

Kneel on the floor.

Place the feet together and separate the knees.

Lean forward and place both palms between the knees on the floor with the fingers pointing towards the feet. The hand position will have to be adjusted according to comfort and flexibility.

Bring the elbows and forearms together.

Lean further forward and rest the abdomen on the elbows and the chest on the upper arms.

Stretch the legs backward so they are straight and together. Tense the muscles of the body and slowly elevate the trunk and legs so that they are horizontal to the floor.

Hold the head upward.

The whole body should now be balanced only on the palms of the hands.

Try to elevate the legs and feet higher, keeping them straight by applying more muscular effort and by adjusting the balance of the body.

Do not strain.

In the final position, the weight of the body should be supported by the muscles of the abdomen and not the chest.

347

Maintain the pose for a short period of time, then slowly return to the base position.

This is one round.

The asana may be repeated when the breathing rate has returned to normal.

Breathing: Exhale while raising the body from the floor.

Inhale while lowering the body back to the floor.

To begin with, hold the breath out in the final position. Advanced practitioners may breathe slowly and deeply in the pose.

Allow the breathing to return to normal before attempting a second round.

Duration: Up to 3 rounds. In the beginning, this asana should be held for a few seconds, slowly increasing the duration with practice. Adepts may hold the final position for a few minutes.

Awareness: Physical – on the pressure on the abdomen and on maintaining balance.

Spiritual – on manipura chakra.

Sequence: Perform at the end of an asana session. Mayurasana speeds up the circulation quite vigorously and tends to increase the amount of toxins in the blood as part of the process of purification. Therefore, it should never be practised before any inverted asana as it may direct excess toxins to the brain.

Contra-indications: Mayurasana should not be practised by people with high blood pressure, or any heart ailment, hernia, peptic or duodenal ulcer. This pose should not be attempted if there is any sign of illness or physical weakness. Pregnant women are strongly advised not to practise this asana. Cautions for inverted postures apply.

Benefits: This asana stimulates the metabolic processes which increase secretions from different glands. It stimulates the elimination of toxins from the blood, assisting the removal of skin conditions such as boils. All the digestive organs are massaged and intestinal peristalsis is stimulated. It is useful in managing flatulence, constipation, diabetes and sluggishness of the liver and kidneys. It harmonizes the glands of the endocrine system, develops mental and physical balance, strengthens the muscles of the whole body and develops muscular control. In particular, the toxins accumulated in the body are burnt, bringing the three doshas or humours: *vata*, wind, *kapha*, phlegm, and *pitta*, bile, into balance and harmony.

Practice note: As women have a different muscular system to men in the abdomen and chest areas, they may find mayurasana difficult to perform.

It is very easy to fall forward from the final position and crush the nose on the floor. So be careful and, if necessary, place a small cushion on the floor under the face.

PADMA MAYURASANA

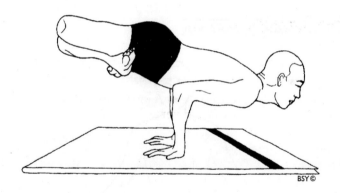

BSY©

Padma Mayurasana (lotus or bound peacock pose)

Sit in padmasana.

Stand on the knees and place the palms flat on the floor in front of the body with the fingers pointing backwards towards the knees.

Bend the elbows and bring them together. Lean forward and place the elbows against each side of the abdomen.

Lean further forward so that the chest rests on the upper arms. Find the balance point of the body.

Lean further forward and slowly raise the folded legs from the floor. Do not strain.

The trunk, head and legs should lie in one horizontal, straight line. This is the final position.

Maintain the position for a comfortable length of time.

Slowly lower the knees and return to the starting position. Change the position of the legs, making the opposite leg uppermost, and perform another round.

Contra-indications: As for mayurasana. In addition, those with sciatica, or weak or injured knees should not practise this asana.

Other details: As for mayurasana.

Practice note: If the practitioner is able to sit comfortably in padmasana, padma mayurasana is easier to perform than the basic mayurasana pose, especially for women.

MOOLABANDHASANA

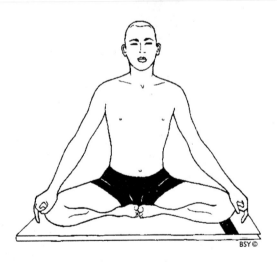

BSY©

Moolabandhasana (perineal contraction pose)
Sit with the legs outstretched in front of the body.

Bend the knees and bring the soles of the feet together.

Draw the heels towards the body.

The outside of the feet should remain on the floor.
Placing the hands behind the buttocks with the fingers pointing backward, raise the buttocks on to the heels, so that the heels press the perineum.
The knees remain on the floor.
Do not strain the ankles.
Place the hands on the knees in either chin or jnana mudra.
Practise nasikagra drishti.
Hold the final position for as long as is comfortable.
Release the legs and stretch them forward.
Repeat when all the tension has left the legs and feet.

Breathing: Breathe normally throughout the practice.

Awareness: Physical – on the pressure of the heels at the perineum.
Spiritual – on mooladhara chakra or the tip of the nose.

Contra-indications: This pose should not be attempted until the knees and ankles have become very flexible.

Benefits: This asana automatically induces moola bandha and is primarily used for awakening mooladhara chakra. It is an important asana for the conservation of sexual energy, and tones the reproductive and eliminatory organs. It also makes the legs and feet exceptionally supple.

Note: Bhadrasana, *the gentle or gracious pose, is a variation of* moolabandhasana.

GORAKSHASANA

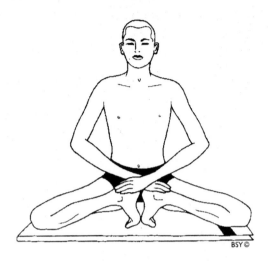

BSY©

Gorakshasana (Yogi Gorakhnath's pose)

Sit with the legs stretched out in front of the body.

Bend the knees, take hold of the feet and place the soles together. Draw the heels up to the perineum.

Raise the heels, keeping the balls of the feet on the floor. Place the hands behind the buttocks, fingers pointing backward, and lever the body forward until the feet become vertical. The knees should remain on the floor.

Do not strain.

Cross the wrists in front of the navel. Hold the left heel with the right hand and the right heel with the left hand.

Straighten the spine and face forward.

Perform nasikagra drishti.

This is the final position.

Hold for as long as is comfortable.

Breathing: Breathe normally throughout the practice.

Awareness: Physical–on maintaining balance or on the feet and knees.

Spiritual–on mooladhara chakra.

Contra-indications: This pose should not be attempted until the knees and ankles have become very flexible.

Benefits: This asana reverses the flow of apana, directing it upward to the higher centres for use in meditative states. It makes the legs and feet extremely supple.

Practice note: To perform this asana, the muscles of the legs and feet need to be slowly stretched over a period of time.

Note: *People who can comfortably remain in the final position may utilize it for meditation. This was the preferred meditation asana of the great yogi, Gorakhnath.*

ASTAVAKRASANA

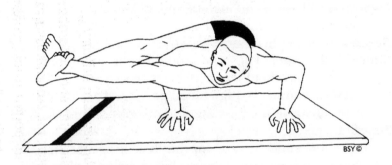

Astavakrasana (eight-twists pose)

Stand with the feet about half a metre apart.

Bend the knees. Place the right palm on the floor between the feet and the left palm a little in front of the left foot.

Place the right leg above the right arm, resting the thigh on the back of the upper right arm, just above the elbow.

Bring the left foot forward between the arms so that it lies close to the right foot.

Lift both legs from the floor and interlock them by placing the left foot on the right ankle.

Stretch both legs to the right side.

Be sure that the right arm is between the thighs.

The right elbow should be slightly bent below the thighs.

353

The left upper arm should be straight.

Balance on the arms.

Bend the elbows, lower the trunk and head until they are parallel to the floor.

This is the final position.

Hold the position for as long as is comfortable.

Straighten the arms and raise the trunk. Release the legs and lower them to the floor.

Return to the starting position.

Repeat on the oposite side.

Breathing: Exhale while lifting the legs off the floor and lowering the head and trunk into the final position.

Breathe normally in the final position.

Inhale while stretching the legs sideways and while raising the trunk to come out of the final position.

Awareness: Physical – on maintaining balance.

Spiritual – on manipura chakra.

Sequence: Follow this asana with either shavasana or advasana.

Contra-indications: This pose should not be attempted until the arms and shoulders have become very strong. People with heart ailments, high blood pressure, back conditions or problems in the hips should not practise this asana.

Benefits: This asana develops nervous control throughout the body and mind. It reverses the flow of apana, directing the energy towards manipura chakra, helping to maintain brahmacharya, 'celibacy'. It strengthens the wrists, the arm and leg muscles, and the muscles of the abdomen.

Note: *Astavakrasana is dedicated to Sage Astavakra, the spiritual preceptor of King Janaka of Mithila. When the sage was in his mother's womb, his father Kagola made several mistakes while reciting the Vedas. Hearing these, the unborn sage laughed. His father became enraged and cursed his son to be born crooked. So it came to pass that he was born twisted in eight places, and was thus named Astavakra.*

354

VRISCHIKASANA

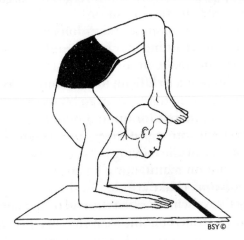

Vrischikasana (scorpion pose)

Place a folded blanket on the floor for the head. Assume the final position of sirshasana.

Relax the whole body, bend the knees and arch the back. After securing the balance, move the forearms carefully so that they lie on each side of the head, parallel with each other, palms flat on the floor.

Transfer the weight on to the forearms and find the balance. Lower the feet as far as possible toward the head.

Slowly raise the head backward and upward.

Raise the upper arms so that they are vertical.

The heels should rest on the crown of the head in the final position.

Try to relax the whole body as much as possible.

Hold the final position for as long as is comfortable.

Slowly return to sirshasana and lower the feet to the floor. Relax in shashankasana for a minute or two before assuming the upright position.

Breathing: Retain the breath inside while assuming sirshasana. Breathe normally in sirshasana.

When learning to practise vrischikasana, the legs may be lowered in stages; inhaling and relaxing the spine, exhaling and lowering a little more each time.

Experienced practitioners would retain the breath inside while going into the final position.

As the neck, shoulders, spine and abdomen are all extended in this pose, the breathing may be fast and heavy. However, try to breathe normally in the final position.

Duration: Vrischikasana is difficult to maintain for long. In the beginning, it may be held for up to 30 seconds, although adepts may maintain it for up to 5 minutes.

Awareness: Physical – on transferring the weight on to the forearms or head while moving between vrischikasana and sirshasana, and on maintaining balance.

Spiritual – on ajna chakra.

Sequence: Practise vrischikasana at the end of an asana session. Follow with a forward bending asana for an equal amount of time. After that, perform tadasana for 30 seconds. Finally, rest in shavasana.

Contra-indications: This asana should not be practised by people with high blood pressure, vertigo, cerebral thrombosis, chronic catarrh or heart disease. Only those who can perform all the inverted poses without the slightest difficulty should attempt it. All cautions for strenuous inverted postures should be observed.

Benefits: Vrischikasana reorganizes prana in the body, arresting the physical ageing process. It improves the blood flow to the brain and pituitary gland, revitalizing all the body's systems. It improves circulation in the lower limbs and abdomen, and tones the reproductive organs. The arched position stretches and loosens the back, toning the nerves of the spine. It strengthens the arms and develops the sense of balance.

Practice note: Practise near a wall until this pose is perfected. There should be no furniture or other objects nearby against which the body may fall, if balance is lost.

Note: Vrischika *means scorpion. In order to sting its victim, the scorpion arches its tail above its back and then strikes beyond its head. This asana resembles a striking scorpion.*

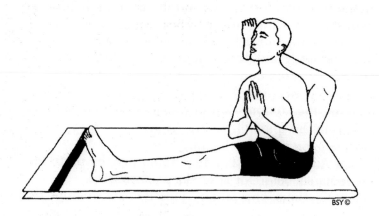

Eka Pada Sirasana (one foot to head pose)

Sit with the legs outstretched in front of the body.

Bend the right knee, turning it slightly out to the side.

Bring the right arm under the calf muscle and hold the outside of the leg just above the ankle.

Raise the left arm and hold the outside of the right ankle.

The right arm should be positioned so that the elbow lies between the thigh and the lower leg.

Raise the right leg using the arms and hands.

As the leg is raised, bend the trunk forward and twist slightly to the left.

Without straining, place the leg on top of the right shoulder.

Release the grip of the right hand.

Raise the right leg higher by using the left arm and by pushing the thigh back using the right upper arm.

Without straining, try to place the right foot behind the head at the nape of the neck.

This is achieved by bending the head forward under the calf muscle, which then rests on the shoulder.

Finally, place the hands in front of the chest at the centre of the sternum.

Try to straighten the spine and hold the head upright.

This is the final position.

Close the eyes and hold the pose for as long as is comfortable.
Slowly release the leg and return to the starting position.
Repeat on the other side.

Breathing: Breathe normally while moving into the pose. Breathe slowly and deeply in the final position.

Duration: 1 or 2 times on each side.

Awareness: Physical – on the stretch in the hip, groin and leg muscles, the compression in the abdomen and the sensations in the spine.
Spiritual – on anahata chakra.

Sequence: Any backward bending asana may be performed immediately before or after eka pada sirasana.

Contra-indications: This posture should not be attempted by people with sciatica, hip problems or hernia. To prevent strained muscles and torn ligaments, this asana should not be attempted unless the body is very flexible. It should be avoided by people with any back ailment.

Benefits: This asana compresses each side of the abdomen, thoroughly massaging the internal organs, stimulating peristalsis and removing constipation. It tones the reproductive organs and improves blood circulation in the legs, relieving varicose veins. It increases the level of energy in the chakras, thus vitalizing the body and mind.

Practice note: The right leg should be raised first in order to massage the internal organs in the natural direction of digestion.
In order to practise this posture, the hips must be extremely flexible.

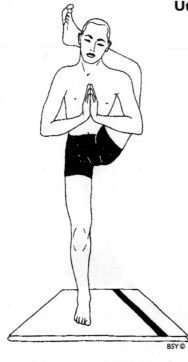

**Utthan Eka Pada Sirasana
(standing foot to head pose)**

Assume eka pada sirasana with the right leg behind the head. Place both palms on the floor, using the hands and arms for support.

Lean back slightly and come into a squatting position on the left leg.

Straighten the knee and stand upright.

Do not strain.

When balance is secured in the standing position, place the palms together in front of the chest.

This is the final position.

Maintain balance in the standing position for as long as is comfortable.

Carefully sit down and release the raised leg. Stretch the legs forward and relax.

Repeat with the other leg behind the head.

Breathing: Inhale as the body is raised. Breathe normally in the final position. Exhale as the body is lowered.

Awareness: Physical–on raising the body to the upright position, on normal breathing in the final position, and on maintaining balance.

Spiritual–on anahata chakra.

Sequence: This asana should only be attempted after mastering eka pada sirasana.

Contra-indications: As for eka pada sirasana. In addition, it is very strenuous for the knees and ankles. Those with high blood pressure or vertigo should avoid this asana.

359

Benefits: As for eka pada sirasana. In addition, this asana strengthens the thigh and back muscles, and improves concentration.

DWI PADA SIRASANA

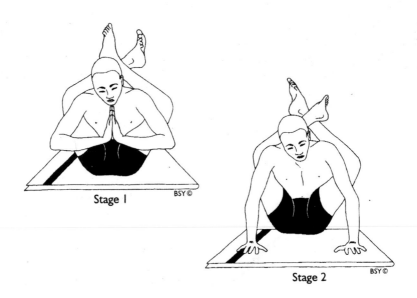

Stage 1 · BSY©

Stage 2 · BSY©

Dwi Pada Sirasana (two feet to head pose)

Perform eka pada sirasana and relax.

Similarly, carefully and without straining, place the leg behind the shoulder.

Lock the feet behind the neck by crossing the ankles.

Place the hands on the floor by the side of the hips and balance on the coccyx.

Once balance is achieved, proceed to the following stages.

Stage 1: Place the palms together at the chest.

Maintain this position for 10 to 30 seconds, then again place the palms beside the hips.

Stage 2: Straighten the elbows, exhale, and lift the whole body off the floor, balancing on the hands.

Do not release the ankle lock.

Maintain this position for a comfortable length of time and then gently lower the body to the ground and release.

Breathing: Exhale while placing the second foot behind the neck, otherwise breathe normally throughout.

Other details: As for dwi pada kandharasana.

DWI PADA KANDHARASANA

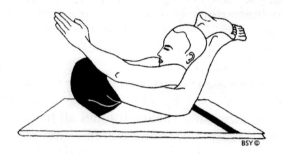

BSY©

Dwi Pada Kandharasana (two-legged shoulder pose)

Lie on the back with the legs straight and the arms by the sides. Relax the whole body.

Bend one leg and bring the foot behind the head and the leg under the armpit.

Repeat the process with the other leg so that both arms rest above the legs.

Gently press the legs downward with the arms.

Try to cross the feet behind the head, but do not strain.

In the final position, point the arms forward and place the palms together.

Relax the whole body.

Close the eyes and maintain the position for as long as is comfortable.

Release the legs and return to the starting position.

Breathing: Breathe normally while assuming the final position.

Breathe slowly and deeply in the final position.

Inhale deeply, then exhale as the legs are released.

361

Duration: Practise once during an asana program.

Awareness: Physical – on the stretch in the groin, hips and legs, the sensations along the spine and at the back of the neck, on the compression of the abdomen and chest, and on relaxing with the breath.

Spiritual – on swadhisthana chakra.

Sequence: Dwi pada kandharasana should not be attempted before eka pada sirasana is mastered. It should be practised towards the end of the asana program and followed by a backward bending asana such as dhanurasana, bhujangasana or matsyasana.

Contra-indications: To prevent strained muscles and torn ligaments, this asana should not be attempted unless the body is very flexible. It should be avoided by persons with any back ailment.

Benefits: This asana helps to control the nervous system. The solar plexus and the adrenal glands are powerfully massaged, increasing vitality. It tones all the abdominal and pelvic organs, improving the efficiency of the digestive, reproductive and eliminatory systems.

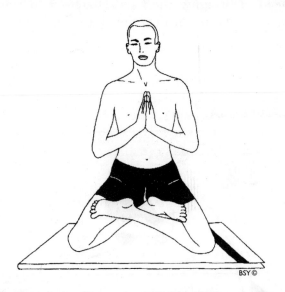

BSY©

Padma Parvatasana (lotus mountain pose)

Perform padmasana. Relax the whole body.

Firstly, supporting the weight with the hands, stand on the knees.

Focus the gaze on a fixed point, lift the hands from the floor and, when balanced, bring the palms of the hands together in front of the chest in the prayer pose.

Hold the final position for as long as is comfortable.

To release, slowly lower the hands and then the buttocks to the floor and sit in padmasana.

Release the legs, change their position and repeat the pose for the same length of time.

Breathing: Exhale while initially raising the buttocks.

Breathe normally in the final position.

Exhale while lowering the body to the floor.

Awareness: Physical – on maintaining balance and on the breath.

Spiritual – on swadhisthana chakra.

Benefits: In addition to the benefits of padmasana, this asana develops the sense of balance.

363

Variation: Santolan Parvatasana (standing mountain pose)
Instead of bringing the hands together in front of the chest, raise both arms overhead, one at a time, keeping the elbows straight.

KASHYAPASANA

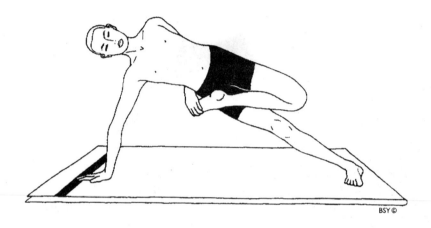

BSY ©

Kashyapasana (Sage Kashyapa's pose)
Assume santolanasana, variation 1.
Bend the left knee and place the foot on the right thigh as in ardha padmasana.
Take the left arm behind the back and hold the left foot or big toe with the left hand.
The chest and extended right arm should be in one plane. This is the final position.
Hold for as long as is comfortable.
Release the left foot and return to santolanasana.
Repeat on the other side.
Practise once on each side and then relax in shashankasana.
Breathing: Normal throughout.
Awareness: Physical – on the alignment of trunk and limbs, and on maintaining balance.
Spiritual – on manipura chakra.

364

Benefits: This asana strengthens the shoulders, arms and legs and opens the chest. Anahata and manipura chakras are activated, along with samana vayu. A sense of balance and concentration is developed.

Note: *This asana is dedicated to Sage Kashyapa, son of Sage Marichi. He is also said to be the father of all living beings and is called Prajapati, the progenitor.*

VISHWAMITRASANA

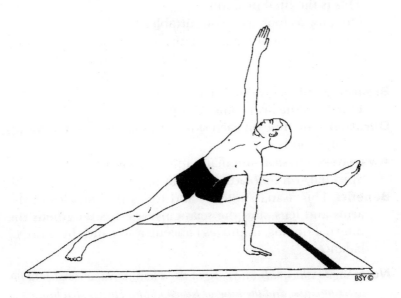

BSY ©

Vishwamitrasana (Sage Vishwamitra's pose)

Stand upright with the arms by the sides and the feet together.

Close the eyes and mentally relax the whole body.

Open the eyes, slowly bend forward from the hips and place the palms on the floor beside the feet.

Without moving the hands, take the legs back about 120 to 150 cm and rest the crown of the head on the floor with the buttocks raised.

Raise the head, swing the right leg over the right hand and place the back of the right thigh on the back of the upper part of the right arm.

The right foot should not touch the floor.

Immediately, turn the body to the left, place the left arm along the left thigh and balance.

Turn the left foot sideways and press the heel on the floor.

Straighten the right leg.

Stretch the left arm up vertically from the shoulder and gaze at the upstretched left hand.

This is the final position.

Hold for as long as is comfortable.

Release the right leg and return to the starting position.

Repeat the pose for the same length of time on the other side.

Breathing: Inhale as the arm moves up.

Exhale as the arm comes down.

Duration: One time on each side, holding the position for up to 30 seconds.

Awareness: Physical – on maintaining balance.

Spiritual – on mooladhara chakra.

Benefits: This asana stretches and tones the muscles of the arms and legs, and the sciatic nerves. It strengthens the internal organs, improves concentration and the sense of balance.

Note: *Sage Vishwamitra was originally a* kshatriya, *a member of the warrior class, and the king of Kanyakubja. He devoted himself to the most rigorous yogic austerities until he successfully achieved the titles of* rajarishi, *royal sage,* rishi, *sage or seer,* maharishi, *great sage or patriarch of mankind, and finally* brahmarishi, *brahmanical sage. This asana is dedicated to him.*

Pranayama

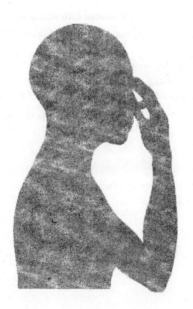

अथासने दृढे योगी वशी हितमिताशन: ।
गुरूपदिष्टमार्गे प्राणायामान्समभ्यसेत् ॥ 2:1 ॥

Athaasane dridhe yogee vashee hitamitaashanaha.
Guroopadishtamaargena praanaayaamaansamabhyset.

Thus being established in asana and having control (of
the body), taking a balanced diet; pranayamas should be
practised according to the instructions of the guru.

Hatha Yoga Pradipika

Introduction to Pranayama

Pranayama is generally defined as breath control. Although this interpretation may seem correct in view of the practices involved, it does not convey the full meaning of the term. The word pranayama is comprised of two roots: 'prana' plus 'ayama'. *Prana* means 'vital energy' or 'life force'. It is the force which exists in all things, whether animate or inanimate. Although closely related to the air we breathe, it is more subtle than air or oxygen. Therefore, pranayama should not be considered as mere breathing exercises aimed at introducing extra oxygen into the lungs. Pranayama utilizes breathing to influence the flow of prana in the *nadis* or energy channels of the *pranamaya kosha* or energy body.

The word *yama* means 'control' and is used to denote various rules or codes of conduct. However, this is not the word which is joined to prana to form pranayama; the correct word is 'ayama' which has far more implications. *Ayama* is defined as 'extension' or 'expansion'. Thus, the word *pranayama* means 'extension or expansion of the dimension of prana'. The techniques of pranayama provide the method whereby the life force can be activated and regulated in order to go beyond one's normal boundaries or limitations and attain a higher state of vibratory energy and awareness.

Four aspects of pranayama

In the pranayama practices there are four important aspects of breathing which are utilized. These are:

1. *Pooraka* or inhalation
2. *Rechaka* or exhalation
3. *Antar kumbhaka* or internal breath retention
4. *Bahir kumbhaka* or external breath retention.

The different practices of pranayama involve various techniques which utilize these four aspects of breathing. There is another mode of pranayama, which is called *kevala kumbhaka* or spontaneous breath retention. This is an advanced stage of pranayama which occurs during high states of meditation. During this state, the fluctuation of prana ceases. At this time, the veil which prevents one from seeing the subtle aspect of existence is lifted and a higher vision of reality is attained.

The most important part of pranayama is actually kumbhaka or breath retention. However, in order to perform kumbhaka successfully, there must be a gradual development of control over the function of respiration. Therefore, in the pranayama practices more emphasis is given to inhalation and exhalation at the beginning, in order to strengthen the lungs and balance the nervous and pranic systems in preparation for the practice of kumbhaka. These initial practices influence the flow of prana in the nadis, purifying, regulating and activating them, thereby inducing physical and mental stability.

The pranic body

According to yogic physiology, the human framework is comprised of five bodies or sheaths, which account for the different aspects or dimensions of human existence. These five sheaths are known as:
1. *Annamaya kosha*, the food or material body
2. *Manomaya kosha*, the mental body
3. *Pranamaya kosha*, the bioplasmic or vital energy body
4. *Vijnanamaya kosha*, the psychic or higher mental body
5. *Anandamaya kosha*, the transcendental or bliss body.

Although these five sheaths function together to form an integral whole, the practices of pranayama work mainly with pranamaya kosha. Pranamaya kosha is made up of five major pranas, which are collectively known as the *pancha*, or five, pranas: *prana, apana, samana, udana* and *vyana*.

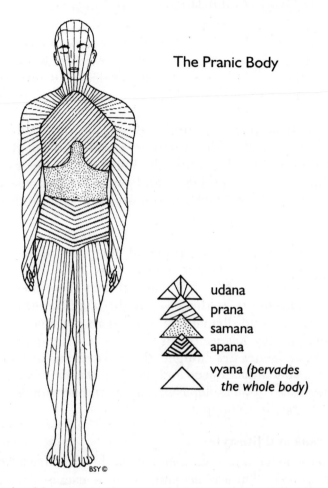

The Pranic Body

udana
prana
samana
apana
vyana *(pervades
the whole body)*

BSY©

Prana in this context does not refer to cosmic prana, but rather to just one flow of energy, governing the thoracic area between the larynx and the top of the diaphragm. It is associated with the heart and organs of respiration together with the muscles and nerves that activate them. It is the force by which the breath is drawn inside.

Apana governs the abdomen, below the navel region, and provides energy for the large intestine, kidneys, anus and genitals. It is concerned with the expulsion of waste from the body and is the force which expels the breath.

Samana is located between the heart and the navel. It activates and controls the digestive system: the liver, intestines, pancreas and stomach, and their secretions. Samana is responsible for transformation. On a physical level this relates to the assimilation and distribution of nutrients. On an evolutionary level it relates to kundalini and expansion of consciousness.

Udana governs the neck and head, activating all the sensory receptors such as the eyes, tongue, nose and ears. Udana also harmonizes and activates the limbs and all their associated muscles, ligaments, nerves and joints. It is responsible for the erect posture of the body, sensory awareness, and the ability to respond to the outside world.

Vyana pervades the whole body, regulating and controlling all movement, and coordinating the other pranas. It acts as the reserve force for the other pranas.

Along with these five major pranas there are five minor pranas known as the *upa-pranas*: naga, koorma, krikara, devadatta and dhananjaya. *Naga* is responsible for belching and hiccups. *Koorma* opens the eyes and stimulates blinking. *Krikara* generates hunger, thirst, sneezing and coughing. *Devadatta* induces sleep and yawning. *Dhananjaya* lingers after death and upon its departure, decay and decomposition of the body begins to happen.

Prana and lifestyle

Lifestyle has a profound impact on the pranamaya kosha and its pranas. Physical activities such as exercise, work, sleep, intake of food and sexual relations all affect the distribution and flow of prana in the body. Faculties of the mind such as emotion, thought and imagination affect the pranic body even more. Irregularities in lifestyle, dietary indiscretions and stress deplete and obstruct the pranic flow. This results in what people experience as being 'drained of energy'. Depletion of energy in a particular prana leads to the devitalization of the organs and limbs it governs and ultimately to disease or metabolic dysfunction. The techniques of pranayama reverse this process, energizing and balancing the different pranas within pranamaya kosha. Pranayama practices should be performed after asanas in an integrated yoga program.

Breath, health and pranayama

The breath is the most vital process of the body. It influences the activities of each and every cell and, most importantly, is intimately linked with the performance of the brain. Human beings breathe about 15 times per minute and 21,600 times per day. Respiration fuels the burning of oxygen and glucose, producing energy to power every muscular contraction, glandular secretion and mental process. The breath is intimately linked to all aspects of human experience.

Most people breathe incorrectly, using only a small part of their lung capacity. The breathing is then generally shallow, depriving the body of oxygen and prana essential to its good health. The first five practices given in this section are preparatory techniques which introduce correct breathing habits. In addition, they help focus the awareness on the breathing process, which is otherwise normally ignored. Practitioners develop sensitivity to the respiratory process and retrain the muscles of the pulmonary cavity, enhancing their vital capacity and preparing them for pranayama.

Rhythmic, deep and slow respiration stimulates and is stimulated by calm, content, states of mind. Irregular breathing disrupts the rhythms of the brain and leads to physical, emotional and mental blocks. These, in turn, lead to inner conflict, an unbalanced personality, a disordered lifestyle and disease. Pranayama establishes regular breathing patterns, breaking this negative cycle and reversing the debilitating process. It does so by giving us control of the breath and re-establishing the natural, relaxed rhythms of the body and mind.

Although breathing is mainly an unconscious process, conscious control of it may be taken at any time. Consequently, it forms a bridge between the conscious and unconscious areas of the mind. Through the practice of pranayama, the energy trapped in neurotic, unconscious mental patterns may be released for use in more creative and joyful activity.

Breathing and life span

In addition to influencing the quality of life, the length or quantity of life is also dictated by the rhythm of the respiration. The ancient yogis and rishis studied nature in great detail. They noticed that animals with a slow breath rate such as pythons, elephants and tortoises have long life spans, whereas those with a fast breathing rate such as birds, dogs and rabbits live for only a few years. From this observation they realized the importance of slow breathing for increasing the human lifespan. Those who breathe in short, quick gasps are likely to have a shorter life span than those who breathe slowly and deeply. On the physical level, this is because the respiration is directly related to the heart. A slow breathing rate keeps the heart stronger and better nourished and contributes to a longer life. Deep breathing also increases the absorption of energy by pranamaya kosha, enhancing dynamism, vitality and general wellbeing.

Pranayama and the spiritual aspirant

Pranayama practices establish a healthy body by removing blockages in the pranamaya kosha, enabling increased absorption and retention of prana. The spiritual seeker requires tranquillity of mind as an essential prelude to spiritual practice. To this end, many pranayama techniques utilize kumbhaka, breath retention, to establish control over the flow of prana, calming the mind and controlling the thought process.

Once the mind has been stilled and prana flows freely in the nadis and chakras, the doorway to the evolution of consciousness opens, leading the aspirant into higher dimensions of spiritual experience. In *The Science of Pranayama*, Swami Sivananda writes, "There is an intimate connection between the breath, nerve currents and control of the inner prana or vital forces. Prana becomes visible on the physical plane as motion and action, and on the mental plane as thought. Pranayama is the means by which a yogi tries to realize within his individual body the whole cosmic nature, and attempts to attain perfection by attaining all the powers of the universe."

General notes for the practitioner

In the traditional texts, there are innumerable rules and regulations pertaining to pranayama. The main points are to exercise moderation, balance and common sense with regard to inner and outer thinking and living. However, for those who seriously wish to take up the advanced practices of pranayama, the guidance of a guru or competent teacher is essential.

Contra-indications: Pranayama should not be practised during illness, although simple techniques such as breath awareness and abdominal breathing in shavasana may be performed. Carefully observe the contra-indications given for individual practices.

Time of practice: The best time to practise pranayama is at dawn, when the body is fresh and the mind has very few impressions. If this is not possible, another good time is just after sunset. Tranquillizing pranayamas may be performed before sleep. Try to practise regularly at the same time and place each day. Regularity in practice increases strength and willpower as well as acclimatizing the body and mind to the increased pranic force. Do not be in a hurry; slow, steady progress is essential.

Bathing: Take a bath or shower before commencing the practice, or at least wash the hands, face and feet. Do not take a bath for at least half an hour after the practice to allow the body temperature to normalize.

Clothes: Loose, comfortable clothing made of natural fibres should be worn during the practice. The body may be covered with a sheet or blanket when it is cold or to keep insects away.

Empty stomach: Practise before eating in the morning or wait at least three to four hours after meals before starting pranayama. Food in the stomach places pressure on the diaphragm and lungs, making full, deep respiration difficult.

Diet: A balanced diet of protein, carbohydrates, fats, vitamins and minerals is suitable for most pranayama practices. A combination of grains, pulses, fresh fruit and vegetables, with some milk products if necessary, is recommended.

When commencing pranayama practice, constipation and a reduction in the quantity of urine may be experienced. In the case of dry motions, stop taking salt and spices, and drink plenty of water. In the case of loose motions, stop the practices for a few days and go on a diet of rice and curd or yoghurt.

The more advanced stages of pranayama require a change in diet and a guru should be consulted for guidance on this.

Place of practice: Practise in a quiet, clean and pleasant room, which is well ventilated but not draughty. Generally, avoid practising in direct sunlight as the body will become overheated, except at dawn when the soft rays of the early morning sun are beneficial. Practising in a draught or wind, in air-conditioning or under a fan may upset the body temperature and cause chills.

Breathing: Always breathe through the nose and not the mouth unless specifically instructed otherwise. Both nostrils must be clear and flowing freely. Mucous blockages may be removed through the practice of neti or kapalbhati. If the flow of breath in the nostrils is unequal, it may be balanced by practising padadhirasana as a breath balancing technique.

Sequence: Pranayama should be performed after shatkarmas and asanas, and before meditation practice. Nadi shodhana pranayama should be practised in each pranayama session as its balancing and purifying effects form the basis for successful pranayama. After practising pranayama, one may lie down in shavasana for a few minutes.

Sitting position: A comfortable, sustainable meditation posture is necessary to enable efficient breathing and body steadiness during the practice. Siddha/siddha yoni asana or padmasana are the best postures for pranayama. The body should be as relaxed as possible throughout the practice with the spine, neck and head erect. Sit on a folded blanket or cloth of natural fibre to ensure the maximum conduction of energy during the practice. Those who cannot sit in a meditation posture may sit against a wall with the legs outstretched or in a chair which has a straight back.

Avoid strain: With all pranayama practices, it is important to remember that the instruction not to strain, not to try to increase your capacity too fast, applies just as it does to asana practice. If one is advised to practise a pranayama technique until it is mastered, and it can be practised without any strain or discomfort, it is wise to follow that instruction before moving on to a more advanced practice or ratio. Furthermore, breath retention should only be practised for as long as is comfortable. The lungs are very delicate organs and any misuse can easily cause them injury. Not only the physical body, but also the mental and emotional aspects of the personality need time to adjust. Never strain in any way.

Side effects: Various symptoms may manifest in normally healthy people. These are caused by the process of purification and the expulsion of toxins. Sensations of itching, tingling, heat or cold, and feelings of lightness or heaviness may occur. Such experiences are generally temporary, but if they persist, check with a competent teacher. Energy levels may increase or fluctuate; interests may change. If such changes cause difficulty in lifestyle, decrease or stop the practice until a competent teacher or guru gives guidance.

NATURAL BREATHING

This is a simple technique which introduces practitioners to their own respiratory system and breathing patterns. It is very relaxing and may be practised at any time. Awareness of the breathing process is itself sufficient to slow down the respiratory rate and establish a more relaxed rhythm.

Natural breathing

Sit in a comfortable meditation posture or lie in shavasana and relax the whole body.

Observe the natural and spontaneous breathing process.

Develop total awareness of the rhythmic flow of the breath.

Feel the breath flowing in and out of the nose.

Do not control the breath in any way.

Notice that the breath is cool as it enters the nostrils and warm as it flows out.

Observe this with the attitude of a detached witness.

Feel the breath flowing in and out at the back of the mouth above the throat.

Bring the awareness down to the region of the throat and feel the breath flowing in the throat.

Bring the awareness down to the region of the chest and feel the breath flowing in the trachea and bronchial tubes.

Next, feel the breath flowing in the lungs.

Be aware of the lungs expanding and relaxing.

Shift the attention to the ribcage and observe the expansion and relaxation of this area.

Bring the awareness down to the abdomen. Feel the abdomen move upward on inhalation and downward on exhalation.

Finally, become aware of the whole breathing process from the nostrils to the abdomen and continue observing it for some time.

Bring the awareness back to observing the physical body as one unit and open the eyes.

378

Abdominal or diaphragmatic breathing is practised by enhancing the action of the diaphragm and minimizing the action of the ribcage. The diaphragm is a domed sheet of muscle that separates the lungs from the abdominal cavity and, when functioning correctly, promotes the most efficient type of breathing. It is the effect of the diaphragm rather than the diaphragm itself that is experienced as the stomach rises and falls, but sensitivity will come with practice. During inhalation the diaphragm moves downward, pushing the abdominal contents downward and outward. During exhalation the diaphragm moves upward and the abdominal contents move inward.

Movement of the diaphragm signifies that the lower lobes of the lungs are being utilized. The proper use of the diaphragm causes equal expansion of the alveoli, improves lymphatic drainage from basal parts of the lungs, massages the liver, stomach, intestines and other organs that lie immediately beneath it, exerts a positive effect on the cardiac functions and coronary supply, and improves oxygenation of the blood and circulation.

Abdominal breathing is the most natural and efficient way to breathe. However, due to tension, poor posture, restrictive clothing and lack of training, it is often forgotten. Once this technique again becomes a part of daily life and correct breathing is restored, there will be a great improvement in the state of physical and mental wellbeing.

Abdominal (or diaphragmatic) breathing

Lie in shavasana and relax the whole body.

Place the right hand on the abdomen just above the navel and the left hand over the centre of the chest.

Observe the spontaneous breath without controlling it in any way. Let it be absolutely natural.

To practise abdominal breathing, feel as though you are

drawing the energy and breath in and out directly through the navel.

The right hand will move up with inhalation and down with exhalation. The left hand remains almost still.

Let the abdomen relax. Do not try to force the movement in any way.

Do not expand the chest or move the shoulders.

Feel the abdomen expanding and contracting.

Continue breathing slowly and deeply.

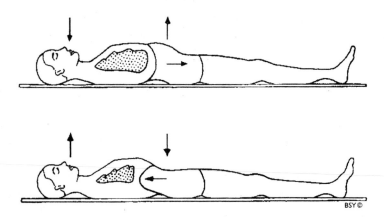

Inhale while expanding the abdomen as much as is comfortable, without expanding the ribcage.

At the end of the inhalation, the diaphragm will be compressing the abdomen and the navel will be at its highest point.

On exhalation, the diaphragm moves upward and the abdomen moves downward.

At the end of the exhalation, the abdomen will be contracted and the navel compressed towards the spine.

Continue for a few minutes.

Relax any effort and once again watch the spontaneous breathing pattern.

Bring the awareness back to observing the physical body as a whole. Be aware of the surroundings and gently open the eyes.

Thoracic breathing utilizes the middle lobes of the lungs by
expanding and contracting the ribcage. It expends more
energy than abdominal breathing for the same quantity of
air exchange. It is often associated with physical exercise and
exertion, as well as stress and tension; when combined with
abdominal breathing, it helps the body to obtain more oxygen.
However, the tendency in many people is to continue this type
of breathing instead of abdominal breathing long after the
stressful situation has passed, creating bad breathing habits
and continued tension.

Thoracic breathing
Sit in a meditation posture or lie in shavasana and relax
the whole body.
Maintain unbroken awareness of the natural breath for
some time, concentrating on the sides of the chest.
Discontinue any further use of the diaphragm and begin
to inhale by slowly expanding the ribcage.
Feel the movement of the individual ribs outward and
upward, and be aware of this expansion drawing air into
the lungs.
Expand the chest as much as possible.
Exhale by relaxing the chest muscles. Feel the ribcage
contracting and forcing the air out of the lungs.
Breathe slowly and deeply through the chest with total
awareness. Do not use the diaphragm.
Continue thoracic breathing for a few minutes, pausing
slightly after each inhalation and exhalation.
Relax any effort and once again watch the spontaneous
breathing pattern.
Bring the awareness back to observing the physical body
as a whole. Be aware of the surroundings and gently open
the eyes.

CLAVICULAR BREATHING

Clavicular breathing is the final stage of total ribcage expansion. It occurs after the thoracic inhalation has been completed. In order to absorb a little more air into the lungs, the upper ribs and the collar bone are pulled upwards by the muscles of the neck, throat and sternum. This requires maximum expansion on inhalation and only the upper lobes of the lungs are ventilated. In daily life, clavicular breathing is only used under conditions of extreme physical exertion and when experiencing obstructive airway diseases such as asthma.

Clavicular breathing

Lie in shavasana and relax the whole body.

Maintain unbroken awareness of the natural breath for some time, concentrating on the sides of the chest.

Perform thoracic breathing for a few minutes.

Inhale, fully expanding the ribcage.

When the ribs are fully expanded, inhale a little more until expansion is felt in the upper portion of the lungs around the base of the neck. The shoulders and collar bone should also move up slightly.

This will take some effort.

Exhale slowly, first releasing the lower neck and upper chest, then relaxing the rest of the ribcage back to its starting position.

Continue for a few more breaths, observing the effect of this type of breathing.

Relax any effort and once again watch the spontaneous breathing pattern.

Bring the awareness back to observing the physical body as a whole. Be aware of the surroundings and gently open the eyes.

YOGIC BREATHING

Yogic breathing combines the previous three techniques. It is used to maximize inhalation and exhalation. Its purpose is to gain control of the breath, correct poor breathing habits and increase oxygen intake.

It may be practised at any time and is especially useful in situations of high stress or anger for calming the nerves. However, while its inclusion in a daily yoga program will correct and deepen natural breathing patterns, yogic breathing itself should not be performed continually.

Yogic breathing
Sit in a meditation posture or lie in shavasana and relax the whole body.
Inhale slowly and deeply, allowing the abdomen to expand fully.
Try to breathe so slowly that little or no sound of the breath can be heard.
Feel the air reaching into the bottom of the lungs.
At the end of abdominal expansion, start to expand the chest outward and upward.
When the ribs are fully expanded, inhale a little more until expansion is felt in the upper portion of the lungs around the base of the neck. The shoulders and collar bone should also move up slightly. Some tension will be felt in the neck muscles.
The rest of the body should be relaxed.
Feel the air filling the upper lobes of the lungs.
This completes one inhalation.
The whole process should be one continuous movement, each phase of breathing merging into the next without any obvious transition point. There should be no jerks or unnecessary strain. The breathing should be like the swell of the sea.
Now start to exhale.

383

First, relax the lower neck and upper chest, then allow the chest to contract downward and then inward.

Next, allow the diaphragm to push upward and toward the chest.

Without straining, try to empty the lungs as much as possible by drawing or pulling the abdominal wall as near as possible to the spine.

The entire movement should be harmonious and flowing. Hold the breath for a few seconds at the end of exhalation. This completes one round of yogic breathing.

At first perform 5 to 10 rounds and slowly increase to 10 minutes daily.

Relax any effort and once again watch the spontaneous breathing pattern.

Bring the awareness back to observing the physical body as a whole. Be aware of the surroundings and gently open the eyes.

Practice note: The main requirement in pranayama is that respiration be comfortable and relaxed. Consequently, once awareness and control of the breathing process has been established, the clavicular technique is dropped and yogic breathing is modified to become a combination of abdominal and thoracic breathing. The breath should flow naturally and not be forced.

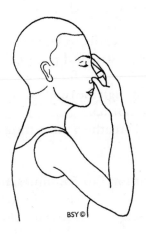

Hand position: Nasagra Mudra (nosetip position)

Hold the fingers of the right hand in front of the face. Rest the index and middle fingers gently on the eyebrow centre. Both fingers should be relaxed.

The thumb is above the right nostril and the ring finger above the left. These two digits control the flow of breath in the nostrils by alternately pressing on one nostril, blocking the flow of breath, and then the other.

The little finger is comfortably folded. When practising for long periods, the elbow may be supported in the palm of the left hand, although care is needed to prevent chest restriction.

Nadi Shodhana Pranayama (psychic network purification)
Technique 1: Preparatory practice

Stage 1: Sit in any comfortable meditation posture, preferably siddha/siddha yoni asana or padmasana.

Keep the head and spine upright.

Relax the whole body and close the eyes.

Practise yogic breathing for some time.

Adopt nasagra mudra with the right hand and place the left hand on the knee in chin or jnana mudra.

Close the right nostril with the thumb.

Inhale and exhale through the left nostril 5 times.

The rate of inhalation and exhalation should be normal.

Be aware of each breath.

After completing 5 breaths, release the pressure of the thumb on the right nostril and press the left nostril with the ring finger, blocking the flow of air.

Inhale and exhale through the right nostril 5 times, keeping the respiration rate normal.

Lower the hand and breathe 5 times through both nostrils together.

This is one round.

Practise 5 rounds or for 3 to 5 minutes, making sure that there is no sound as the air passes through the nostrils.

Practise until this stage is mastered before commencing the next stage.

Stage 2: Begin to control the duration of each breath.

Count the length of the inhalation and exhalation through the left, right and both nostrils. Breathe deeply without strain.

While inhaling, count mentally, "1, Om; 2, Om; 3, Om", until the inhalation ends comfortably.

While exhaling, simultaneously count, "1, Om; 2, Om; 3, Om". Inhalation and exhalation should be equal.

Practise 5 rounds or for 3 to 5 minutes, making sure that there is no sound as the air passes through the nostrils.

Extension: Notice that the length of the breath will spontaneously increase after some days of practice.

When the count reaches 10 without any strain, go on to technique 2.

Contra-indications: Nadi shodhana is not to be practised while suffering from colds, flu or fever.

Benefits: Technique 1 increases awareness of and sensitivity to the breath in the nostrils. Minor blockages are removed and the flow of breath in both nostrils becomes more balanced. Breathing through the left nostril tends to activate the right brain hemisphere; breathing through the right nostril activates the left hemisphere. The long, slow, balanced breathing of stage 2 has profound effects, calming and balancing the energies.

Practice note: Both nostrils must be clear and flowing freely. Mucous blockages may be removed through the practice of neti (see the section Shatkarma). If the flow of breath in the nostrils is unequal, it may be balanced by practising padadhirasana as a breath balancing technique (see Vajrasana Group of Asanas).

Beginners should be familiar with abdominal breathing before taking up nadi shodhana.

Technique 2: Alternate nostril breathing

In this technique the basic pattern of alternate nostril breathing is established.

Stage I: Begin with equal inhalation and exhalation, using the ratio 1:1.

Close the right nostril with the thumb and inhale through the left nostril.

At the same time count mentally, "1, Om; 2, Om; 3, Om", until the inhalation ends comfortably. This is the basic count.

Breathe deeply without strain.

Close the left nostril with the ring finger and release the pressure of the thumb on the right nostril. While exhaling through the right nostril, simultaneously count, "1, Om; 2, Om; 3, Om". The time for inhalation and exhalation should be equal.

Next, inhale through the right nostril, keeping the same count in the same manner.

At the end of inhalation, close the right nostril and open the left nostril. Exhale through the left nostril, counting as before.

This is one round.

Practise 5 to10 rounds.

Extension: After one week, if there is no difficulty, increase the length of inhalation and exhalation by one count.

Continue to increase the count in this way until the count of 10:10 is reached.

Do not force the breath in any way. Be careful not to speed up the counting during exhalation to compensate for shortage of breath. Reduce the count at the slightest sign of discomfort.

Stage 2: After perfecting the above 1:1 ratio, it may be changed to 1:2.

Initially halve the length of the inhalation. Inhale for a count of 5 and exhale for a count of 10.

Repeat on the other side.

This is one round.

Practise 5 to 10 rounds.

Extension: During the ensuing months of practice, continue extending the breath by adding one count to the inhalation and two to the exhalation, up to the count of 10: 20.

When this technique can be performed with complete ease, move on to technique 3.

Contra-indications: Stage 2 of technique 2 begins the process of introversion, which is not recommended for a depressed or withdrawn person. The extension of stage 2, involving longer counts, is not recommended for people with heart problems.

Benefits: Technique 2 gives more pronounced balancing of the breath and the brain hemispheres. It has calming effects and relieves anxiety, improves concentration and stimulates ajna chakra.

The ratio 1:1 in stage 1 establishes a calming rhythm for the brain and heart, assisting people with cardiovascular and nervous disorders specifically, and stress-related conditions generally.

As the count is extended, the breath slows down. The respiration becomes more efficient because the air flow is smoother and less turbulent. This ratio helps people with respiratory problems such as asthma, emphysema and bronchitis.

The ratio 1:2 in stage 2 gives profound relaxation. The heartbeat and pulse rate slow, and blood pressure drops, but the extension of count should be built up slowly.

Technique 3: with Antar Kumbhaka (inner retention)

In this technique antar kumbhaka or internal breath retention is introduced. The inhalation and exhalation should be silent, smooth and controlled.

Stage 1: Begin with equal inhalation, inner retention and exhalation, using the ratio 1:1:1.

Close the right nostril and inhale slowly through the left nostril for a count of 5.

At the end of inhalation, close both nostrils and retain the air in the lungs for a count of 5.

Open the right nostril and exhale for a count of 5.

At the end of exhalation, inhale through the right nostril for a count of 5, keeping the left nostril closed.

Again, retain the breath for a count of 5 with both nostrils closed.

Open the left nostril and exhale for a count of 5.

This is one round using the ratio 5:5:5.

Maintain constant awareness of the count and of the breath.

Practise up to 10 rounds.

Extension: After becoming comfortable with the count of 5:5:5, the breath and kumbhaka can be lengthened. Gradually increase the count by adding 1 unit to the inhalation, 1 unit to the retention and 1 unit to the exhalation. The count of one round will then be 6:6:6.

When this has been perfected and there is no discomfort, increase the count to 7:7:7.

Continue in this way until the count of 10:10:10 is reached. Do not force the breath. At the slightest sign of strain reduce the count.

Stage 2: After perfecting the ratio of 1:1:1, increase the ratio to 1:1:2. Initially use a short count. Inhale for a count of 5, perform internal kumbhaka for a count of 5 and exhale for a count of 10.

Extension: After mastering the count of 5:5:10, gradually increase the count by adding one unit to the inhalation, one unit to the retention and two units to the exhalation. The count of one round will then be 6:6:12. When this has been perfected and there is no discomfort, increase the count to

7:7:14. Gradually increase the count over several months of practice until the count of 10:10:20 is reached.

Stage 3: Change the ratio to 1:2:2. Inhale for a count of 5, do internal kumbhaka for a count of 10 and exhale for a count of 10. Practise until the ratio is comfortable and there is no tendency to speed up the count during retention or exhalation due to shortness of breath.

Extension: When this has been perfected, the count can be gradually increased by adding 1 unit to the inhalation, 2 units to the retention and 2 units to the exhalation. The count of one round will then be 6:12:12. In this manner, gradually increase the count to 10:20:20.

Stage 4: The next ratio, 1:3:2, is intermediary. First reduce the count, inhale for a count of 5, do internal kumbhaka for a count of 15 and exhale for a count of 10.

Practise until the ratio is comfortable and there is no tendency to speed up the count during retention or exhalation due to shortness of breath.

Extension: When this has been perfected and there is no discomfort, the count can be gradually increased by adding 1 unit to the inhalation, 3 units to the retention and 2 units to the exhalation. The count of one round will then be 6:18:12. In this manner, gradually increase the count to 10:30:20.

Stage 5: The final ratio is 1:4:2. Begin with 5:20:10. Once the ratio has been established, the count can gradually increase.

Extension: Add 1 unit to the inhalation, 4 units to the retention and 2 units to the exhalation. The count of one round will then be 6:24:12. In this manner, gradually increase the count to 10:40:20.

Contra-indications: Technique 3 is not suitable for women in the later half of pregnancy. It is not recommended for people with heart problems, high blood pressure, emphysema or any major disorders.

Stage 2 is not recommended for asthmatics.

Benefits: The inner retention of breath, which characterizes technique 3, activates various brain centres and harmonizes the pranas. The benefits increase with the progression of the ratios. The ratio 1:4:2 is most widely recommended in the yogic texts. It gives profound psychological and pranic effects and is used as a preparation for kundalini awakening.

Advanced practice: (addition of bandhas)

Before applying the bandhas in this practice, they should be perfected as individual practices. For details of these practices refer to the section on Bandha.

When adding bandhas, reduce the ratio and count so that it is effortless. Extend the count gradually as previously instructed.

Jalandhara bandha: First practise jalandhara bandha with internal breath retention.

Inhale through the left nostril, hold the breath and practise jalandhara bandha with internal retention.

Release jalandhara and exhale through the right nostril.

Inhale through the right nostril.

Practise jalandhara bandha with internal retention.

Release jalandhara and exhale through the left nostril.

This is one round, practise 5 rounds.

Extension: Once the bandha can be held without strain, gradually build up the count.

Jalandhara and moola bandhas: Reduce the count and combine jalandhara bandha with moola bandha.

Inhale through the left nostril.

Close both nostrils and hold the breath inside.

Practise jalandhara bandha and then moola bandha.

After the required count of retention, release moola bandha and then jalandhara.

Exhale through the right nostril.

Inhale through the right nostril and hold the breath inside.

Practise jalandhara bandha and moola bandha.

Release mool bandha and then jalandhara.

Exhale through the left nostril.

This is one round. Practise 5 rounds.

Extension: When the bandhas can be held without strain, gradually build up the count and then the ratio.

Precaution: Do not practise pranayama with bandhas without the guidance of a competent teacher or guru.

Benefits: The ratio 1:4:2 with bandhas purifies and balances the pranic forces.

Technique 4: Antar and Bahir Kumbhaka (internal and external retention)

In this technique bahir kumbhaka or outer breath retention is introduced. Do not try to hold the breath outside for long at first, even though it may seem easy.

Stage 1: Begin with the ratio 1:1:1:1 and a count such as 5:5:5:5.

Inhale through the left nostril, counting to 5.

Retain the breath in antar kumbhaka, counting to 5.

Exhale through the right nostril, counting to 5.

After exhalation, close both nostrils and hold the breath outside, counting to 5.

The glottis may be slightly contracted to hold the air outside. Exhale slightly through the right nostril immediately before inhaling. This will release the lock on the lungs and the glottis and bring the respiratory system smoothly back into operation.

Inhale slowly through the right nostril, counting to 5.

Retain the breath, counting to 5.

Exhale through the left nostril, counting to 5.

Again, hold the breath outside, counting to 5 with both nostrils closed. If necessary, exhale slightly through the left nostril before breathing in at the start of the next round. This is one round.

Practise 5 rounds.

Extension: When the ratio has been perfected at this count, gradually increase by adding 1 unit to the inhalation, internal retention, exhalation and external retention. The count should slowly be increased from 5 to 6, 6 to 7 and so on, until the count of 10:10:10:10 is reached.

Do not increase the count for inhalation until the counts for exhalation and breath retentions are comfortable.

Stage 2: The next ratio is 1:1:2:1. It should be commenced with a low count and extended gradually as previously instructed. Begin with 5:5:10:5.

Extension: Once the ratio has been established, the count can be gradually increased. Add one unit to the inhalation, one unit to the internal retention, 2 units to the exhalation and one unit to the external retention. The count for one round would thus become 6:6:12:6. Over time, the count can be slowly increased. Do not increase the count for inhalation until the relative counts for exhalation and breath retentions are comfortable.

Stage 3: The next ratio is 1:2:2:1. Begin with the count of 5:10:10:5. Do not increase the count for inhalation until the relative counts for exhalation and breath retentions are comfortable.

Stage 4: The next ratio is 1:2:2:2. Begin with the count of 5:10:10:10. Build up the count gradually without strain.

Stage 5: The next ratio is 1:3:2:2. Begin with the count of 5:15:10:10. Each time the ratio is changed, use the same care to start with a low count, which is allowed to build up gradually without strain.

Stage 6: The final ratio is 1:4:2:2. Begin with the count of 5:20:10:10.

Advanced practice: (addition of bandhas)

When technique 4 has been mastered, it may be practised in conjunction with jalandhara, moola and uddiyana bandhas. First practise jalandhara bandha with internal breath retention only. When this has been perfected, combine jalandhara bandha with external breath retention also.

When this has been mastered, combine jalandhara and moola bandha with internal and external retention.

When this has been perfected, maha bandha can be added during external retention. At the end of the exhalation, practise jalandhara, moola and uddiyana bandhas. Maintain the bandhas throughout the external retention.

Release jalandhara, moola and uddiyana, in this order, at the end of external retention.

Adjust the ratio of the breath to suit individual capacity.

Breathing: Breathing should be silent in all techniques of nadi shodhana, ensuring that it is not forced or restricted in any way.

393

As the ratio and duration increases, the breath becomes very light and subtle. Increased ratios and breath duration should not be attained at the expense of relaxation, rhythm and awareness. The flow of breath must be smooth, with no jerks, throughout the practice.

Awareness: Physical–on the breath and the counting.

Mental–it is easy for the mind to wander during nadi shodhana. Simply be aware of this wandering tendency of the mind while continuing the practice and the count. This will automatically encourage the awareness to return to the practice.

Spiritual–on ajna chakra.

Precautions: Under no circumstance should the breath be forced. Never breathe through the mouth. Proceed carefully and only under the guidance of a competent teacher. At the slightest sign of discomfort, reduce the duration of inhalation, exhalation and retention and, if necessary, discontinue the practice. Nadi shodhana should never be rushed or forced.

Sequence: If one of the nostrils is blocked, perform jala neti or breath balancing exercises before commencing.

Nadi shodhana should be practised after shatkarma and asanas, and before other pranayamas. The best time to practise is around sunrise; however, it may be performed at any time during the day, except after meals.

Duration: 5 to 10 rounds or 10 to 15 minutes daily.

Benefits: Nadi shodhana ensures that the whole body is nourished by an extra supply of oxygen. Carbon dioxide is efficiently expelled and the blood is purified of toxins. The brain centres are stimulated to work nearer to their optimum capacity. It also induces tranquillity, clarity of thought and concentration, and is recommended for those engaged in mental work. It increases vitality and lowers levels of stress and anxiety by harmonizing the pranas. It clears pranic blockages and balances ida and pingala nadis, causing sushumna nadi to flow, which leads to deep states of meditation and spiritual awakening.

Practice note: Development of nadi shodhana is intended to take place over a long period of time. Each technique should be practised until perfected. Developing the ratios and counts in each technique may take many years.

Each time the ratio is changed, start with a low count and build up gradually without strain. Practise a given ratio until perfected. The length of the breath should increase spontaneously without the use of force.

The point is not how long the breath can be held, but rather to give the mind, body and lifestyle time to adapt to psychic and physical repercussions.

Techniques 1 and 2 prepare the lungs and the nervous system for techniques 3 and 4, which introduce antar and bahir kumbhaka (internal and external breath retention). Mastery of the techniques should take time as the body and mind need to adjust to the effects of extended breath retention. The full benefits of this practice will be obtained by systematically perfecting each level, rather than by struggling prematurely with the advanced techniques.

It is important to experience each stage fully and become established in that new pattern of breath and its effects on the nervous system, energy levels, emotions, mental clarity and subtle aspects of the personality.

Note: *The word* nadi *means 'channel' or 'flow' of energy and* shodhana *means 'purification'.* Nadi shodhana, *therefore, means that practice which purifies the nadis.*

The number 24, used for timing the breath, derives from classical texts, which use the Gayatri mantra as a metre to measure the length of pranayamas. The Gayatri mantra is made up of 24 individual matras *or sound syllables.*

395

SHEETALI PRANAYAMA

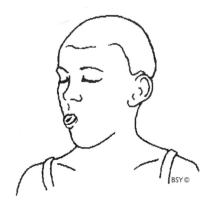

Sheetali Pranayama (cooling breath)
Technique I

Sit in any comfortable meditation posture.

Close the eyes and relax the whole body.

Extend the tongue outside the mouth as far as possible without strain. Roll the sides of the tongue up so that it forms a tube. Practise a long, smooth and controlled inhalation through the rolled tongue.

At the end of inhalation, draw the tongue in, close the mouth and exhale through the nose.

Practise yogic breathing throughout.

The breath should produce a sucking sound.

A feeling of icy coldness will be experienced on the tongue and the roof of the mouth. This is one round.

Duration: With practice, the duration of the inhalation should gradually become longer to increase the cooling effect.

Gradually increase the number of rounds from 9 to 15. For general purposes 15 rounds is sufficient; however, up to 60 rounds may be performed in very hot weather.

Awareness: On the tongue, the sound and the cooling sensation of the inhaled breath.

Sequence: Practise after asanas and other yogic practices which heat the body in order to restore temperature balance.

Technique 2: with Antar Kumbhaka (internal retention)
At the end of inhalation, retain the breath inside for one or two seconds at first. The duration may be gradually increased as the technique is mastered.

Advanced practice: (addition of bandhas)
Once jalandhara bandha is perfected, it may also be combined with this practice during internal retention.

Precaution: Do not practise in a polluted atmosphere or during cold weather. The nose heats up and cleans the inhaled air before it enters the delicate lungs. However, breathing through the mouth bypasses this air-conditioning and the induction of cold or dirty air directly into the lungs may cause harm.
Practise inner retention for a short time only as prolonged kumbhaka has a heating effect.

Contra-indications: People suffering from low blood pressure or respiratory disorders such as asthma, bronchitis and excessive mucus, should not practise this pranayama. Those with heart disease should practise without breath retention.
This practice cools down the activity of the lower energy centres and therefore those suffering from chronic constipation should avoid it. Generally, this pranayama should not be practised in winter or in cool climates.

Benefits: This practice cools the body and affects important brain centres associated with biological drives and temperature regulation. It cools and reduces mental and emotional excitation, and encourages the free flow of prana throughout the body. It induces muscular relaxation, mental tranquillity and may be used as a tranquillizer before sleep. It gives control over hunger and thirst, and generates a feeling of satisfaction.

Practice note: About one-third of the population is genetically unable to roll the sides of the tongue into a tube. However, the practice of sheetkari pranayama gives similar benefits.

Note: *Sheetali is derived from the root* sheet, *which means 'cold'.* Sheetal *means 'that which is calm, passionless and soothing'.*

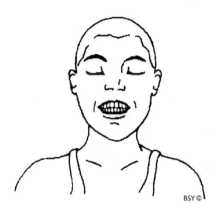

Sheetkari Pranayama (hissing breath)
Sit in any comfortable meditation posture.
Close the eyes and relax the whole body.
Hold the teeth lightly together.
Separate the lips, exposing the teeth.
The tongue may be kept flat or folded against the soft palate in khechari mudra.
Inhale slowly and deeply through the teeth.
At the end of the inhalation, close the mouth.
Exhale slowly through the nose in a controlled manner
This is one round.

Awareness: On the hissing sound and the cooling sensation of the inhaled breath.

Contra-indications: As for sheetali pranayama. Practitioners with sensitive teeth, missing teeth or dentures should practise sheetali pranayama instead.

Other details: As for sheetali pranayama.

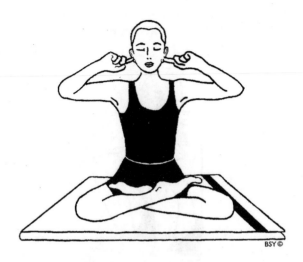

BSY©

Bhramari Pranayama (humming bee breath)
Technique I

Sit in a comfortable meditation asana, preferably padmasana or siddha/siddha yoni asana with the hands resting
on the knees in jnana or chin mudra.

Close the eyes and relax the whole body.

The lips should remain gently closed with the teeth slightly
separated throughout the practice. This allows the sound
vibration to be heard and felt more distinctly.

Raise the arms sideways and bend the elbows, bringing the
hands to the ears. Use the index or middle fingers to plug
the ears or the flaps of the ears may be pressed without
inserting the fingers.

Bring the awareness to the centre of the head, where ajna
chakra is located, and keep the body absolutely still.

Inhale through the nose.

Exhale slowly and in a controlled manner while making a
deep, steady humming sound like that of the black bee.

The humming should be smooth, even and continuous for
the duration of the exhalation. The sound should be soft
and mellow, making the front of the skull reverberate.

At the end of exhalation, the hands can be kept steady or returned to the knee and then raised again for the next round. The inhalation and exhalation should be smooth and controlled. This is one round.

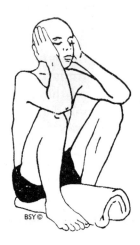

Variation: Nadanusandhana Asana (exploration of sound pose)
Sit on a rolled blanket with the heels drawn up to the buttocks. Place the feet flat on the floor with the knees raised and the elbows resting on the knees. Plug the ears with the thumbs, resting the other four fingers on the head. This position gives increased stability without strain when practising for long periods of time as a preparatory practice for nada yoga, which uses subtle sound vibration to attune the practitioners with their true nature.

Awareness: Physical – on the humming sound within the head and on the steady, even breath.
Spiritual – on ajna chakra.

Duration: 5 to 10 rounds is sufficient in the beginning, then slowly increase to 10 to 15 minutes. In cases of extreme mental tension or anxiety, or when used to assist the healing process, practise for up to 30 minutes.

Time of practice: The best time to practise is late at night or in the early morning as there are fewer external noises to interfere with internal perception. Practising at this time awakens psychic sensitivity. However, bhramari may be practised at any time to relieve mental tension.

Contra-indications: Bhramari should not be performed while lying down. People suffering from severe ear infections should not practise this pranayama.

Benefits: Bhramari relieves stress and cerebral tension, and so helps in alleviating anger, anxiety and insomnia, increasing the healing capacity of the body. It strengthens and improves the voice. Bhramari induces a meditative state by harmonizing the mind and directing the awareness inward. The vibration of the humming sound creates a soothing effect on the mind and nervous system.

Technique 2: with Antar Kumbhaka (inner retention)

Inhale slowly and deeply through the nose.

Retain the breath inside with awareness at ajna or bindu. The exhalation should be as long as is comfortable to enhance the mind's absorption in the humming sound.

Contra-indications: People with heart disease must practise without breath retention.

Practice note: Inner retention should be gradually increased as it helps in increasing introversion and concentration. Do not strain when performing kumbhaka; one or two seconds is sufficient at first. The duration may be increased gradually as the technique is mastered.

Advanced practice: (addition of bandhas)

Before applying the bandhas in this practice, they should be perfected as individual practices.

Once antar kumbhaka has been mastered, jalandhara and moola bandhas may be incorporated.

For details of these practices refer to the section on Bandha. The full form of jalandhara can be practised if the hands are returned to the knees between rounds. If the hands remain raised, plugging the ears, then practise the simple variation of jalandhara.

Inhale for a long smooth breath.

Practise jalandhara and then moola bandha during internal retention for a comfortable duration.

401

Release moola bandha and then jalandhara bandha, and exhale through the nose with the humming sound.
This is one round.
Once the bandhas can be held without strain, gradually build up the number of rounds.

Precaution: Do not practise pranayama with bandhas without the guidance of a competent teacher or guru.

Note: *The word* bhramari *means 'bee' and the practice is so called because a sound is produced which imitates that of the black bee.*

UJJAYI PRANAYAMA

Ujjayi Pranayama (the psychic breath)
Technique I
Sit in any comfortable meditation asana.
Close the eyes and relax the whole body.
Take the awareness to the breath in the nostrils and allow the breathing to become calm and rhythmic.
After some time, transfer the awareness to the throat.
Feel or imagine that the breath is being drawn in and out through the throat and not through the nostrils, as if it is taking place through a small hole in the throat.
As the breathing becomes slower and deeper, gently contract the glottis so that a soft snoring sound, like the breathing of a sleeping baby, is produced in the throat. If practised correctly, there will be a spontaneous contraction of the abdomen, without any effort being made.
Both inhalation and exhalation should be long, deep and controlled.
Practise yogic breathing while concentrating on the sound produced by the breath in the throat.
The sound of the breath should be audible to the practitioner alone.

Extension: When this breathing has been mastered, fold the tongue back into khechari mudra (refer to the section on Mudra).

If the tongue becomes tired, release it, while continuing the ujjayi breathing. When the tongue is rested, again fold it back.

Duration: Begin with 10 breaths and slowly increase to 5 minutes for general benefits.

As an adjunct to meditation or mantra repetition, practise for 10 to 20 minutes.

Contra-indications: People who are too introverted by nature should not perform this practice.

Benefits: Ujjayi is classified as a tranquillizing pranayama and it also has a heating effect on the body. This practice soothes the nervous system and calms the mind. It has a profoundly relaxing effect at the psychic level. It helps to relieve insomnia and may be practised in shavasana just before sleep. It slows down the heart rate and is useful for people suffering from high blood pressure.

Practice note: Ujjayi may be performed in any position, standing, sitting or lying. Those suffering from slipped disc or vertebral spondylitis may practise ujjayi in vajrasana or makarasana.

Relax the face as much as possible. Do not contract the throat too strongly. The contraction should be slight and applied continuously throughout the practice.

Technique 2: with Antar Kumbhaka (inner retention)

The inhalation and exhalation should be smooth and controlled.

Inhale slowly and deeply through the nose.

Retain the breath inside with awareness at ajna or bindu.

The exhalation should be as long as is comfortable. Do not strain when performing kumbhaka; one or two seconds is sufficient at first. The duration may be increased gradually as the technique is mastered.

Contra-indications: Those suffering from heart disease should not combine bandhas or breath retention with ujjayi.

403

Practice note: Inner retention should be gradually increased as it helps in increasing introversion and concentration.

Advanced practice: (addition of bandhas)

Before applying the bandhas in this practice, they should be perfected as individual practices. For details of these practices refer to the section on Bandha.

Once antar kumbhaka has been mastered, bandhas may be incorporated.

Jalandhara bandha: Inhale for a long, smooth breath.

Practise jalandhara bandha with internal retention for a comfortable duration.

Release jalandhara and exhale.

This is one round.

Jalandhara and moola bandhas: Inhale. Practise jalandhara and then moola bandha, holding the breath inside for a comfortable duration.

Release moola bandha and then jalandhara and exhale.

This is one round.

Once the bandha can be held without strain, gradually build up the number of rounds.

Note: *The Sanskrit word* ujjayi *means 'victorious'. It is derived from the root* ji, *which means 'to conquer' or 'to acquire by conquest', and the prefix* ud, *which means 'bondage'. Ujjayi is therefore the pranayama which gives freedom from bondage. It is also known as the psychic breath, as it leads to subtle states of mind and is used together with khechari mudra, the tongue lock, in tantric meditation techniques such as mantra japa, ajapa japa, kriya yoga and prana vidya.*

Bhastrika Pranayama (bellows breath)
Technique I: Preparatory practice

Sit in a comfortable meditation posture with the hands resting on the knees in either chin or jnana mudra.

Keep the head and spine straight, close the eyes and relax the whole body.

Take a deep breath in and breathe out forcefully through the nose. Immediately afterwards breathe in with the same force. Forceful inhalation results from fully expanding the abdominal muscles and forceful exhalation from firm contraction of the abdominal muscles. Do not strain.

During inhalation, the diaphragm descends and the abdomen moves outward. During exhalation, the diaphragm moves upward and the abdomen moves inward. The movements should be slightly exaggerated.

Continue in this manner, counting 10 breaths.

Take a deep breath in and breathe out slowly.

This is one round. Practise up to 5 rounds.

Practice note: When accustomed to this style of breathing, gradually increase the speed, always keeping the breath rhythmical. The force of inhalation and exhalation must be equal.

Technique 2: Alternate nostrils

Sit in a comfortable meditation asana, preferably padmasana or siddha/siddha yoni asana.

Keep the head and spine straight. Close the eyes and relax the whole body.

Raise the right hand and perform nasagra mudra.

Left nostril: Close the right nostril with the thumb.

Breathe in and out forcefully, without straining, through the left nostril 10 times. There should be a snuffing sound in the nose, but no sound should come from the throat or chest.

405

The abdomen should expand and contract rhythmically with the breath. The pumping action should be performed by the abdomen alone; the chest, shoulders and face remain relaxed.

After 10 breaths, take a deep breath in and breathe out through the left nostril.

Right nostril: Close the left nostril and repeat the same process through the right nostril.

Both nostrils: Replace the raised hand on the knee.

Repeat the same process through both nostrils.

Duration: Ten breaths through the left, the right and both nostrils, as above, forms one complete round.

Practise up to 5 rounds.

Breathing: Beginners may take several free breaths between rounds so that there is no strain.

Breathing may be practised at 3 breath rates: slow, medium and fast, depending on individual capacity.

Slow bhastrika is approximately one breath every 2 seconds, with no undue force on inhalation or exhalation. It is like amplified normal breathing. It is especially useful for beginners, but may also be practised at all stages.

Medium breathing increases the speed of respiration to approximately one breath every second.

Fast breathing means a speed of around 2 breaths per second. Both medium and fast breathing are suitable for intermediate and advanced practitioners.

As abdominal muscles become stronger with regular practice, the number of respirations may be increased by 5 per month until the count of 50 respirations is attained.

Awareness: Physical – on the breathing process and the physical movement of the abdomen.

Spiritual – on manipura chakra.

Precautions: Bhastrika is a dynamic practice requiring a large expenditure of physical energy. Beginners are advised to take a short rest after each round. Avoid violent respiration, facial contortions and excessive shaking of the body. A feeling of faintness, excessive perspiration or vomiting indicates that the practice is being performed incorrectly.

If any of these symptoms are experienced, the advice of a competent teacher should be sought.

This practice purifies the blood. However, if the stages are rushed, all the impurities will be ejected from the body in a rush, which may exacerbate conditions caused by detoxification. A slow, conscientious approach to this practice is therefore recommended.

Contra-indications: Bhastrika should not be practised by people with high blood pressure, heart disease, hernia, gastric ulcer, stroke, epilepsy, retinal problems, glaucoma or vertigo. The elderly, those suffering from lung diseases such as asthma and chronic bronchitis, those recovering from tuberculosis, or in the first trimester of pregnancy are recommended to practise only under the guidance of a competent teacher.

Benefits: This practice burns up toxins and helps balance the *doshas* or humours: *kapha*, phlegm; *pitta*, bile; and *vata*, wind. It is a useful practice for women during labour after a few months of proper preparation.

Because of the rapid exchange of air in the lungs, there is an increase in the exchange of oxygen and carbon dioxide into and out of the bloodstream. This stimulates the metabolic rate, producing heat and flushing out wastes and toxins. The rapid and rhythmic movement of the diaphragm also massages and stimulates the visceral organs, toning the digestive system.

Bhastrika reduces the level of carbon dioxide in the blood. It helps to alleviate inflammation in the throat and any accumulation of phlegm. It balances and strengthens the nervous system, inducing peace, tranquillity and one-pointedness of mind in preparation for meditation.

Technique 3: with Antar Kumbhaka (inner retention)

Once technique 2 has been mastered.

Left nostril: Close the right nostril with the thumb.

Breathe in and out forcefully through the left nostril.

The abdomen should expand and contract rhythmically with the breath.

407

After completing the forceful breaths, take a deep breath in, expanding both the abdomen and the chest, close both nostrils and retain the breath for a few seconds.

Exhale through the left nostril

Right nostril: Close the left nostril and repeat the same process through the right nostril.

Both nostrils: After completing the forceful breaths through both nostrils, inhale slowly and deeply, close both nostrils and retain the breath for a few seconds.

Breathe out slowly through both nostrils.

This is one round. Practise up to 5 rounds.

Practice note: If the exhalation seems locked after retention, a slight inhalation before exhalation releases the locked condition of the glottis and brings the respiratory muscles back into action.

Advanced practice: (addition of bandhas)

Jalandhara bandha and moola bandha should be perfected as individual practices before being applied in this practice. After antar kumbhaka has been mastered, jalandhara and moola bandha may be practised during internal breath retention.

At the end of each round, inhale deeply and hold the breath inside.

Practise jalandhara bandha and then moola bandha.

After the required count of retention, release moola bandha, jalandhara bandha, and then exhale.

Duration: Up to 5 rounds. The duration of inner retention can gradually be increased up to 30 seconds.

Do not strain.

Precaution: Before practising pranayama with bandhas seek the guidance of a competent teacher.

Contra-indications: The contra-indications for jalandhara and moola bandhas apply as well as those for bhastrika technique 2.

Technique 4: with Bahir Kumbhaka (external retention)

After technique 3 has been mastered, external retention may be commenced.

After perfecting the practice with external retention, maha bandha may be applied. Maha bandha should first be perfected as an individual practice.

At the end of each round, inhale deeply through both nostrils and then exhale completely.

Hold the breath outside for a few seconds.

Practise maha bandha.

Release maha bandha and inhale.

Duration: Up to 5 rounds.

The duration of external retention can be gradually increased up to 30 seconds. Do not strain.

Contra-indications: See the contra-indications for maha bandha as well as for bhastrika.

Benefits: This practice activates the brain and induces clarity of thought and concentration. It increases vitality and lowers levels of stress and anxiety by raising the energy and harmonizing the pranas. It clears pranic blockages, causing sushumna nadi to flow, which leads to deep states of meditation and spiritual awakening. It is reputed to burn through karma.

Note: *The Sanskrit word* bhastrika *means 'bellows'. Thus, bhastrika pranayama is also known as the bellows breath, as air is drawn forcefully in and out of the lungs like the bellows of a village blacksmith. The bellows increases the flow of air into the fire, producing more heat. Similarly, bhastrika pranayama increases the flow of air into the body to produce inner heat at both the physical and subtle levels, stoking the inner fire of mind and body.*

KAPALBHATI PRANAYAMA

Kapalbhati Pranayama (frontal brain cleansing breath)
Technique I: Preparatory practice (shatkarma method)
Sit in a comfortable meditation asana. The head and spine should be straight with the hands resting on the knees in either chin or jnana mudra.

Close the eyes and relax the whole body.

Exhale through both nostrils with a forceful contraction of the abdominal muscles. The following inhalation should take place passively by allowing the abdominal muscles to relax.

Inhalation should be a spontaneous recoil, involving no effort.

After completing 10 rapid breaths in succession, inhale and exhale deeply. Allow the breath to return to normal.

This is one round. Practise up to 5 rounds.

Breathing: The rapid breathing should be from the abdomen; the shoulders and face remain relaxed.

Beginners may take several free breaths between rounds. The number of respirations may be increased from the initial count of 10 up to 50, as the abdominal muscles become stronger. Advanced practitioners can increase up to 60 or 100 breaths per round.

Sequence: As a shatkarma to clear excess mucus from the nasal passages, kapalbhati should be practised before pranayama.

Precautions: Kapalbhati should be performed on an empty stomach, 3 to 4 hours after meals. If practised late at night, it can prevent sleep.

If pain or dizziness are experienced, stop the practice and sit quietly for some time. Practise with more awareness and less force. If the problem continues, consult a competent teacher.

Contra-indications: Kapalbhati should not be practised by those suffering from heart disease, high blood pressure, vertigo, epilepsy, stroke, hernia or gastric ulcer. It is not recommended during pregnancy.

Benefits: Kapalbhati has a cleansing effect on the lungs and is a good practice for respiratory disorders. It balances and strengthens the nervous system and tones the digestive organs. It purifies the nadis, and removes sensory distractions. It energizes the mind for mental work and removes sleepiness.

Practice note: Although kapalbhati is similar to bhastrika, there are important differences. Bhastrika uses force on both inhalation and exhalation, expanding and contracting the lungs above and below their resting or basic volume. Kapalbhati, on the other hand, actively reduces the volume of air in the lungs below this level through forced exhalation. In this practice, inhalation remains a passive process, which brings the level of air in the lungs back to the basic volume only. Kapalbhati reverses the normal breathing process, which involves active inhalation and passive exhalation. It has profound effects on the nervous system.

Technique 2: Alternate nostrils

Sit in a comfortable meditation asana, preferably padmasana, or siddha/siddha yoni asana.

Raise the right hand and perform nasagra mudra.

Left nostril: Close the right nostril with the thumb.

Exhale forcefully and inhale passively through the left nostril 10 times. The pumping action should be performed by the abdomen alone; the chest, shoulders and face remain relaxed.

After the 10 breaths, take a deep breath in and out through the left nostril.

Right nostril: Close the left nostril and repeat the same process through the right nostril.

Both nostrils: Replace the raised hand on the knee.

Repeat the same process through both nostrils.

Duration: Ten breaths through the left, the right and both nostrils forms one complete round.

Practise up to 5 rounds.

Breathing: Beginners may take several free breaths between rounds. The number of respirations may be gradually increased from 10 up to 50, as the abdominal muscles become stronger.

Technique 3: with Antar Kumbhaka (inner retention)

After perfecting technique 2, antar kumbhaka may be commenced.

At the end of the round, inhale deeply and retain the breath for a comfortable length of time without straining. Exhale slowly with control. Practise up to 5 rounds.

Sequence: Practise just before meditation techniques.

Advanced practice: (addition of bandhas)

Before applying bandhas in this practice, they should first be perfected as individual practices. After antar kumbhaka has been mastered, jalandhara and moola bandhas may be combined during internal retention.

At the end of each round, inhale deeply. Practise jalandhara bandha and then moola bandha during internal retention. Hold the breath inside without straining.

After the required count of retention, release moola bandha, jalandhara bandha, and then exhale.

Precaution: Before practising pranayama with bandhas seek the guidance of a competent teacher.

Contra-indications: The contra-indications for jalandhara bandha and moola bandha apply, as well as those for kapalbhati technique 1.

Technique 4: with Bahir Kumbhaka (external retention)

After perfecting technique 3, bahir kumbhaka may be commenced.

At the end of the round, inhale deeply and retain the breath for a comfortable length of time. Exhale slowly.

Retain the breath outside for a comfortable length of time.

Advanced practice: (addition of bandhas)

After perfecting maha bandha as an independent practice, it can be incorporated into the practice of kapalbhati during external retention.

After completing one round, inhale deeply and retain the

breath inside for a few seconds.

Exhale completely and practise maha bandha.

Retain the bandha, and the breath outside for a comfortable length of time without straining.

Release maha bandha and inhale.

Maintain awareness of the eyebrow centre, feeling an all-pervading calmness.

Duration: Up to 5 rounds.

Experienced practitioners can gradually increase the number of respirations to 60, and slowly increase the duration of external retention up to 30 seconds.

Further rounds should be practised only under the guidance of a competent teacher. Do not strain.

Awareness: Physical – on rhythmic, forceful exhalation.

Spiritual – on the void at the eyebrow centre.

Precaution: Proceed slowly with awareness of the effects of the practice. Build up the number of breaths, number of rounds and length of retention gradually. Do not strain by practising for extended periods. If breathlessness is experienced, discontinue the practice or reduce the number of rounds to a comfortable level.

Contra-indications: The contra-indications for maha bandha apply, as well as those for kapalbhati technique 1.

Benefits: This practice is useful for spiritual aspirants as it arrests thoughts and visions. It calms the mind in preparation for meditation. At the same time, it energizes the mind so one is not overcome by sleep while sitting for meditation.

Practice note: If the inhalation seems locked after external retention in maha bandha, a slight exhalation before inhalation relieves the locked condition of the glottis and brings the respiratory muscles back into action.

Note: *The Sanskrit word* kapal *means 'cranium' or 'forehead' and* bhati *means 'light' or 'splendour' and also 'perception' or 'knowledge'. Hence* kapalbhati *is the practice which brings a state of light or clarity to the frontal region of the brain. Another name for this practice is* kapalshodhana, *the word* shodhana *meaning 'to purify'.*

MOORCHHA PRANAYAMA

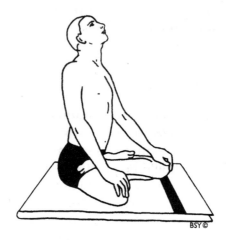

Moorchha Pranayama (swooning or fainting breath)

Sit in any comfortable meditation asana, preferably padmasana or siddha/siddha yoni asana.

Keep the head and spine straight. Relax the whole body. Observe the breath until it becomes slow and deep.

Adopt khechari mudra, then slowly inhale through both nostrils with ujjayi pranayama, while gently and smoothly bending the head slightly back.

Perform shambhavi mudra.

Straighten the arms by locking the elbows and pressing the knees with the hands.

Reta'n the breath inside for as long as is comfortable, maintaining shambhavi mudra.

Exhale and relax the arms. Close the eyes and slowly bring the head back to the upright position.

Relax the whole body for a few seconds, keeping the eyes closed. Experience the lightness and tranquillity in the mind and body. This is one round.

Duration: Practise until a fainting sensation is felt.

Awareness: Physical – on the breath, head movement and eyebrow centre.

Spiritual – on the void behind the eyebrow centre.

Sequence: After asanas and other pranayamas and before meditation. It is also beneficial before sleep.

Precautions: This technique induces the sensation of light-headedness or swooning. It should only be practised under the guidance of a competent teacher.

Contra-indications: This technique should not be practised by those suffering from heart disease, high blood pressure, epilepsy, brain disorders or atherosclerosis of the carotid or basilar arteries. Discontinue the practice as soon as the fainting sensation is felt. The aim is to induce a swooning sensation, not complete unconsciousness.

Benefits: Moorchha pranayama is an excellent preparation for meditation as it draws the mind inwards and enables a psychic state to be experienced. It cuts out the distractions of the outside world, inhibits identification with the physical body and brings about mental tranquillity. It helps alleviate tension, anxiety, anger and neuroses, and raises the level of prana.

Practice note: The essence of moorchha pranayama is internal breath retention. It is possible to slowly develop the capacity to hold the breath for long periods of time. Stopping the breath acts directly on the mind via the pranic body to induce a state of void.

The sensation of fainting and light-headedness arises for two reasons. Firstly, pressure on the blood vessels in the neck causes fluctuations in the pressure within the cranial cavity. Secondly, the carotid sinuses, vital to maintaining autonomic control of the body's circulation, are continuously compressed, changing the tone of the autonomic nervous system and inducing a swooning sensation. The practice of antar kumbhaka further reduces the oxygen supply to the brain, especially if held for a long time.

415

SURYA BHEDA PRANAYAMA

Surya Bheda Pranayama (vitality stimulating breath)
Technique I
> Assume a comfortable meditation asana. Place the hands on the knees in either chin or jnana mudra. Close the eyes and relax the whole body.
> When the body is comfortable and still, watch the breath until it spontaneously becomes slow and deep.
> Adopt nasagra mudra.
> Close the left nostril with the ring finger and inhale slowly and deeply through the right nostril.
> Exhale slowly through the right nostril, keeping the left nostril closed with the ring finger.
> This is one round.

Technique 2: with Antar Kumbhaka (inner retention)
> At the end of inhalation close both nostrils. Maintain the internal retention for a comfortable length of time.
> Exhale slowly through the right nostril, keeping the left nostril closed with the ring finger.
> Slowly increase the duration of the inhalation, retention and exhalation without straining.

Advanced practice: (addition of bandhas)
> Before applying jalandhara and moola bandhas with antar kumbhaka, they should be perfected as individual practices.
> Perform jalandhara and then moola bandha after the inhalation.
> Hold for a comfortable length of time.
> Release moola bandha, then jalandhara and slowly raise the head.
> When the head is upright, exhale slowly through the right nostril.

Awareness: On the breath in the right nostril.

Duration: When first practising surya bheda pranayama, 10 rounds are sufficient. Over time, however, as the practice becomes comfortable, the duration may be increased to

10 minutes. Slowly increase the length of retention over a matter of months.

A ratio of 1:1:1 may be introduced to stabilize the practice. Once this is mastered, it may be increased to 1:1:2 and then 1:2:2.

Precautions: Never practise surya bheda pranayama after eating, as it will interfere with the natural flow of energy associated with digestion.

This pranayama may cause imbalance in the breathing cycle if performed for prolonged periods.

Surya bheda is a very powerful pranayama and should only be performed under the guidance of a competent teacher.

Do not practise pranayama with bandhas without the guidance of a competent teacher.

Contra-indications: People suffering from heart disease, hypertension, epilepsy, hyperthyroid, peptic ulcer, acidity or anxiety should not practise this pranayama.

Benefits: This practice creates heat in the body and counteracts imbalances of the *vata* (wind) and *kapha* (phlegm) *doshas* (humours). It stimulates and awakens the pranic energy by activating pingala nadi. By increasing extroversion and dynamism, it enables physical activities to be performed more efficiently and helps to alleviate depression. It is especially recommended for those who are dull and lethargic or who find it difficult to communicate with the external world. It makes the mind more alert and perceptive and is an excellent pre-meditation pranayama.

Note: *The Sanskrit word* surya *means 'sun', which refers to pingala nadi, while* bheda *means 'to pierce', 'pass through' or 'awaken'. Surya bheda, then, means to pierce or purify pingala nadi.*

Mudra

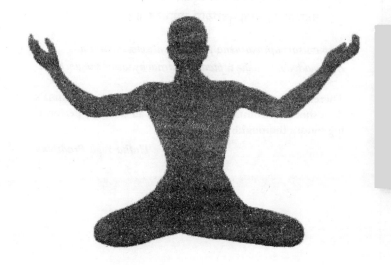

तस्मात्सर्वप्रयत्नेन प्रबोधयितुमीश्वरीम् ।
ब्रह्मद्वारमुखे सुप्तां मुद्राभ्यासं समाचरेत् ॥ 3:5 ॥

Tasmaatsarvaprayatnena prabodhayitumeeshvareem.
Brahmadvaaramukhe suptaam mudraabhyaasam samaacharet.

Therefore, the goddess sleeping at the entrance of Brahma's
door should be constantly aroused with all effort, by performing mudra thoroughly.

Hatha Yoga Pradipika

Introduction to Mudra

The Sanskrit word *mudra* is translated as 'gesture' or 'attitude'. Mudras can be described as psychic, emotional, devotional and aesthetic gestures or attitudes. Yogis have experienced mudras as attitudes of energy flow, intended to link individual pranic force with universal or cosmic force. The *Kularnava Tantra* traces the word mudra to the root *mud*, meaning 'delight' or 'pleasure', and *dravay*, the causal form of *dru*, which means 'to draw forth'. Mudra is also defined as a 'seal', 'short-cut' or 'circuit bypass'.

Mudras are a combination of subtle physical movements which alter mood, attitude and perception, and which deepen awareness and concentration. A mudra may involve the whole body in a combination of asana, pranayama, bandha and visualization techniques, or it may be a simple hand position. The *Hatha Yoga Pradipika* and other yogic texts consider mudra to be a *yoganga*, an independent branch of yoga, requiring a very subtle awareness. Mudras are introduced after some proficiency has been attained in asana, pranayama and bandha, and gross blockages have been removed.

Mudras have been described in various texts from antiquity to the present day in order to preserve them for posterity. However, such references were never detailed or clearly delineated as these techniques were not intended to be learned from a book. Practical instruction from a guru was always considered to be a necessary requisite before attempting them. Mudras are higher practices which lead to awakening of the pranas, chakras and

421

kundalini, and which can bestow major *siddhis*, psychic powers, on the advanced practitioner.

Mudras and prana

The attitudes and postures adopted during mudra practices establish a direct link between *annamaya kosha*, the physical body, *manomaya kosha*, the mental body and *pranamaya kosha*, the energy body. Initially, this enables the practitioner to develop awareness of the flow of prana in the body. Ultimately, it establishes pranic balance within the koshas and enables the redirection of subtle energy to the upper chakras, inducing higher states of consciousness.

Mudras manipulate prana in much the same way that energy in the form of light or sound waves is diverted by a mirror or a cliff face. The nadis and chakras constantly radiate prana which normally escapes from the body and dissipates into the external world. By creating barriers within the body through the practice of mudra, the energy is redirected within. For example, by closing the eyes with the fingers in shanmukhi mudra, the prana being radiated through the eyes is reflected back. In the same way, the sexual energy emitted through vajra nadi is redirected to the brain through the practice of vajroli mudra.

Tantric literature states that once the dissipation of prana is arrested through the practice of mudra, the mind becomes introverted, inducing states of *pratyahara*, sense withdrawal, and *dharana*, concentration. Because of their ability to redirect prana, mudras are important techniques for awakening kundalini. For this reason they are incorporated extensively in kriya and kundalini yoga practices.

A scientific look at mudras

In scientific terms, mudras provide a means to access and influence the unconscious reflexes and primal, instinctive habit patterns that originate in the primitive areas of the brain around the brain stem. They establish a subtle, non-intellectual connection with these areas. Each mudra sets up a different link and has a correspondingly different effect on the body, mind and prana. The aim is to create fixed, repetitive postures and gestures which can snap the practitioner out of instinctive habit patterns and establish a more refined consciousness.

FIVE GROUPS OF YOGA MUDRAS

The yoga mudras can be categorized into approximately five groups, which are described as follows.

1. Hasta (hand mudras)

The hand mudras presented in this book are meditative mudras. They redirect the prana emitted by the hands back into the body. Mudras which join the thumb and index finger engage the motor cortex at a very subtle level. They generate a loop of energy which moves from the brain down to the hand and then back again. Conscious awareness of this process rapidly leads to internalization. Techniques included in this category are:
Jnana mudra
Chin mudra
Yoni mudra
Bhairava mudra
Hridaya mudra.

2. Mana (head mudras)

These practices form an integral part of kundalini yoga and many are meditation techniques in their own right. They utilize the eyes, ears, nose, tongue and lips. Techniques included in this category are:
Shambhavi mudra
Nasikagra drishti
Khechari mudra
Kaki mudra
Bhujangini mudra
Bhoochari mudra
Akashi mudra
Shanmukhi mudra
Unmani mudra.

3. Kaya (postural mudras)

These practices utilize physical postures combined with breathing and concentration. Techniques included in this category are:
Vipareeta karani mudra
Pashinee mudra
Prana mudra
Yoga mudra
Manduki mudra
Tadagi mudra.

4. Bandha (lock mudras)

These practices combine mudra and bandha. They charge the system with prana and prepare it for kundalini awakening. Techniques included in this category are:
Maha mudra
Maha bheda mudra
Maha vedha mudra.

5. Adhara (perineal mudras)

These techniques redirect prana from the lower centres to the brain. Mudras concerned with sublimating sexual energy are in this group. Techniques included in this category are:
Ashwini mudra
Vajroli/sahajoli mudra.

Between them these five groups engage substantial areas of the cerebral cortex. The comparatively large number of head and hand mudras reflects the fact that the operation and interpretation of information coming in from these two areas occupies approximately fifty percent of the cortex.

Mudras are performed either in combination with or after asana and pranayama. The mudras presented in this book represent a small selection of those discussed in the yogic texts.

424

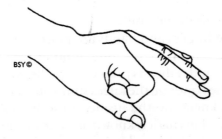

Jnana Mudra (psychic gesture of knowledge)

Assume a comfortable meditation posture.

Fold the index fingers so that they touch the inside root of the thumbs. Straighten the other three fingers of each hand so that they are relaxed and slightly apart.

Place the hands on the knees with the palms facing down. Relax the hands and arms.

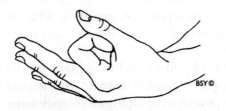

Chin Mudra (psychic gesture of consciousness)

Chin mudra is performed in the same way as jnana mudra, except that the palms of both hands face upwards, with the backs of the hands resting on the knees.

Relax the hands and arms.

Sequence: One of these two mudras should be adopted whenever practising meditation, unless otherwise specified.

Benefits: Jnana mudra and chin mudra are simple but important psycho-neural finger locks which make meditation asanas more powerful. The palms and fingers of the hands

425

have many nerve root endings which constantly emit energy. When the index finger touches the thumb, a circuit is produced which allows the energy that would normally dissipate into the environment to travel back through the body and up to the brain.

When the fingers and hands are placed on the knees, the knees are sensitized, creating another pranic circuit that maintains and redirects prana within the body. In addition, placing the hands on the knees stimulates a nadi which runs from the knees, up the inside of the thighs and into the perineum. This nadi is known as *gupta* or the hidden nadi. Sensitizing this channel helps to stimulate the energies at mooladhara chakra.

When the palms face upward in chin mudra, the chest area is opened up. The practitioner may experience this as a sense of lightness and receptivity, which is absent in the practice of jnana mudra.

Variation: Jnana and chin mudras are often performed with the tip of the thumb and index finger touching and forming a circle. Beginners may find this variation less secure for prolonged periods of meditation, as the thumb and index finger tend to separate more easily when body awareness is lost. Otherwise, this variation is as effective as the basic position.

Practice note: The effect of chin or jnana mudras is very subtle and it requires great sensitivity on the part of the practitioner to perceive the change in consciousness established. With practice, however, the mind becomes conditioned to the mudra and when it is adopted, the signal to enter a meditative state is transmitted.

Note: *The word* jnana *means 'wisdom' or 'knowledge', and thus* jnana mudra *is the gesture of intuitive knowledge.* Chin, *on the other hand, is derived from the word* chit *or* chitta, *which means 'consciousness'.* Chin mudra, *therefore, is the psychic gesture of consciousness.*

Symbolically, the small, ring and middle fingers represent the three gunas *or qualities of nature:* tamas, *stability;* rajas, *activity*

426

and creativity; and sattwa, *luminosity and harmony. In order for consciousness to pass from ignorance to knowledge, these three states must be transcended. The index finger represents individual consciousness, the* jivatma, *while the thumb symbolizes supreme consciousness. In jnana and chin mudras the individual (index finger) is bowing down to the supreme consciousness (the thumb), acknowledging its unsurpassed power. The index finger, however, is touching the thumb, symbolizing the ultimate unity of the two experiences and the culmination of yoga.*

YONI MUDRA

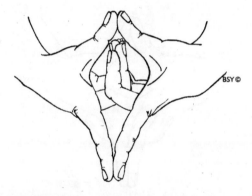

Yoni Mudra (attitude of the womb or source)
Assume a comfortable meditation posture with the head and spine straight.
Place the palms of the hands together with the fingers and thumbs straight and pointing away from the body.
Keeping the pads of the index fingers together, turn the little, ring and middle fingers inwards so that the backs of the fingers are touching.
Interlock the little, ring and middle fingers.
Bring the thumbs towards the body and join the pads of the fingers together to form the base of a yoni or womb shape.

427

Benefits: The interlocking of the fingers in this practice creates a complete cross-connection of energies from the right hand into the left and vice versa. As well as balancing the energies in the body, it helps to balance the activities of the right and left hemispheres of the brain. Placing the tips of the index fingers and thumbs together further intensifies the flow of prana.

This mudra makes the body and mind more stable in meditation and develops greater concentration, awareness and internal physical relaxation.

It redirects prana back into the body which would otherwise be dispersed through the hands and fingers. The elbows naturally tend to point to the side when performing this mudra which helps open up the chest area.

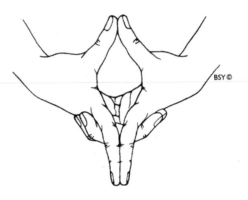

Variation: Yoni mudra may also be performed by interlocking the middle, ring and little fingers without turning them inward. The thumbs may be crossed in front of the outstretched index fingers, or outstretched with the pads touching towards the body.

Note: *The word* yoni *means 'womb' or 'source'. Yoni mudra invokes the primal energy inherent in the womb or source of creation.*

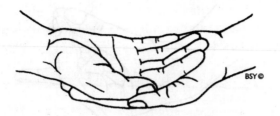

Bhairava Mudra (fierce or terrifying attitude)
Assume a comfortable meditation posture with the head
and spine straight.
Place the right hand on top of the left, so that the palms of
both hands are facing upward. Both hands rest in the lap.
Close the eyes and relax the whole body, keeping it
motionless.
Variation: When the left hand is placed on top of the right, the
practice is called Bhairavi mudra. Bhairavi is the female
counterpart of Bhairava.

Note: *The two hands represent ida and pingala nadis, and the union
of the individual with the supreme consciousness.*
*Bhairava mudra is used in prana mudra. It may also be used
during pranayama and meditation practice.*

HRIDAYA MUDRA

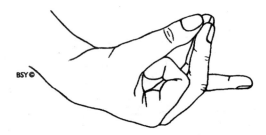

Hridaya Mudra (heart gesture)

Sit in any comfortable meditation asana with the head and spine straight.

Place the tips of the index fingers at the root of the thumbs, as in chin and jnana mudras, and join the tips of the middle and ring fingers to the tips of the thumbs. The little finger remains straight.

Place the hands on the knees with the palms facing upward. Close the eyes and relax the whole body, keeping it motionless.

Duration: This practice may be performed for up to 30 minutes.

Awareness: Physical – on the breath in the chest area.

Spiritual – on anahata chakra.

Benefits: This mudra diverts the flow of prana from the hands to the heart area, improving the vitality of the heart. The middle and ring fingers relate directly to nadis connected with the heart, while the thumb closes the pranic circuit and acts as an energizer, diverting the flow of prana from the hands to these nadis. Hridaya mudra is therefore beneficial for the heart. It is very simple and may be used safely and easily, even in acute situations. The heart is the centre of emotion. Hridaya mudra helps to release pent-up emotion and unburden the heart. It may be practised during emotional conflict and crisis.

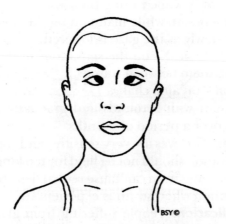

Shambhavi Mudra (eyebrow centre gazing)

Sit in any comfortable meditation asana.

Keep the head and spine upright and straight, and place the hands on the knees in either chin or jnana mudra.

Close the eyes and relax the whole body.

Relax all the muscles of the face, including the forehead, the eyes and behind the eyes.

Slowly open the eyes and look ahead at a fixed point, keeping the head and the whole body absolutely still.

Next, look upward and inward, focusing the eyes at the eyebrow centre.

The head should not move.

When performed correctly, the curve of the eyebrows will form a V-shaped image. The apex of the V is located at the eyebrow centre.

If the V-formation is not seen, the gaze is not directed upward and inward correctly.

Release the gaze at the slightest sensation of strain.

Hold the gaze for only a few seconds at first.

Close the eyes and relax them.

Suspend the thought processes and meditate on the stillness in the dark space in front of the closed eyes.

431

Breathing: After mastering the eye movement, coordinate it with the breath.

Inhale slowly while raising the gaze.

Hold the breath while maintaining the upward gaze.

Exhale slowly as the gaze is lowered.

Awareness: Physical – on the sensations in the eyes, and on relaxing them between rounds.

Spiritual – on ajna chakra.

Duration: Start with 5 rounds and gradually increase to 10 rounds over a period of months.

Precautions: The eyes are very sensitive and consequently the final position should not be held for too long. If the nerves are weak, any strain can cause retinal detachment. Release the position when strain is experienced.

Contra-indications: People suffering from glaucoma should not practise this mudra. Those with diabetic retinopathy or those who have just had cataract surgery, lens implant or other eye operations, should not perform shambhavi without the guidance of a competent teacher.

Benefits: Physically, shambhavi mudra strengthens the eye muscles and releases accumulated tension in this area. Mentally, it calms the mind, removing emotional stress and anger. It develops concentration, mental stability and the state of thoughtlessness.

Advanced practice: (internal shambhavi mudra)

Once shambhavi mudra has been mastered with the eyes open, it may be performed with the eyes closed. This is a more powerful practice because the awareness is more internalized. Be careful not to lose awareness of the eyebrow centre during the practice. Always ensure that the inner gaze is directed upward, although the eyes are closed.

Practice note: Shambhavi mudra is a powerful technique for awakening ajna chakra and is a meditation practice in its own right. It may produce profound experiences and should only be performed under the guidance of a competent teacher. Shambhavi mudra is also incorporated in asanas such as simhasana, the lion pose.

Note: *Shambhavi mudra is a means of attaining higher awareness and inducing higher consciousness within the practitioner. The practice is also known as* bhrumadhya drishti; bhru *means 'eyebrow centre' and* drishti *means 'gazing', hence this is the practice of eyebrow centre gazing.*

NASIKAGRA DRISHTI

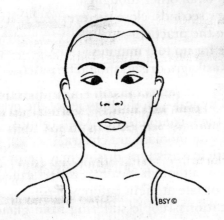

Technique 1: Preparatory practice

It may be difficult at first to focus the eyes on the nosetip. To overcome this, hold the index finger up at arm's length from the eyes and focus the gaze upon it.

Slowly bring the finger towards the nose, keeping the gaze steadily fixed upon it.

When the finger touches the tip of the nose, the eyes should still be focused on the finger.

Transfer the focus of the eyes to the nosetip.

Eventually this method becomes superfluous and the eyes readily fix on the nosetip at will.

Technique 2: Nasikagra Drishti (nosetip gazing)

Sit in any comfortable meditation posture with the head and spine straight.

Rest the hands on the knees in chin or jnana mudra.
Close the eyes and relax the whole body.
Open the eyes and focus them on the nosetip.
Do not strain the eyes in any way.
When the eyes are correctly focused a refraction of light, forming a V is seen just above the nosetip.
Concentrate on the apex of the V.
Become completely absorbed in the practice to the exclusion of all other thoughts.
After a few seconds, close the eyes and relax them before repeating the practice.
Continue for up to 5 minutes.

Breathing: Nasikagra drishti should be practised with normal breathing.

Awareness: Physical – on the muscles of the eyes, and on relaxing them completely between rounds.
Spiritual – on mooladhara chakra.

Time of practice: Nasikagra drishti may be practised at any time of day, although ideally it is performed early in the morning or late at night before sleep.

Contra-indications: People suffering from glaucoma should not practice this mudra. Those with diabetic retinopathy or who have just had cataract surgery, lens implant or other eye operations, should not perform nasikagra drishti without the guidance of a competent teacher.
Those suffering from depression should avoid this practice.

Benefits: Nasikagra drishti is an excellent technique for calming anger and disturbed states of mind. Although the eyes are open, the aim of this practice is to create introspection. The open eyes should not be aware of the outside world. Focusing them on the nosetip concentrates the mind.
This mudra develops the powers of concentration and induces meditative states. It takes the practitioner into the psychic and spiritual planes of consciousness.

Note: *The word* nasika *means 'nose',* agra *means 'tip' and* drishti *means 'gazing'. Another name for this practice is* agochari mudra, *which comes from the Sanskrit word* agocharam, *meaning 'beyond* *sensory perception', 'unknown' or 'invisible'. This mudra, therefore, enables the practitioner to transcend normal awareness.*

Symbolically, in nasikagra drishti the bridge of the nose is related to the spinal cord. At the top is the eyebrow centre, ajna chakra, while at the bottom is the nosetip, mooladhara chakra. Just as shambhavi mudra aims to activate ajna chakra by gazing at the eyebrow centre, nasikagra drishti aims to activate mooladhara chakra by gazing at the nosetip.

KHECHARI MUDRA

Khechari Mudra (tongue lock)

Sit in any comfortable meditation pose, preferably padmasana or siddha/siddha yoni asana, with the head and spine straight and the hands in chin or jnana mudra.

Relax the whole body and close the eyes.

Fold the tongue upward and backward, so that the lower surface lies in contact with the upper palate.

Stretch the tip of the tongue backward as far as is comfortable. Do not strain.

Perform ujjayi pranayama.

Breathe slowly and deeply.

Hold the tongue lock for as long as possible without straining.

At first there may be some discomfort and ujjayi pranayama may irritate the throat, but with practice it will become more comfortable.

When the tongue becomes tired, release and relax it, then repeat the practice.

Breathing: Gradually reduce the respiration rate over a period of months until the number of breaths per minute is 5 or 6. This may be reduced further under the guidance of a competent teacher.

Duration: Practise for 5 to 10 minutes. Khechari mudra may also be performed with other yoga practices.

Awareness: Physical—on the stretch of the tongue and the light pressure against the upper palate.

Spiritual—at vishuddhi chakra.

Precaution: Discontinue this mudra if a bitter secretion is tasted. Such a secretion is a sign of toxins in the system.

Contra-indications: Tongue ulcers and other common mouth ailments will temporarily preclude performance of this practice.

Benefits: Khechari mudra stimulates a number of pressure points located in the back of the mouth and the nasal cavity. These points influence the whole body. A number of glands are also massaged, stimulating the secretion of certain hormones and of saliva. This practice reduces the sensations of hunger and thirst, and induces a state of inner calm and stillness. It preserves the vitality of the body and is especially beneficial for inner healing.

Ultimately, this mudra has the potential to stimulate prana and awaken kundalini shakti.

Practice note: The advanced hatha yoga form of this practice involves the careful severing of the frenum beneath the tongue so that it can move right into the nasal cavity and stimulate important psychic centres situated there. This form of khechari mudra is not recommended here, as the effects make it unsuitable for interaction with the outside world.

Note: *The word khechari comes from two Sanskrit roots:* khe, *meaning 'sky', and* charya, *meaning 'one who moves'. Khechari mudra is associated with* amrita, *the nectar or elixir of life which is secreted from* bindu, *a point situated at the posterior fontanel, and then collected at vishuddhi chakra. Perfection of this practice enables the yogi to trap the descending drops of amrita at vishuddhi, overcoming hunger and thirst, and rejuvenating the entire body.*

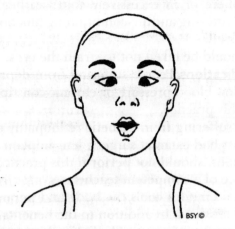

Kaki Mudra (the crow's beak)

Sit in any comfortable meditation asana with the head and spine straight and the hands resting on the knees in either chin or jnana mudra.

Close the eyes and relax the whole body for a few minutes.

Open the eyes and perform nasikagra drishti by focusing both eyes on the nosetip.

Try not to blink the eyes throughout this practice.

Purse the lips, forming a beak through which air may be inhaled.

The tongue should be relaxed.

Inhale slowly and deeply through the pursed lips.

At the end of inhalation close the lips and exhale slowly through the nose.

Repeat the process for 3 to 5 minutes.

Awareness: On the flow and sound of the breath, and on the nosetip.

Sequence: This mudra is a cooling practice. It balances the temperature of the body when performed after heating pranayamas.

Time of practice: It may be performed at any time of day, although it is best performed early in the morning or late at night. It should not be performed in cold weather.

Precautions: Kaki mudra should not be practised in a polluted atmosphere or in excessively cold weather because the normal filtering and air-conditioning function of the nose is bypassed.

Care should be taken not to strain the eyes.

Contra-indications: People suffering from depression, glaucoma, low blood pressure or chronic constipation should avoid this practice.

People suffering from diabetic retinopathy or those who have just had cataract surgery, lens implant or other eye operations, should not perform this practice without the guidance of a competent teacher.

Benefits: Kaki mudra cools the body and mind and soothes mental tensions. In addition to the benefits of nasikagra drishti, the act of pursing the lips in this practice, together with the contact of the indrawn air with the membranes of the mouth, stimulates digestive secretions, aiding the digestive process generally.

Practice note: Practitioners should be thoroughly familiar with nasikagra drishti prior to commencing this technique. The eyes must be kept open throughout the practice and nasikagra drishti should be continuous. If the eyes become tired, relax them for as long as necessary before recommencing the practice.

Note: *The word* kaki *means 'crow'. Kaki mudra is so called because during inhalation the mouth is shaped like a crow's beak. It is claimed that regular practice of this mudra leads to the disease-free, long life that is associated with the crow.*

This mudra is also considered to be a pranayama practice because of its close similarity to sheetali and sheetkari pranayamas.

Bhujangini Mudra (cobra respiration)
Sit in any comfortable meditation asana.
Close the eyes and relax the whole body, especially the abdomen.
Push the chin forward and a little upward.
Suck in air through the mouth and draw it into the stomach, not the lungs, in a series of gulps as though drinking water.
Expand the stomach as much as possible.
Hold the air inside for as long as comfortable, then expel the air by belching.

Duration: For general purposes, 3 to 5 rounds is sufficient. For specific ailments, further rounds may be performed.

Sequence: This mudra may be practised at any time, but is particularly beneficial after the technique of shankha-prakshalana.

Benefits: Bhujangini mudra tones the whole stomach, removes stagnant wind and helps alleviate abdominal disorders. Retaining air in the stomach enables the practitioner to float in water for any length of time.

Practice note: This practice is similar to the shatkarma, vatsara dhauti, and can be used as a cleansing practice. However, in vatsara dhauti the air is expelled from the anus rather than by belching.

439

BHOOCHARI MUDRA

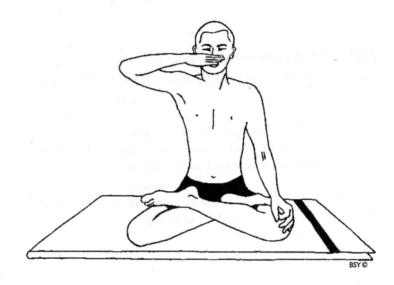

Bhoochari Mudra (gazing into nothingness)

Sit in any comfortable meditation asana with the head and spine straight and the hands in chin or jnana mudra.

Close the eyes and relax the whole body.

Open the eyes and raise the right hand in front of the face. The elbow should point to the side of the body.

Hold the hand horizontally, palm down, with the fingers together.

The side of the thumb should be in contact with the top of the upper lip.

Focus the eyes on the tip of the little finger and gaze at it intently for a minute or so, without blinking or flickering the eyes.

Try to maintain continuous awareness of the little fingertip. After a minute or so lower the hand. Continue to gaze into the place where the little finger was, without blinking.

Become fully engrossed in this point of nothingness.

Simultaneously, be aware of any thought processes.

When the focus dissipates, raise the hand and again concentrate on the tip of the little finger. After some time lower the hand and continue to gaze intently into the space, the nothingness.

Be aware of space only; there should be no registration of outer events in the field of conscious perception.

Continue the practice for 5 to 10 minutes.

Awareness: Physical – on the sensation of complete relaxation and stillness.

Spiritual – on ajna chakra.

Contra-indications: People suffering from glaucoma, diabetic retinopathy or those who have just had cataract surgery, lens implant or other eye operations should not perform bhoochari mudra without the guidance of a competent teacher.

Benefits: Bhoochari mudra develops the power of concentration and memory. It tranquillizes and introverts the mind and is particularly beneficial for calming anger and stress. It develops mental stability and the state of thoughtlessness. It helps to awaken ajna chakra and induce meditative states. It takes the practitioner into the psychic and spiritual planes of consciousness.

Practice note: Bhoochari mudra should be practised in a meditative asana. It is best performed facing a blank wall or an open space, such as the sky or a body of still water. This ensures that there are no visual obstructions to distract the attention.

Note: *Bhoochari mudra may be performed as a preparation for meditation and as a meditation technique in its own right. It belongs to a group of techniques featuring gazing at an external focal point as a means to achieve* dharana *or the meditative state of relaxed concentration. It is allied to nasikagra drishti and shambhavi mudras, all three being forms of trataka.*

AKASHI MUDRA

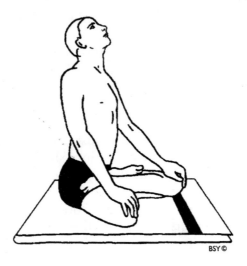

BSY©

Akashi Mudra (awareness of inner space)

Sit in any comfortable meditation asana.

Close the eyes and relax the whole body for a few minutes.

Fold the tongue back against the palate in khechari mudra.

Practise ujjayi pranayama and shambhavi mudra.

Bend the head backward about 45 degrees.

Straighten the arms and lock the elbows, pressing the knees with the hands.

Breathe slowly and deeply in ujjayi.

Continue for as long as feels comfortable.

End the practice by bending the elbows and releasing khechari and shambhavi mudras.

Raise the head to the upright position.

Resume normal breathing and be aware of the inner space.

Duration: Begin with one round and gradually increase to 5. Maintain the final position for as long as is comfortable, increasing the length of time in the mudra very slowly.

Awareness: On ajna chakra.

Precaution: As soon as faintness is felt, stop the practice. This technique must be practised slowly under the guidance of a competent teacher.

Contra-indications: People suffering from high blood pressure, vertigo, brain disorders or epilepsy should not practise this mudra.

Benefits: This practice combines the benefits of kumbhaka, ujjayi, shambhavi and khechari. It induces calmness and tranquillity, and develops control over the senses. When perfected, it arrests the thought processes and induces higher states of consciousness.

Variation: Akashi mudra may also be practised with breath retention. Perform the practice as described above. Inhale while bending the head backwards. Hold the breath inside in the final position. Exhale while slowly raising the head to the starting position.

Practice note: It is recommended that the practitioner be completely familiar with the practices of ujjayi, khechari and shambhavi before commencing akashi mudra. At first ujjayi pranayama may irritate the throat when performed with the head back. However, with practice, it will become more comfortable.

Note: *Akashi mudra belongs to the group of techniques featuring gazing at an external focal point as a means to achieving* dharana *or the meditative state of relaxed concentration.*

SHANMUKHI MUDRA

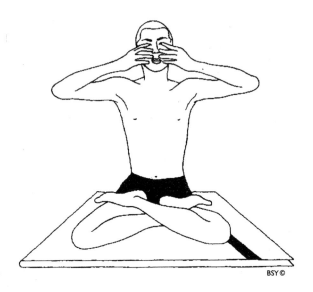

BSY©

Shanmukhi Mudra (closing the seven gates)
    If possible sit in siddha/siddha yoni asana or padmasana.
Otherwise take a comfortable meditation asana and place
a small cushion beneath the perineum to provide pressure
in this area.
    Hold the head and spine straight.
    Close the eyes and place the hands on the knees.
    Relax the whole body.
    Raise the arms in front of the face with the elbows pointing
sideways.
    Close the ears with the thumbs, the eyes with the index
fingers, the nostrils with the middle fingers, and the mouth
by placing the ring fingers above and little fingers below
the lips.
    Release the pressure of the middle fingers and open
the nostrils. Inhale slowly and deeply, using full yogic
breathing.
    At the end of inhalation, close the nostrils with the middle
fingers.

Retain the breath inside for as long as is comfortable.
After some time, release the pressure of the middle fingers and slowly exhale.
This is one round.
Inhale again immediately to start another round.
To end the practice, lower the hands to the knees, keeping the eyes closed, and slowly externalize the mind, becoming aware of external sounds and the physical body.

Breathing: This technique gives greater benefits when the practitioner can retain the breath for extended periods.

Duration: Practise for 5 minutes to begin with. Gradually build the duration up over a period of months to 30 minutes.

Awareness: Physical – on synchronizing the hand mudra with the breath.

Spiritual – bindu, ajna or anahata chakra may be used for concentration. The important point is to introvert the senses.

Time of practice: Shanmukhi mudra is best practised early in the morning or late at night when there is maximum quiet. Practising at this time awakens psychic sensitivity.

Contra-indications: People suffering from depression should avoid this practice.

Benefits: Physically, the energy and heat from the hands and fingers stimulate and relax the nerves and muscles of the face. Mentally, it introverts the awareness. Spiritually, it induces the state of pratyahara or sense withdrawal.

Practice note: Shanmukhi mudra is a practice used in nada yoga to hear any internal manifestation of sound in the region of bindu chakra. There may be many sounds or none at all; just listen. Do not expect to hear subtle sounds immediately; practice is necessary. At first there may be no sound or a confused jumble of sounds. Upon hearing one distinct sound, focus the awareness totally upon it. This may take a few weeks of practice. As sensitivity develops, subtler sounds will be heard.

Shanmukhi mudra is also used to enhance visualization in other branches of yoga such as swara yoga, tattwa shuddhi and kriya yoga.

Note: *The word shanmukhi is comprised of two roots:* shat *means 'six' and* mukhi *means 'gates' or 'faces'. Shanmukhi mudra involves redirecting the awareness inside by closing the six doors of outer perception: the two eyes, the two ears, the nose and the mouth. This practice is also known as* baddha yoni asana, *the locked source pose;* devi mudra, *attitude of the great goddess;* parangmukhi mudra, *the gesture of inner focusing;* sambhava mudra, *the gesture of equipoise; and* yoni mudra, *attitude of the source.*

UNMANI MUDRA

Unmani Mudra (the attitude of mindlessness)

Sit in any comfortable meditation asana.

Open the eyes fully, but without straining.

Inhale slowly and deeply. Hold the breath inside. Focus the awareness at bindu in the back of the head for a few seconds.

Exhale slowly, allowing the awareness to descend with the breath from bindu through the chakras in the spine: ajna, vishuddhi, anahata, manipura, swadhisthana, mooladhara. The eyes should slowly close as the awareness descends. By the time the awareness reaches mooladhara, the eyes should be fully closed.

Even when the eyes are open, the awareness is looking within.

Do not try too hard, but allow the process to occur spontaneously.

Inhale deeply and begin the next round.

Continue for 5 to 10 minutes.

Contra-indications: Those who have just had eye operations, or who have glaucoma or diabetic retinopathy should not perform unmani without the guidance of a competent teacher.

Benefits: Unmani mudra calms stress and agitation, and induces a meditative state.

VIPAREETA KARANI MUDRA

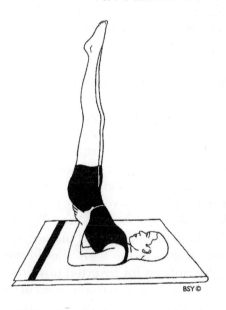

Vipareeta Karani Mudra (inverted psychic attitude)

Assume vipareeta karani asana.

Bring the legs over the head so that the eyes look straight up at the feet.

Close the eyes and relax the whole body.

This is the starting position.

Fix the awareness at manipura chakra in the spine, directly behind the navel.

Inhale slowly and deeply with ujjayi pranayama.

447

Simultaneously, feel the breath and consciousness moving from manipura to vishuddhi chakra.

While exhaling, maintain the awareness at vishuddhi.

At the end of exhalation, immediately bring the awareness back to manipura and repeat the same process.

Duration: Practise up to 7 rounds at first, or until discomfort arises. If pressure builds up in the head, end the practice. Gradually increase the number of rounds up to 21 over a period of months.

The length of the inhalation and exhalation will increase spontaneously over time, as the practice becomes more comfortable.

Awareness: Physical – on the inverted posture and the movement of the breath.

Spiritual – on manipura and vishuddhi chakras.

Sequence: At the end of the daily practice program and before meditation. Do not perform after vigorous exercise or for at least 3 hours after meals. Upon completion of the practice, it is advisable to do a counterpose such as matsyasana, bhujangasana or ushtrasana.

Time of practice: Vipareeta karani mudra should be practised daily at the same time, preferably in the early morning.

Contra-indications: This inverted practice should not be performed unless the body is healthy. People suffering from high blood pressure, heart disease, enlarged thyroid or excessive toxins in the body should not perform this practice. Precautions for inverted postures apply.

Benefits: This practice gives all the benefits of vipareeta karani asana. It balances the activities of the thyroid.

The posture reverses the downward and outward movement of energy, revitalizing and expanding the awareness. The flow of prana in ida and pingala nadis is balanced, resulting in an equal flow of breath in the nostrils. The balancing effect also helps to prevent disease on the physical and mental planes.

Practice note: The metabolic rate may increase when this mudra is practised for extended periods. If this happens, the food intake should be adjusted accordingly.

Note: *The Sanskrit word* vipareeta *means 'inverted' and* karani *means 'one who does'. Vipareeta karani mudra provides the basis for the kriya of the same name.*

PASHINEE MUDRA

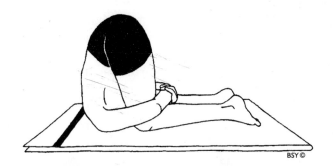

Pashinee Mudra (folded psychic attitude)
   Assume halasana. Separate the feet by about half a metre.
   Bend the knees and bring the thighs towards the chest
   until the knees touch the ears, shoulders and floor.
   Wrap the arms tightly around the back of the legs.
   Relax the whole body in this position and close the eyes.
   Breathe slowly and deeply.
   Maintain the position for as long as is comfortable.
   Slowly release the arms and come back into halasana.
   Lower the legs and relax in shavasana.
Awareness: Physical–on the stretch of the neck.
   Spiritual–on mooladhara or vishuddhi chakra.
Sequence: This mudra should be followed by a backward
   bending asana.
Contra-indications: As for sarvangasana and halasana. People
   suffering from any spinal condition should avoid this
   practice. Precautions for inverted postures apply
Benefits: Pashinee mudra brings balance and tranquillity
   to the nervous system and induces pratyahara, sensory

449

withdrawal. It stretches the spine and back muscles, and stimulates all the spinal nerves. It massages the abdominal organs.

Note: *The word* pash *means 'noose'.* Pashinee, *therefore, means 'bound in a noose'.*

TADAGI MUDRA

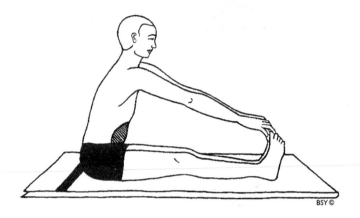

Tadagi Mudra (barrelled abdomen technique)
Sit with the legs stretched out in front of the body and the feet slightly apart. The legs should remain straight throughout the practice. Place the hands on the knees, keeping the head and spine straight.

Close the eyes and relax the whole body, especially the abdominal area.

Lean forward and grasp the big toes with the thumbs, index and second fingers. Keep the head facing forward.

Inhale slowly and deeply, expanding the abdominal muscles to their fullest extent.

Retain the breath inside for a comfortable length of time without straining the lungs in any way.

Exhale slowly and deeply while relaxing the abdomen.

Maintain the hold on the the toes.

450

Repeat the breathing up to 10 times.
Then release the toes and return to the starting position.
This is one round.

Duration: Practise 3 to 5 rounds.

Awareness: Physical – on the abdomen.
Spiritual – on manipura chakra.

Contra-indications: Pregnant women and those suffering from hernia or prolapse should avoid this practice.

Benefits: Tadagi mudra relieves tension stored in the diaphragm and pelvic floor, tones the abdominal organs and stimulates blood circulation to these areas. The nerve plexuses in the visceral area are stimulated and toned.
Bending forward and extending the stomach stretches the diaphragm and pelvic floor, and creates pressure throughout the trunk of the body. This stimulates manipura chakra, the centre of energy distribution, and raises the level of prana generally.

Practice note: Release the hold on the toes between breaths if the position becomes uncomfortable.

Note: *The word* tadagi *literally means 'water pot', which resembles the shape of the extended abdomen.*

PRANA MUDRA

Prana Mudra (invocation of energy)
Sit in any comfortable meditation posture, preferably padmasana or siddha/siddha yoni asana with the hands in bhairava mudra.
Close the eyes and relax the whole body, especially the abdomen, arms and hands.

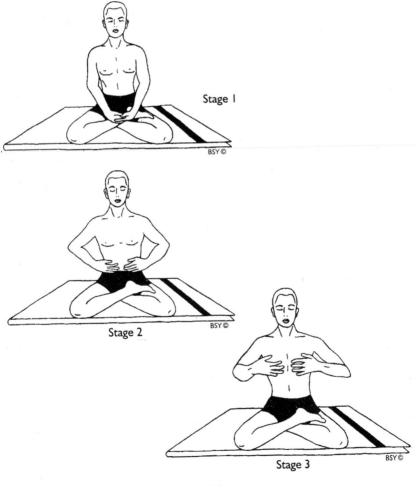

Stage 1

Stage 2

Stage 3

Stage I: Keeping the eyes closed, inhale and exhale as deeply as possible, contracting the abdominal muscles to expel the maximum amount of air from the lungs.

With the breath held outside, perform moola bandha while concentrating on mooladhara chakra in the perineum.

Retain the breath outside for as long as is comfortable.

Stage 2: Release moola bandha.

Inhale slowly and deeply, expanding the abdomen fully. Draw as much air into the lungs as possible.

Simultaneously, raise the hands until they are in front of the navel. The hands should be open with the palms facing the body, the fingers pointing towards each other, but not touching.

The upward movement of the hands should be coordinated with the abdominal inhalation.

The arms and hands should be relaxed.

While inhaling from the abdomen, feel the prana or vital energy being drawn from mooladhara chakra to manipura chakra.

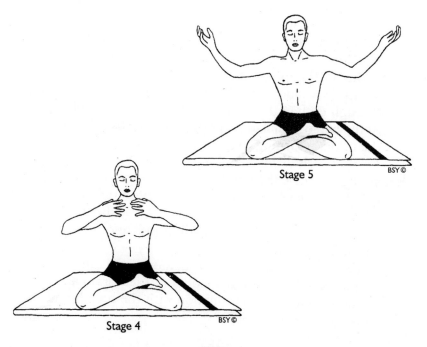

Stage 5

Stage 4

453

Stage 3: Continue the inhalation by expanding the chest and raising the hands until they are directly in front of the sternum at the centre of the chest.

Feel the pranic energy being drawn up from manipura to anahata chakra while inhaling.

Stage 4: Draw even more air into the lungs by slightly raising the shoulders and raise the hands to the front of the throat in coordination with the breath.

Feel the prana being drawn up to vishuddhi.

Stage 5: Retain the breath inside while spreading the arms out to the sides.

Feel the prana spreading in a wave through ajna, bindu and sahasrara chakras.

In the final position, the hands are level with the ears. The arms are outstretched but not straight, and the palms are turned upward.

Concentrate on sahasrara chakra and visualize an aura of pure light emanating from the head.

Feel that the whole being is radiating vibrations of peace to all beings.

Retain this position, with the breath held inside, for as long as possible without straining the lungs in any way.

While exhaling, repeat stages 4, 3, 2, 1, and slowly return to the starting position.

During exhalation, feel the prana progressively descending through each of the chakras until it reaches mooladhara.

At the end of exhalation, perform moola bandha and feel the prana returning to mooladhara chakra.

Relax the whole body and breathe normally.

Breathing: Increase the duration of inhalation, retention and exhalation slowly. Be careful not to strain the lungs.

When the practice has been perfected, visualize the breath as a stream of white light ascending and descending within sushumna nadi.

Awareness: The awareness should move in a smooth and continuous flow from mooladhara to sahasrara and back to mooladhara, in coordination with the breath and the movement of the hands.

Sequence: Prana mudra is best practised after asana and pranayama and before meditation, but it may be performed at any time.

Time of practice: Ideally, practise at sunrise while facing the sun.

Benefits: Prana mudra awakens the dormant prana shakti, vital energy, and distributes it throughout the body, increasing strength, health and confidence. It develops awareness of the nadis and chakras, and the subtle flow of prana in the body. It instils an inner attitude of peace and equanimity by adopting an external attitude of offering and receiving energy to and from the cosmic source.

Note: *This practice is also known as* shanti mudra, *the peace mudra.*

YOGA MUDRA

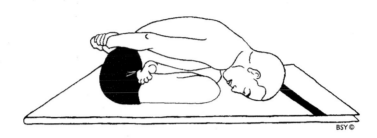

BSY ©

Yoga Mudra (attitude of psychic union)

Sit in padmasana.

Take hold of one wrist behind the back.

Close the eyes and relax the whole body.

Bring the awareness to mooladhara chakra (slight moola bandha may also be performed).

Inhale slowly and feel the breath gradually rising from mooladhara to ajna chakra. Retain the breath for a few seconds and concentrate on ajna chakra.

Exhale slowly while bending forward from the hips.

Synchronize the movement with the breath, so that the forehead just touches the floor in yogamudrasana as the air is fully expelled from the lungs.

Simultaneously, feel the breath gradually descending from ajna to mooladhara chakra.

Retain the breath outside for a few seconds while concentrating at mooladhara chakra.

Inhaling, raise the trunk to the vertical position. Be aware of the breath moving upward from mooladhara to ajna chakra.

All the movements should be performed in a harmonious, smooth and synchronized manner.

Remain in the upright position, holding the breath for a few seconds and concentrate on ajna chakra.

Exhale slowly, moving the awareness back down the spine to mooladhara chakra.

This is one round.

Immediately start another round, performing a light moola bandha with the breath held outside and the awareness at mooladhara chakra. Beginners may take a few normal breaths before starting the next round.

Perform 3 to 10 rounds.

Breathing: The respiration should be as slow as possible without the slightest strain.

Sequence: This practice may be followed by any backward bending asana such as bhujangasana or ushtrasana.

Awareness: Physical – on synchronizing the movement of the body with the breath.

Spiritual – on mooladhara and ajna chakras.

Contra-indications: People suffering from sciatica, high blood pressure, pelvic inflammatory disease or any other serious abdominal ailment should avoid this practice.

Benefits: The practice massages the abdominal organs and stretches the back, contributing to good general health. In addition, it is an excellent preparatory practice for meditation, engendering a sense of relaxation. It relieves anger and tension, inducing tranquillity. It develops awareness and control of psychic energy and is used to awaken manipura chakra.

Variations: The hands may also be placed:
a) on the heels of the feet, with the elbows pointing out to the sides,
b) palms down on the soles of the feet,
c) palm to palm with the fingers pointing upward in the middle of the back (this is *hamsa* or swan mudra).

Practice note: People with stiff backs and those unable to sit in padmasana comfortably may perform the practice from sukhasana or vajrasana. If adopting the latter, bend forward into shashankasana with the hands clasped behind the back. If vajrasana is still uncomfortable, the knees may be separated slightly, allowing the chest to come closer to the floor.

Note: *Yoga mudra is so called because it unites the individual consciousness with the supreme consciousness, or the outer nature with the inner nature.*

457

MANDUKI MUDRA

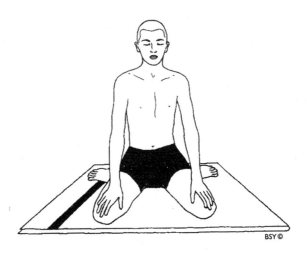

Manduki Mudra (gesture of the frog)

Sit in bhadrasana. If possible without straining, adjust so that the toes are pointing outward.

The buttocks should rest on the floor. A folded blanket may also be placed underneath the buttocks to apply firm pressure to the perineum, stimulating the region of mooladhara chakra.

Place the hands on the knees, holding the spine and head straight.

Close the eyes and relax the whole body.

This is manduki asana.

Open the eyes and perform nasikagra drishti.

When the eyes become tired, close them for a few seconds.

Continue the practice for 5 minutes, until the mind and senses become introverted.

Breathing: Breathing should be slow and rhythmic.

Awareness: Physical – on the nosetip.

Spiritual – on mooladhara chakra.

Contra-indications: People with glaucoma should not practise this much. Those with diabetic retinopathy or those who have just had cataract surgery, lens implant or other eye operations should not perform nasikagra drishti without

458

the guidance of a competent teacher. Manduki asana should not be practised unless the ankles, knees and hips are very flexible.

Benefits: Manduki asana is a counterpose for cross-legged meditative asanas. Manduki mudra activates mooladhara chakra. It calms the disturbances and fluctuations of the mind and balances ida and pingala nadis, leading directly to meditation.

Practice note: Manduki mudra is an advanced variation of nasikagra drishti. It should be performed in mild light so that the tip of the nose can be seen clearly.

Note: *The word* manduki *means 'frog'. This mudra is so named because the sitting posture resembles a frog at rest. This practice also gives the basis for the kriya of the same name.*

MAHA MUDRA

Base position: Utthanpadasana (stretched leg pose)
Sit with the legs outstretched.
Bend the left knee and press the left heel firmly into the perineum at the location point of mooladhara chakra. The right leg remains outstretched.
Place both hands on the right knee.
Adjust the position so that it is comfortable.
Bend forward just enough to be able to clasp the right big toe with both hands.
Hold the position for a comfortable duration.
Return to the upright position with both hands resting on the right knee.
Repeat on the other side, and then with both legs outstretched.
This is one round.
Practise 3 rounds.

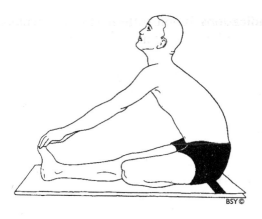

Maha Mudra (great psychic attitude)

Sit in utthanpadasana with the right leg outstretched.

Keep the back straight.

Relax the whole body.

Practise khechari mudra.

Take a deep breath in.

Exhale and bend forward. Clasp the right big toe with both hands.

Keep the head erect, and the back straight.

Slowly inhale, tilting the head slightly back.

Perform shambhavi mudra and then moola bandha.

Hold the breath inside and rotate the awareness from the eyebrow centre, to the throat, to the perineum. Mentally repeat, 'ajna, vishuddhi, mooladhara'. The concentration should remain at each chakra for only 1 or 2 seconds.

Release shambhavi and moola bandha.

Slowly exhale, returning to the upright position.

This is one round.

Breathing: One round is equivalent to 2 complete breaths. The length of the breath should be extended gradually.

Duration: Practise 3 rounds with the left leg folded, then with the right leg folded, and then with both legs outstretched.

Sequence: This practice should ideally be practised after asana and pranayama and before meditation.

Time of practice: In the early morning while the stomach is completely empty.

460

Contra-indications: People suffering from high blood pressure, heart complaints or glaucoma should not perform this practice. Those with diabetic retinopathy or who have just had cataract surgery, lens implant or other eye operations should not perform the practice without the guidance of a competent teacher.

Maha mudra should not be performed without prior purification of the body. Impurity is indicated by any symptoms of accumulated toxins, such as skin eruptions. The practise of maha mudra generates heat and should be avoided in hot summers.

Do not practise during menstruation or pregnancy.

Benefits: Maha mudra combines the benefits of shambhavi mudra, khechari mudra, moola bandha and kumbhaka.

It stimulates the energy circuit, linking mooladhara with ajna chakra. The whole system is charged with prana which intensifies awareness and induces spontaneous meditation. Energy blockages are removed.

Practice note: Before commencing maha mudra, the practitioner should be thoroughly proficient in the techniques of shambhavi mudra, khechari mudra, moola bandha and kumbhaka.

This practice should only be attempted under the guidance of a competent teacher.

MAHA BHEDA MUDRA

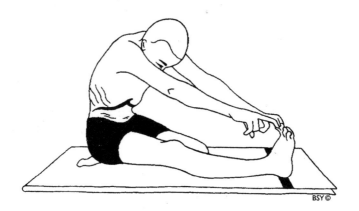

Maha Bheda Mudra (the great separating attitude)
Assume utthanpadasana as described for maha mudra.
Keep the back straight.
Relax the whole body.
Take a deep breath in.
While exhaling, lean forward and clasp the right big toe
with both hands.
Retain the breath outside and perform jalandhara,
uddiyana and moola bandhas.
Rotate the awareness successively from the throat, to the
abdomen, to the perineum, mentally repeating, 'vishuddhi,
manipura, mooladhara'. The awareness should rest on each
chakra for only one or two seconds and then move to the
next in a smooth flow.
Release moola bandha, uddiyana and jalandhara.
When the head is raised, inhale and return to the upright
postion.
Exhale and relax.
This is one round.
Breathing: One round is equivalent to two complete breaths.
The length of the breath should be extended gradually.
Duration: Practise 3 times with the left leg folded, then with the
right leg folded and then with both legs outstretched.

462

Sequence: After asana and pranayama and before meditation.

Time of practice: In the early morning while the stomach is completely empty.

Contra-indications: Precautions and contra-indications for kumbhaka, moola, uddiyana and jalandhara bandhas apply. People suffering from high blood pressure or heart complaints, cervical spondylosis, high intracranial pressure, vertigo, colitis, stomach or intestinal ulcer, diaphragmatic hernia or abdominal problems should not perform this practice.

It should not be performed without prior purification of the body. Maha bheda mudra generates a lot of heat and should be avoided in hot summers.

Do not practise during active menstruation or during pregnancy.

Benefits: Maha bheda mudra has a profound influence at a pranic level. It influences mooladhara, manipura and vishuddhi chakras, harnessing their energies to induce concentration of mind and meditation. Maha bheda supplements and follows maha mudra; together they supercharge the whole body-mind complex.

Practice note: Before commencing this practice, the practitioner should be familiar with the techniques of jalandhara, uddiyana and moola bandhas and bahir kumbhaka.

This practice should be attempted only under the guidance of a competent teacher.

MAHA VEDHA MUDRA

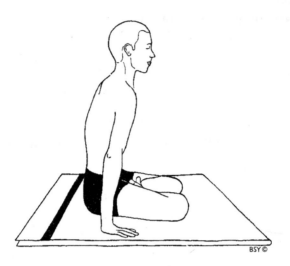

Maha Vedha Mudra (the great piercing attitude)

Sit in padmasana. Relax the body and close the eyes.

Place the palms of the hands on the floor beside the thighs with the fingers pointing forward or make fists with the knuckles facing down.

The arms should be straight but relaxed.

Inhale slowly and deeply.

Retain the breath inside.

Raise the body by placing all the weight on the hands and straightening the arms.

Gently beat the buttocks on the ground 3 times, keeping the awareness at the perineum. The buttocks and the back of the thighs should touch the ground simultaneously. The spine must be kept straight.

Gently rest the buttocks back on the floor. Exhale.

This is one round.

When the breathing returns to normal, repeat the process. Practise 3 rounds.

Breathing: Inhale deeply in the starting position.

Retain the breath inside while raising and lowering the buttocks.

464

Exhale only after the body has been finally lowered to the floor.

Awareness: Physical – on retaining the breath while lightly beating the buttocks.

Spiritual – on mooladhara chakra.

Sequence: After asana and before meditation.

Precautions: Beat the buttocks very gently. It is important to use a thick mat to avoid injury. Do not let the coccyx (tailbone) land directly on the floor. The backs of the legs and buttocks should hit the floor simultaneously. This cushions and distributes the impact over a wide area.

Contra-indications: People who have any inflammatory disease, infection or general complaints in or around the pelvic area should avoid this practice. Those with heart problems, high blood pressure, sciatica or weak or injured knees should not attempt this practice. Do not practise during active menstruation or pregnancy.

Benefits: This is a powerful practice for introverting the mind. It awakens psychic faculties and the kundalini which resides in mooladhara chakra.

Practice note: If padmasana has not been mastered this practice can be performed with the legs outstretched, although this method is less effective.

Note: *The Sanskrit word* maha *means 'great' and* vedha *means 'piercing'. The purpose of maha vedha mudra is to pierce mooladhara chakra and channel the kundalini energy upwards. This technique belongs to hatha yoga and is a preparatory technique for the kriya yoga practice of tadan kriya.*

ASHWINI MUDRA

Ashwini Mudra (horse gesture)
Technique 1: Rapid contraction
Sit in any comfortable meditation asana.
Close the eyes and relax the whole body.
Become aware of the natural breathing process.
Take the awareness to the anus.
Rapidly contract the anal sphincter muscles for a few seconds without straining, then relax them.
Confine the action to the anal area.
Contraction and relaxation should be performed 10 to 20 times, smoothly and rhythmically.
Gradually make the contractions more rapid.

Technique 2: Contraction with antar kumbhaka
Sit in any comfortable meditation asana.
Close the eyes and relax the whole body.
Inhale slowly and deeply while simultaneously contracting the anal sphincter muscles.
Practise antar kumbhaka (internal breath retention) while holding the contraction of the anal sphincter muscles as tightly as possible without strain.
Exhale while releasing the contraction of the anus.
Perform 5 to 10 rounds.
Awareness: Physical–on anal contraction and relaxation.
Spiritual–on mooladhara chakra.
Contra-indications: People with high blood pressure or heart disease should not practise with antar kumbhaka.
Benefits: This practice strengthens the anal muscles. It prevents the escape of pranic energy and redirects it upward for spiritual purposes.

Note: Ashwini *means 'horse'. The practice resembles the movement a horse makes with its sphincter immediately after evacuation of the bowels.*

Vajroli Mudra (for men) and Sahajoli Mudra (for women) (thunderbolt/spontaneous psychic attitude)

Sit in siddha/siddha yoni asana, or any comfortable meditation posture with the head and spine straight.

Place the hands on the knees in chin or jnana mudra.

Close the eyes and relax the whole body.

Take the awareness to the urethra.

Inhale, hold the breath inside and draw the urethra upward. This action is similar to holding back an intense urge to urinate. The testes in men and the labia in women should move slightly upward during this contraction.

Confine the contraction to the urethra.

Hold the contraction for as long as comfortable, starting with a few seconds, and gradually increasing.

Exhale, releasing the contraction, and relax.

Duration: Begin with 3 contractions Slowly increase to 10.

Awareness: Physical – on isolating the point of contraction, avoiding generalized contraction of the pelvic floor.
Spiritual – on swadhisthana chakra.

Contra-indications: Vajroli and sahajoli mudras should not be practised by people suffering from urethritis as the irritation and pain may increase.

Benefits: Vajroli and sahajoli mudras regulate and tones the entire uro-genital system. It helps overcome psycho-sexual conflicts and unwanted sexual thoughts. It conserves and redirects energy, enhancing meditative states.

Note: *The word vajroli is derived from the Sanskrit root* vajra, *which means 'thunderbolt', 'lightning' or 'mighty one'. Vajra is also the name of the nadi which conducts sexual energy. Sahajoli is from the root* sahaj, *meaning 'spontaneous'. Vajroli is therefore the force which moves upward with the power of lightning, and sahajoli is the psychic attitude of spontaneous arousing.*

Bandha

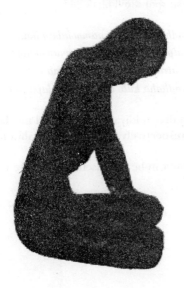

जालन्धरोड्याणनमूलबन्धा-
ज्ज्वलपन्ति कण्ठोदरपायुमूलान् ।
बन्धत्रयेऽस्मिन्परिचीयमाने
बन्ध: कुतो दारुणकालपाशात् ॥ 5 ॥

Jaalandharoddyaananamoolabandhaa
njalpanti kanthodarapaayumoolaan.
Bandhatrayesminparicheeyamaane
bandhaha kuto daarunakaalapaashaat.

Jalandhara bandha, uddiyana bandha and moola bandha
are situated respectively in the throat, abdomen and
perineum.
If their duration can be increased, then where is the fear
of death?

Yogataravali (Sri Adi Shankaracharya)

Introduction to Bandha

Traditionally, bandhas were classified as part of mudras, and were handed down by word of mouth from guru to disciple. The *Hatha Yoga Pradipika* deals with bandhas and mudras together and the ancient tantric texts also make no distinction between the two. Bandhas are extensively incorporated in mudra as well as pranayama techniques. Their locking action, however, reveals them as a fundamentally important group of practices in their own right.

The Sanskrit word *bandha* means to 'hold', 'tighten' or 'lock'. These definitions precisely describe the physical action involved in the bandha practices and their effect on the pranic body. The bandhas aim to lock the pranas in particular areas and redirect their flow into sushumna nadi for the purpose of spiritual awakening.

Bandhas should first be practised and mastered individually. Only then can they be beneficially incorporated with mudra and pranayama practices. When combined in this way, they awaken the psychic faculties and form an adjunct to higher yogic practices. However, it is important to observe the contra-indications.

Bandhas and the granthis

There are four bandhas: *jalandhara*, *moola*, *uddiyana* and *maha*. The last of these is a combination of the first three. These three bandhas act directly on the three *granthis* or psychic knots. Moola bandha is associated with *brahma granthi*, uddiyana

471

bandha with *vishnu granthi* and jalandhara bandha with *rudra granthi*. The granthis prevent the free flow of prana along sushumna nadi and thus impede the awakening of the chakras and the rising of kundalini.

Brahma granthi is the first knot and it is associated with mooladhara and swadhisthana chakras. It is linked with the survival instinct, the urge to procreate and with deep, instinctive knowledge, awareness and desire. When brahma granthi is transcended, the *kundalini* or primal energy is able to rise beyond mooladhara and swadhisthana without being pulled back down by the attractions and instinctual patterns of the personality.

The second knot is vishnu granthi, associated with manipura and anahata chakras. These two chakras deal with the sustenance of the physical, emotional and mental aspects of human existence. Manipura sustains *pranamaya kosha*, the energy body, governing the digestion and metabolism of food. Anahata sustains *manomaya kosha*, the mental body, and they both affect *annamaya kosha*, the physical body. Once vishnu granthi is transcended, one is no longer bound by physical, mental and emotional attachments. Relationships and energy become more univeral, rather than being limited by personal preferences or aversions.

The final knot is rudra granthi, which is associated with vishuddhi and ajna chakras. Vishuddhi and ajna sustain *vijnanamaya kosha*, the intuitive or higher mental body, and represent the transformation of an existing form, idea or concept into its universal aspect. When rudra granthi is pierced, individuality is dropped. The old ego identification is left behind and the experience of unmanifest consciousness, beyond the phenomenal universe, emerges at ajna and sahasrara chakras.

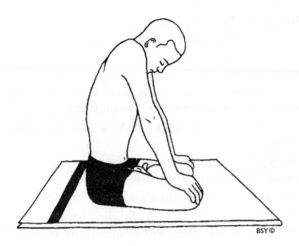

BSY©

Jalandhara Bandha (throat lock)

Sit in padmasana or siddha/siddha yoni asana with the head and spine straight. The knees should be in firm contact with the floor.

Place the palms of the hands on the knees.

Close the eyes and relax the whole body.

Inhale slowly and deeply, and retain the breath inside.

While retaining the breath, bend the head forward and press the chin tightly against the chest.

Straighten the arms and lock them firmly into position, pressing the knees down with the hands.

Simultaneously, hunch the shoulders upward and forward. This will ensure that the arms stay locked, thus intensifying the pressure applied to the neck.

Stay in the final position for a few seconds to begin with. Do not strain.

Relax the shoulders, bend the arms and slowly release the lock. Raise the head and then exhale.

Repeat when the respiration has returned to normal.

Variation: In kriya yoga a more simple and subtle form of jalandhara bandha is practised where the head is simply

473

bent forward so that the chin presses the neck. This variation is commonly used in association with pranayama practices.

Breathing: The practice is performed during internal retention. It may also be performed with external breath retention.

Duration: Jalandhara bandha can be held for as long as the practitioner is able to comfortably retain the breath. Maintain a count while retaining the breath and gradually increase the count. This practice may be repeated up to 5 times.

Awareness: Physical – on the throat pit and sensations connected with breath retention.

Spiritual – on vishuddhi chakra.

Sequence: This bandha is ideally performed in conjunction with mudras, bandhas and pranayamas. If practised on its own, it should be performed after asanas and pranayamas and before meditation.

Contra-indications: People suffering from cervical spondylosis, high intracranial pressure, vertigo, high blood pressure or heart disease should not practise jalandhara bandha. Although the neck lock reduces blood pressure, long retention of the breath strains the heart.

Jalandhara is the first bandha to be taught as the effects are light and soothing. Refrain from the practice if any vertigo or dizziness arises.

Benefits: The full form of jalandhara bandha compresses the carotid sinuses, which are located on the carotid arteries, the main arteries in the neck. The simple variation exerts a subtler pressure. These sinuses help to regulate the circulatory and respiratory systems. Normally, a decrease in oxygen and increase in carbon dioxide in the body leads to an increased heart rate and heavier breathing. This process is initiated by the carotid sinuses. By exerting pressure on these sinuses, this tendency is prevented, allowing for decreased heart rate and increased breath retention. This practice produces mental relaxation, relieving stress, anxiety and anger. It develops meditative introversion and òne-pointedness. The stimulus on the throat helps to balance thyroid function and regulate the metabolism.

Practice note: Do not exhale or inhale until the chin lock and arm lock have been released and the head is fully upright. If suffocation is felt, end the practice and rest. Once the sensation has passed, resume the practice.

Note: *The Sanskrit word* jalan *means 'net' and* dhara *means 'stream' or 'flow'. One interpretation of jalandhara bandha is the lock which controls the network of nadis in the neck. The physical manifestation of these nadis is the blood vessels and nerves of the neck.*

An alternative definition is that jal *means 'water'. Jalandhara bandha is therefore the throat lock which holds the nectar or fluid flowing down to vishuddhi from bindu, and prevents it from falling into the digestive fire. In this way, prana is conserved.*

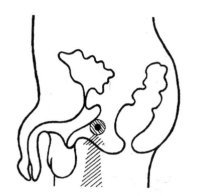 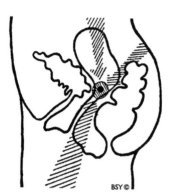

Technique 1: Moola Bandha (perineum contraction)

Stage 1: Sit in a comfortable meditative asana, preferably siddha/siddha yoni asana, so that pressure is applied to the perineal/vaginal region.

Close the eyes and relax the whole body.

Be aware of the natural breath.

Focus the awareness on the perineal/vaginal region.

Contract this region by pulling up on the muscles of the pelvic floor and then relaxing them.

Continue to briefly contract and relax the perineal/vaginal region as rhythmically and evenly as possible.

Breathe normally throughout the practice.

Stage 2: Continue to breathe normally; do not hold the breath.

Slowly contract the perineal/vaginal region and hold the contraction.

Be totally aware of the physical sensation.

Contract a little tighter, but keep the rest of the body relaxed.

Contract only those muscles related to the mooladhara region.

In the beginning the anal and urinary sphincters will also contract, but as greater awareness and control is developed, this will minimize and eventually cease. Ultimately, only one point of contraction will be felt.

Relax the muscles slowly and evenly.

Adjust the tension in the spine to help focus on the point of contraction.

Repeat 10 times with maximum contraction and total relaxation.

Technique 2: with internal breath retention and jalandhara bandha

Close the eyes and relax the whole body for a few minutes.

Inhale deeply, retain the breath inside and perform jalandhara bandha.

Perform moola bandha and hold the contraction as tightly as possible. Do not strain.

This is the final lock.

Hold the contraction for as long as the breath can comfortably be retained.

Slowly release moola bandha, then jalandhara, raising the head to the upright position, and exhale.

Practise up to 10 times.

Breathing: The above practice may also be performed with external breath retention.

Awareness: Physical – at the point of perineal contraction.
Spiritual – on mooladhara chakra.

Sequence: Moola bandha is ideally performed in conjunction with mudras, bandhas and pranayamas. If practised on its own, it should be performed after asanas and pranayamas and before meditation.

Contra-indications: This practice should only be performed under the guidance of a competent teacher. Moola bandha raises the energy, and may precipitate hyperactivity. Do not practise during menstruation.

Benefits: Moola bandha bestows many physical, mental and spiritual benefits. It stimulates the pelvic nerves and tones the uro-genital and excretory systems.

It is helpful in psychosomatic and degenerative illnesses. It relieves depression and promotes good health. It helps

477

to realign the physical, mental and psychic bodies in preparation for spiritual awakening.

Moola bandha is a means to attain sexual control. It may be used to sublimate sexual energy for spiritual development (brahmacharya), or for enhancement of marital relations.

Practice note: Moola bandha is the contraction of specific muscles in the pelvic floor, not the whole perineum. In the male body, the area of contraction is between the anus and the testes. In the female body, the point of contraction is behind the cervix, where the uterus projects into the vagina. On the subtle level, it is the energizing of mooladhara chakra. The perineal body, which is the convergence of many muscles in the groin, acts as a trigger point for the location of mooladhara chakra. Initially, this area is difficult to isolate, so it is recommended that ashwini and vajroli mudras be performed in preparation for moola bandha.

Note: *The Sanskrit word* moola *means 'root', 'firmly fixed', 'source' or 'cause'. In this context it refers to the root of the spine or the perineum where mooladhara chakra, the seat of kundalini, the primal energy, is located. Moola bandha is effective for locating and awakening mooladhara chakra.*

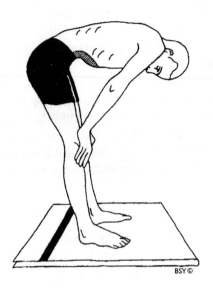

Preparatory practice: Standing abdominal contraction

Stand erect with the feet about half a metre apart.

Inhale deeply through the nostrils.

Bend forward from the waist and exhale all the air through the mouth.

Empty the lungs as much as possible.

Hold the breath outside.

Keep the spine horizontal and bend the knees slightly.

Place the palms of the hands on the thighs just above the knees, so that the knees are supporting the weight of the upper body. The fingers can point either downward or inwards. Make sure the arms are straight.

In this position there is an automatic contraction of the abdominal region.

Bend the head forward, but do not press the chin against the chest.

Make a false inhalation, keeping the glottis closed and expanding the chest, as though breathing in but not actually taking in air.

479

Straighten the knees.

This movement will automatically draw the abdomen upward and inward towards the spine to form uddiyana bandha.

Hold this position for a comfortable length of time.

Do not strain.

Release the abdominal lock and relax the chest.

Raise the head and torso to the upright position.

Exhale slightly to release the lock on the lungs and finally inhale slowly through the nose.

Remain in the standing position until the breath returns to normal before beginning the next round.

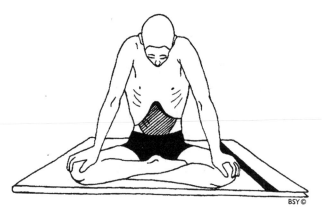

Uddiyana Bandha (abdominal contraction)

Sit in siddha/siddha yoni asana or padmasana with the spine erect and the knees in contact with the floor.

Place the palms of the hands flat on the knees.

Close the eyes and relax the whole body.

Inhale deeply through the nostrils.

Exhale fully.

Hold the breath outside.

Lean forward and press down on the knees with the palms of the hands. Straighten the elbows and raise the shoulders, allowing further extension of the spinal cord.

Practise jalandhara bandha, pressing the chin against the chest.

Contract the abdominal muscles inward and upward.
Hold the abdominal lock and the breath outside for as long as you can without straining.
Then release the abdominal lock, bend the elbows and lower the shoulders.
Raise the head and then slowly inhale.
Remain in this position until the respiration returns to normal, then begin the next round.

Breathing: Uddiyana bandha is performed with external breath retention only.

Duration: Practise 3 rounds in the beginning and gradually increase to 10 rounds over a few months as the system becomes accustomed to the practice.

Awareness: Physical – on the abdomen and breath.
Spiritual – on manipura chakra.

Sequence: Uddiyana bandha is easier to perform if preceded by an inverted asana. It is ideally performed in conjunction with mudras, bandhas and pranayamas. If practised on its own, it should be performed after asanas and pranayamas and before meditation.

Precaution: Uddiyana bandha is an advanced technique and should be attempted only under the guidance of a competent teacher. It should be practised after attaining proficiency in external breath retention, and jalandhara and moola bandhas.

Contra-indications: Persons suffering from colitis, stomach or intestinal ulcer, diaphragmatic hernia, major abdominal problems, high blood pressure, heart disease, glaucoma and raised intracranial pressure should not perform this practice. It should also be avoided during pregnancy.

Benefits: Uddiyana bandha is a panacea for the abdomen. It stimulates the function of the pancreas and liver and strengthens the internal organs. The digestive fire is stimulated and the abdominal organs are massaged and toned. The adrenal glands are balanced, removing lethargy and soothing anxiety and tension. It improves blood circulation throughout the torso.

Uddiyana bandha stimulates the solar plexus, which has many subtle influences on the distribution of energy throughout the body. It creates a suction pressure which reverses the energy flow of apana and prana, uniting them with samana and stimulating manipura chakra.

Practice note: Uddiyana bandha must be practised on an empty stomach. The bowels should also be empty. Agnisara kriya is an excellent preparatory practice.

Note: *The Sanskrit word* uddiyana *means 'to rise up' or 'to fly upward'. This practice is so called because the physical lock applied to the body causes the diaphragm to rise towards the chest. Uddiyana is therefore often translated as the stomach lift. Another meaning is that the physical lock helps to direct prana into sushumna nadi so that it flows upward to sahasrara chakra.*

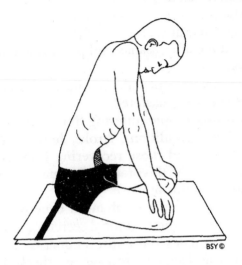

BSY©

Maha Bandha (the great lock)

Sit in siddha/siddha yoni asana or padmasana with the hands on the knees. The spine should be erect and the head straight. Close the eyes and relax the whole body.

Inhale slowly and deeply through the nose.

Exhale forcefully and completely.

Retain the breath outside.

Successively perform jalandhara, uddiyana and moola bandhas in this order.

Hold the bandhas and the breath for as long as is comfortable without straining.

Then release moola, uddiyana and jalandhara bandhas in this order.

Inhale slowly when the head is upright.

This is one round.

Keep the eyes closed, relax the body and let the breath return to normal before commencing the next round.

Awareness: Physical – on the perineal, abdominal and throat regions. Be aware of each region for a few seconds.

Spiritual – on mooladhara, manipura and vishuddhi chakras. Be aware of each chakra for a few seconds.

Duration: Once proficiency is attained, increase by one round until 9 rounds can be performed.

Sequence: Maha bandha is ideally performed in conjunction with pranayamas and mudras. If practised on its own, it should be done after asanas and pranayamas and before meditation.

Precaution: Do not attempt maha bandha until the other three bandhas have been mastered.

Contra-indications: People suffering from high or low blood pressure, heart conditions, stroke, hernia, stomach or intestinal ulcer, and those recovering from any visceral ailment should avoid this practice. Pregnant women should also not attempt this practice.

Benefits: Maha bandha gives enhanced benefits of all three bandhas. It affects the hormonal secretions of the pineal gland and regulates the entire endocrine system. The degenerative and ageing processes are checked and every cell of the body is rejuvenated. It introverts the mind prior to meditation. When perfected, it can fully awaken prana in the main chakras. It leads to the merger of prana, apana and samana in manipura chakra, which is the culmination of all pranayamas.

Practice note: Maha bandha can also be performed from utthanpadasana.

Note: The Sanskrit word maha *means 'great'. Maha bandha is called the great lock as it combines all the three bandhas in one practice.*

Shatkarma

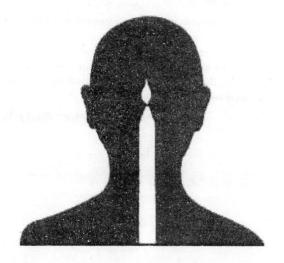

मेदश्लेष्माधिक: पूर्वं षट्कर्माणि समाचरेत् ।
अन्यस्तु नाचरेत्तानि दोषाणां समभावत: ॥ 2:21॥

Medashleshmaadhikaha poorvam shatkarmaani samaacharet.
Anyastu naacharettaani doshaanaam samabhaavataha.

When fat or mucus is excessive, the shatkarmas or six cleansing techniques should be practised before (pranayama). Others, in whom the doshas (i.e. phlegm, wind and bile) are balanced, need not do them.

Hatha Yoga Pradipika

Introduction to Shatkarma

Hatha yoga, as described in the early Yoga Upanishads, was made up of the shatkarmas and is a very precise and systematic science. *Shat* means 'six' and *karma* means 'action'; the shatkarmas consist of six groups of purification practices. The aim of hatha yoga and, therefore, of the shatkarmas is to create harmony between the two major pranic flows, ida and pingala, thereby attaining physical and mental purification and balance.

The shatkarmas are also used to balance the three doshas or humours in the body: *kapha*, mucus; *pitta*, bile; and *vata*, wind. According to both ayurveda and hatha yoga, an imbalance in the doshas will result in illness. These practices are also used before pranayama and other higher yoga practices in order to purify the body of toxins and to ensure safe and successful progression along the spiritual path.

These powerful techniques should never be learned from books or taught by inexperienced people. According to the tradition, only those instructed by a guru may teach others. It is essential to be personally instructed as to how and when to perform the shatkarmas, according to individual limitations and needs.

The six shatkarmas are as follows:

1. *Neti*: A process of cleansing and purifying the nasal passages. Practices included in this category are: jala neti and sutra neti.

2. *Dhauti*: A series of cleansing techniques which are divided into three main groups: *antar dhauti* or internal cleansing,

sirsha dhauti or head cleansing, and *hrid dhauti* or thoracic cleansing. The dhauti techniques which are given in this section clean the entire alimentary canal from the mouth to the anus. There are four practices:

a) *Shankhaprakshalana (varisara dhauti)* and *laghoo shankha-prakshalana,* cleansing of the intestines
b) *Agnisar kriya (vahnisara dhauti),* activating the digestive fire
c) *Kunjal (vaman dhauti),* cleansing the stomach with water
d) *Vatsara dhauti,* cleansing the intestines with air.

All of these practices require the guidance of a competent teacher.

3. **Nauli**: A method of massaging and strengthening the abdominal organs.
4. **Basti**: Techniques for washing and toning the large intestine.
5. **Kapalbhati**: A breathing technique for purifying the frontal region of the brain.
6. **Trataka**: The practice of intense gazing at one point or object which develops the power of concentration.

Although there are six shatkarmas, each one consists of a variety of practices. In this chapter only the most commonly used practices are described in detail.

Advice, precautions and contra-indications are given for each practice individually and should be carefully observed. During pregnancy, only jala neti and trataka are recommended.

Although the cleansing and strengthening effects of shatkarmas may be beneficial therapeutically, this is not their purpose. Shatkarmas are practices to promote the health of yoga practitioners and to awaken and direct the energies in the body, mind and deeper psyche. People suffering from any medical condition, who wish to utilize any of these practices, should seek the advice of a competent teacher.

The water used in these practices should be pure. If necessary, use an ultraviolet filter or boil the water for several minutes and then allow it to cool to the desired temperature.

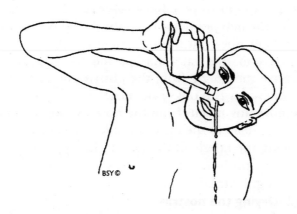

Jala Neti (nasal cleansing with water)

Preparation: A special *neti lota*, 'neti pot' should be used. This pot may be made of plastic, pottery, brass or any other metal which does not contaminate the water. The nozzle on the end of the spout should fit comfortably into the nostril so that the water does not leak out. Even a teapot may be used if the tip of the spout is not too large or sharp.

The water should be pure, at body temperature and thoroughly mixed with salt in the proportion of one teaspoonful per half litre of water. The addition of salt ensures the osmotic pressure of the water is equal to that of the body fluids, thereby minimizing any irritation to the mucous membrane. A painful or burning sensation is an indication of too little or too much salt in the water.

Stage I: Washing the nostrils

Fill the neti pot with the prepared salt water.

Stand squarely, with legs apart so that the body weight is evenly distributed between the feet. Lean forward and tilt the head to one side.

Breathe through the mouth.

Gently insert the nozzle into the uppermost nostril.

There should be no force involved.

The nozzle should press firmly against the side of the

nostril so that no water leakage occurs.
Tilt the neti pot in such a way that water runs into the nostril and not down the face.
Keep the mouth open. Raising the elbow of the hand which holds the neti pot helps to adjust the body position so that the water flows out through the lower nostril.
When half the water has passed through the nostrils, remove the nozzle from the nostril, centre the head and let the water run out of the nose.
Remove any mucus from the nose by blowing gently.
Tilt the head to the opposite side and repeat the process, placing the nozzle of the lota in the upper nostril.
After completing this process, the nostrils must be thoroughly dried.

Stage 2: Drying the nostrils

1. Stand erect.
   Close the right nostril with the right thumb and breathe in and out through the left nostril 10 times in quick succession, as in kapalbhati pranayama.
   Repeat through the right nostril, with the left nostril closed.
   Perform once more through both nostrils.
2. Bend forward from the waist so that the trunk is horizontal.
   Repeat the same process as described above, but tilt the head to the right, closing the right nostril.
   Repeat again, tilting the head to the left and closing the left nostril.
   Finally, repeat again with the head centred, breathing through both nostrils.
   Practice note: This step helps to drain trapped water from the sinus cavities.
3. Stand erect with the feet apart. Close the right nostril and exhale forcefully while bending forward rapidly from the waist. Inhale normally while returning to the upright position. Repeat 5 times.
   Repeat with the right nostril open and then with both nostrils open. Do not blow the nose too hard as the remaining water may be pushed into the ears.

If necessary, perform shashankasana for several minutes to allow the drainage of any remaining water.

Duration: This practice should take about 5 minutes.

Neti may be practised daily, once or twice a week, or as required.

Awareness: Physical – on relaxing and positioning the body, on the flow of water through the nostrils, and on relaxed breathing through the mouth, especially for beginners. Spiritual – on ajna chakra.

Sequence: Jala neti is ideally practised in the morning before asanas and pranayamas. However, if necessary, it may be performed at any time, except after meals.

Precautions: The water should only pass through the nostrils. If any water enters the throat or mouth it causes no harm, but indicates that the position of the head needs to be adjusted. Make sure that the nose is properly dried after the practice, otherwise the nasal passages and sinuses may become irritated and manifest the symptoms of a cold.

Only practise neti when necessary. Prolonged practise is not advisable unless instructed by a competent teacher.

Contra-indications: People who suffer from chronic bleeding in the nose should not do jala neti without the advice of a competent teacher. Those who consistently have great difficulty passing water through the nose may have a structural blockage and should seek expert advice. People prone to or having ear infections should not do neti. During colds, flu or sinusitis, when the nose is totally blocked, neti should be avoided.

Benefits: Jala neti removes mucus and pollution from the nasal passages and sinuses, allowing air to flow without obstruction. It helps prevent and manage respiratory tract diseases. It helps to maintain good health of the ears, eyes and throat.

Jala neti relieves muscular tension of the face and helps the practitioner to maintain a fresh and youthful appearance. It has a calming and soothing influence on the brain. It alleviates anxiety, anger and depression, removes drowsiness and makes the head feel light and fresh.

Jala neti stimulates the various nerve endings in the nose, improving the sense of smell and the overall health of the individual. A balance is brought about between the right and left nostrils and the corresponding left and right brain hemispheres, inducing a state of harmony and balance throughout the body and mind. Most importantly, however, neti helps to awaken ajna chakra.

Practice note: Jala neti may be practised either in a squatting position or standing. The latter is most suitable for doing neti over a sink while the former may be performed outside. After some practice, a full neti pot may be used for each nostril.

Variations: Practitioners may suck water up the nostrils directly from a glass or bowl. This is the original form of the practice called *vyutkrama kapalbhati,* or *usha paan,* which literally means 'water of the dawn'.

Other liquids may also be used instead of water for the practice of neti. These include warm milk – *dugdh neti,* warm clarified butter or ghee – *ghrita neti,* and yoghurt. If oil is used instead of ghee, it must be natural and without added chemicals. The most powerful form of neti is practised with the midflow of one's own urine, and is known as *amaroli neti.* This form is particularly useful for alleviating inflammation of the nasal passages. Each liquid bestows a different benefit. None of these variations should be attempted unless instructed by a competent teacher.

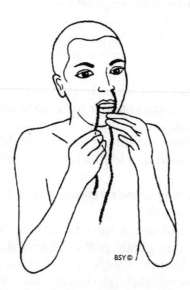

Sutra Neti (nasal cleansing with thread)

Preparation: This practice involves passing a length of cotton thread through the nose. Traditionally, a specially prepared cotton thread, *sutra*, was used. Several strands were tightly wrapped together and dipped in melted beeswax. The width was about 4 mm and the length 36 to 45 cm.

Nowadays, however, the practice is more conveniently performed by using a thin, rubber catheter lubricated with melted ghee, butter, edible oil or one's own saliva, so that it slides easily through the nasal passage. The size of the catheter depends on the individual nasal passage. Beginners may prefer size 4, but progress to size 6.

Technique I: Basic practice

Take any comfortable standing, sitting or squatting position.

Relax the whole body.

Tilt the head slightly back. Gently and slowly insert the narrow end of the catheter or waxed end of the thread into whichever nostril is flowing more freely.

As the thread is inserted, twist it so that it enters the nostril easily. Always keep the tip pointing downward towards the base of the nose. Never push the catheter straight up because the nasal cavity is behind the nose, not at the top of the nose.

When the thread reaches the back of the throat, insert the index finger and thumb, or the middle and index fingers, into the mouth.

Pull the catheter or thread gently and slowly out through the mouth, leaving a few inches of thread hanging out of the nostril.

This action may cause retching at first, but it will become easier with practice.

Hold each end of the sutra or catheter with the fingers. Very slowly and gently pull it backward and forward, no more than 15 times on the first attempt.

Remove it slowly through the nose and repeat the process with the opposite nostril.

Technique 2: Advanced practice

After completing technique 1, leave the thread with one end passing through the mouth and the other through the nostril.

Gently insert the waxed end emerging from one nostril into the other nostril and pull the end through the mouth.

In the final position, both waxed ends emerge from the mouth. Loosen the hard wax at the tip of each end so that the individual strands again become separated.

Push the two ends together so that they merge with one another, and twist the thread so that the two ends become joined. If the join is too thick, some of the threads may be cut away so that the join may pass easily through the nostrils. The thread is now circular.

Slowly draw the join into the mouth, progressively sliding the thread through the nostrils.

Eventually the join should be located between the entrance to the two nostrils.

Disconnect the join.

The thread now enters one nostril and emerges from the other; it no longer passes through the mouth.

Gently pull the sutra to and fro, a few times only to begin with. If there is the slightest discomfort, stop the practice immediately.

Pull one end of the thread and slowly withdraw it from the nose.

Breathing: Breathing is performed through the mouth.

Duration: The practice takes about 10 minutes.

Once every few days or once a week is sufficient.

Awareness: Physical – on relaxing the body and moving the catheter or thread smoothly and slowly.

Spiritual – on ajna chakra.

Sequence: Sutra neti should be performed before jala neti as the latter will flush out all the impurities and particles in the nose which have been dislodged by sutra neti.

Precautions: Do not use force under any circumstances. The interior of the nose is very delicate and any undue force could cause damage. After persistent attempts, if the thread or catheter will not pass through the nose, consult a competent teacher. Make sure that the sutra is perfectly clean before inserting it into the nostril. It is best not to try sutra neti until jala neti has been perfected.

Contra-indications: Those people who suffer from chronic bleeding in the nose should not do sutra neti. Anyone with nasal ulcers, polyps, or severe malformations of the nasal septum or turbinates should first seek the advice of a yogic or ayurvedic doctor.

Benefits: The benefits are the same as for jala neti. In addition, however, sutra neti can rectify the problem of deviated nasal septum. If one or both nostrils are not flowing freely due either to deformed bone or fleshy outgrowths, the regular friction of sutra neti causes these obstructions to disappear within a few months.

Practice note: Although the catheter is easier and quicker, it does not clean the nasal passages as effectively as the cotton thread. Technique 2 is possible with some types of catheter only.

495

SHANKHAPRAKSHALANA

Technique I: Shankhaprakshalana or Varisara Dhauti (cleansing of the entire digestive tract)

Preparation: It is advisable to take a light, semi-liquid meal the night before undertaking this practice.

Plenty of clean, lukewarm water should be available and also extra hot water in case the temperature of the water cools. Add 2 teaspoons of salt per litre to the water, so that it tastes mildly salty.

Prepare a special *khichari* of good quality white rice and mung dal, cooked with *ghee*, clarified butter. The rice and lentils should be cooked together in water until soft. A little *haldi*, turmeric, may be added, but no salt. Finally, the clarified butter should be liberally mixed in so that the final preparation is semi-liquid.

The khichari should be eaten at the end of the practice, after a 45-minute rest period, and again later in the day.

No asana or physical work should be performed, and no food or beverages should be taken before commencing the practice. Not evacuating the bowels prior to the practice helps stimulate the peristaltic movement.

Light and comfortable clothing should be worn.

Complete intestinal wash: Drink 2 glasses of warm salty water as quickly as possible.

Perform the following 5 asanas dynamically, 8 times each in the following sequence:

a) Tadasana
b) Tiryaka tadasana
c) Kati chakrasana (variation: see practice note p 146)
d) Tiryaka bhujangasana
e) Udarakarshanasana.

This is one complete round.

Do not rest between rounds.

Drink 2 more glasses of warm salty water and again repeat the 5 asanas 8 times each.

496

Repeat this process a third time.

After the third round, go to the toilet and see if there is any movement in the bowels, if they have not yet been emptied.

Do not strain.

Resume the practice, regardless of whether there has been any movement or not; it is not essential at this point.

Drink 2 more glasses and repeat the 5 asanas 8 times. Again go to the toilet, but do not use force to produce a bowel movement.

Continue drinking the water, performing the asanas and going to the toilet, allowing the pressure to build up.

Spend as little time in the toilet as possible, a minute or so is enough. The aim is to build up the internal cleansing pressure.

At first solid stool will be evacuated, followed by a mixture of stool and water. As the practice progresses, more water and less solid stool will be excreted. Eventually, cloudy yellow water and, finally, almost clear water will be evacuated.

Sixteen glasses are generally required before clear water is evacuated, but it varies from person to person.

The speed at which one completes the practice should not be compared with that of others.

The practice should be performed in a relaxed way at one's own pace.

Supplementary practices: Kunjal kriya followed by jala neti may be performed 10 minutes after completing the internal wash.

Rest: Total rest is essential after completion of the practice. Do not take a shower or bathe.

Lie down in shavasana for 45 minutes, but do not sleep as a headache or cold may result. It is important to keep warm during this resting period. Try to maintain *mouna*, silence. During this time the whole digestive system is given a chance to revitalize itself.

Passing urine at this time is perfectly normal.

Special meal: Exactly 45 minutes after completing shankha-, prakshalana the specially prepared khichari must be taken.

497

Eating this meal at the correct time is essential. The rhythm of the body has been temporarily disturbed; however, 45 minutes after completion of the practice the digestive functions resume.

The three components of khichari are helpful in the restoration of correct digestive function. The clarified butter is necessary to coat the intestinal walls until the body produces a new lining. The rice provides a simple, easily digestible packing material in the form of carbohydrate, and creates mucus, which also protects the inner lining of the alimentary canal. The lentils supplement the diet by giving the body an easily digestible source of protein, and make for an all-round nutritious meal.

A sufficient quantity of khichari must be eaten to reline the intestines and keep the walls of the gut stretched, otherwise they may cramp due to the absence of the bulk to which they are accustomed. This bulk not only maintains the tone, but aids the intestines to resume peristalsis. It is also important in order to prevent indigestion, diarrhoea, and constipation.

Further rest: Having eaten, further rest is necessary. However, it is important not to sleep for at least three hours after the initial meal. Sleep during this period may lead to physical lethargy and headache. Complete rest should be taken for the remainder of the day. During this period, it is advisable to keep silence, *mouna*, and avoid physical or mental work. Rest the following day also.

Second meal: Khichari should also be prepared for the late afternoon or evening meal, about 6 hours after the first special meal. The stomach must be filled to capacity at both meals, even if there is no feeling of hunger.

Place of practice: The best place to practise shankhaprakshalana is in an ashram, in an open area where there is plenty of fresh air. Ensure that adequate toilet facilities are nearby. The practice is best undertaken with a group of people. The atmosphere should be relaxed, friendly and light-hearted, with no apprehension concerning the practice, as this can create tension and prevent free bowel movement.

Climate: Shankhaprakshalana should not be performed when the weather conditions are extreme. Those who live in cold climates should practise in the summer when the days are warm and dry. This is important, as it is easy for the stomach and intestines to become chilled. On the other hand, do not practise when it is very hot as this would produce too much sweat and the experience would be exhausting.

Very cloudy, windy or rainy weather is also to be avoided. The best time to practise is at the changeover of seasons.

Frequency: This practice should not be performed more than twice a year.

Duration: The whole day should be put aside for this practice and the following day for rest.

Precautions: It is important not to exceed the point beyond which almost clear water without specks of solid matter is being passed, as the system may start producing bile, indicated by bright yellow water. It is better to stop when the water is still slightly cloudy. While resting for 45 minutes after terminating the practice, one should not sleep as a headache or cold may result.

No water or other fluids should be taken until at least 2 hours after the first special meal. Cold liquid will chill the digestive system. Drinking or eating anything before the prescribed period will dilute and wash away the new protective layer which is being reproduced by the body on the stomach and intestinal wall.

Fans and air-conditioning should not be used until the evening as the body must be kept warm to prevent chills and fever. If the room is cool, the body should be covered with a blanket to maintain the inner body temperature. Sitting in the hot sun, near a fire or doing physical exercise should be avoided.

Rest periods should be maintained very carefully.

Mental strain and stressful situations should be avoided.

Food restrictions: For at least one month after the practice, all chemically processed, synthetic, pungent, spicy, acidic, rich and non-vegetarian foods must be strictly avoided.

No pickles, sweets, chocolates, ice cream or soft drinks should be taken. Milk, buttermilk, yoghurt and all fruits, especially acidic fruits such as lemons, grapefruit, oranges or pineapples are restricted. Alcohol, cigarettes, tea, coffee, betel nut preparations such as paan and any type of intoxicant or drug should not be taken.

The diet should be as pure, simple and neutral as possible. It may include foods such as rice, wheat, bread, vegetables with a low acidic content, nuts, lentils and other pulses.

Common sense must be used in this regard. After shankhaprakshalana the digestive system is very vulnerable and extra care should be taken to protect it.

Warning: This practice should only be attempted in an ashram or yoga centre under the guidance of a competent teacher. All guidelines and restrictions must be followed strictly to avoid experiencing harmful side-effects. Those who are unable to follow these restrictions should not practise shankhaprakshalana. They will find the simplified version, laghoo shankhaprakshalana, more appropriate to their needs.

Strong medication such as antibiotics should be avoided for one month. Regular medication can be discontinued during the practice and recommenced 2 or 3 days after the practice.

Contra-indications: People with heart or kidney problems, or high blood pressure, should not practise shankha-prakshalana. Those suffering from any medical condition should seek guidance from their doctor before attempting it, especially those taking medication. This practice should also be avoided during pregnancy.

Benefits: Physically, shankhaprakshalana alleviates digestive problems and tones the liver and other digestive organs and glands. It strengthens the immune system, reduces excessive mucus and purifies the blood.

Shankhaprakshalana recharges the entire pranic body, removes blockages from the nadis and purifies all the chakras. The harmony of the five pranas is restored and the energy level is raised.

Mentally, it calms the mind and prepares the way for higher states of consciousness. Any sadhana performed after this cleansing practice gives manifold results.

Practice note: The five asanas which form the core of the practice activate intestinal peristalsis and enhance the cleansing process. When performed in the correct sequence, they progressively open the pyloric valve at the outlet of the stomach, then the ileocaecal valve at the exit of the small intestine and finally the sphincter which forms the anus.

Tadasana acts mainly on the stomach and stretches the colon; tiryaka tadasana acts on the small intestine and colon; kati chakrasana massages the small intestine; tiryaka bhujangasana and udarakarshanasana squeeze and massage the caecum, sigmoid colon and rectum, and also stimulate the urge to defecate.

Those who have difficulty drinking rapidly or develop a feeling of nausea should reduce the quantity of water from two glasses to one glass before each round. The quantity of salt may also be reduced.

Note: *The word* shankhaprakshalana *comes from two words:* shankha, *meaning 'conch', and* prakshalana, *meaning 'to wash completely'. The word shankha is intended to represent and describe the intestines with their cavernous and coiled shape. Traditionally, this practice was known as* varisara dhauti, *but nowadays it is better known as shankhaprakshalana. The word* varisara *comes from two words:* vari, *meaning 'water', and* sara, *meaning 'essence'. This practice is also a part of* kaya kalpa, *which is an ayurvedic technique for physical purification and transformation,* kaya *meaning 'body' and* kalpa, *'transformation'.*

Technique 2: Laghoo Shankhaprakshalana (short intestinal wash)

Two litres of warm salted water should be prepared as for poorna shankhaprakshalana.

Quickly drink 2 glasses of the prepared water.

Perform the following 5 asanas 8 times each:
a) Tadasana
b) Tiryaka tadasana
c) Kati chakrasana (variation: see practice note p 146)
d) Tiryaka bhujangasana
e) Udarakarshanasana.

Drink 2 more glasses of water and repeat the asanas 8 times each.

Repeat the process for a third and last time.

Go to the toilet, but do not strain, whether there is a bowel movement or not.

If there is no motion immediately, it will come later on.

Additional practices: Kunjal kriya and jala neti may be performed immediately after completing the practice.

Time of practice: Laghoo should be practised in the morning when the stomach is completely empty, before any food or drink is taken.

Duration: Allow an hour for this practice.

Frequency: Once a week is sufficient for general purposes. In cases of constipation, however, it may be practised daily until the condition improves.

Rest: On completion of the practice, rest for half an hour before taking any food or drink.

Restrictions: There are no special food restrictions and no special food has to be taken following this practice, although a light vegetarian diet is preferable for that day.

Precautions: Do not try to force a bowel movement; it should be completely natural.

Contra-indications: As for shankhaprakshalana.

Benefits: The laghoo or short method is intended to encourage normal functioning of the intestines. It is an excellent method of encouraging good bowel movement and is ideal for regular use and for those who are unable to practise the full version. Laghoo is recommended for digestive disorders and to flush out the kidneys.

Practice note: Greater benefits may be derived by combining this practice with light food. Medication may be safely continued.

Technique 3: TTK solution

One litre of warm salted water should be prepared as for shankhaprakshalana, or pure unsalted water at room temperature can be used if the weather is not too cold.

The first 3 asanas of the shankhaprakshalana series are used:

a) Tadasana
b) Tiryaka tadasana
c) Kati chakrasana (variation: see practice note p 146).

Quickly drink one glass of the prepared water.

Practise tadasana 10 times and drink a second glass of water.

Practise tiryaka tadasana 10 times and drink a third glass of water.

Practise kati chakrasana 10 times and drink a fourth glass of water.

Go to the toilet, but do not strain, whether there is a bowel movement or not. If there is no motion immediately, it will come later on.

Time of practice: The TTK solution should be practised in the morning when the stomach is completely empty, before any food or drink is taken and before other asanas.

Frequency: Once a week is sufficient for general purposes. In cases of constipation, however, it may be practised daily until the condition improves.

Restrictions: There are no special food restrictions and no special food has to be taken following this practice.

Precautions: Do not try to force a bowel movement; it should be completely natural.

Benefits: This practice helps to prevent constipation and related digestive problems. It makes the body feel light and ensures a healthy intake of water first thing in the morning.

503

VATSARA DHAUTI

Vatsara Dhauti (cleansing the intestines with air)
Sit in a comfortable position.
Open the mouth and purse the lips like a crow's beak.
Draw air down into the stomach through the open mouth in one sucking action or in a series of gulps. Choose which method is easiest.
Fill the stomach with air as much as possible.
Then relax completely.
Do not try to expel the air.
It will come out through the large intestine in its own time.

Time of practice: This practice may be done at any time of the day, but it is most useful just before a large meal. It should not be done after meals.

Benefits: This practice removes stale gas and wind and stimulates the digestive system.

Practice note: This practice is similar to bhujangini mudra. However, in bhujangini mudra the air is expelled by belching, whereas in vatsara dhauti the air is passed out through the intestines.

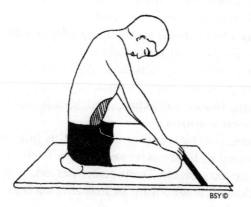

**Agnisara Kriya or Vahnisara Dhauti (activating the digestive
fire or cleansing with the essence of fire)**
Sit in bhadrasana with the big toes touching, or in
padmasana.
Inhale deeply.
Exhale, emptying the lungs as much as possible.
Lean forward slightly, straightening the elbows.
Push down on the knees with the hands and perform
jalandhara bandha.
Contract and expand the abdominal muscles rapidly
for as long as it is possible to hold the breath outside
comfortably.
Do not strain.
Release jalandhara bandha.
When the head is upright, take a slow, deep breath in.
This is one round.
Relax until the breathing normalizes before commencing
the next round.
Duration: Beginners may find this practice difficult and quickly
become tired due to lack of voluntary control over the
abdominal muscles. The muscles must be slowly and
gradually developed over a period of time.
Three rounds of 10 abdominal contractions and expan-
sions are sufficient at first. With regular practice, up to

50 abdominal movements may be performed with each round. The time of breath retention should be gradually increased over a period of time.

Awareness: Physical – on the abdominal movement.

Spiritual – on manipura chakra.

Sequence: Practise after asanas. Agnisara kriya should be practised on an empty stomach, preferably in the early morning before breakfast, and ideally after the bowels have been emptied.

Precautions: During summer months, this practice should be performed with care as it may raise the body heat and blood pressure excessively. During this period, it should always be followed by a cooling pranayama such as sheetkari or sheetali.

Contra-indications: People suffering from high blood pressure, heart disease, acute duodenal or peptic ulcers, overactive thyroid gland or chronic diarrhoea should not perform this kriya.

Women who are pregnant should refrain from this practice.

Benefits: Agnisara kriya stimulates the appetite and improves the digestion. It massages the abdomen, strengthens the abdominal muscles and encourages optimum health of the abdominal organs. Agnisara kriya stimulates the five pranas, especially samana, and raises the energy levels markedly. It alleviates depression, dullness and lethargy.

Preparatory practice: Swana Pranayama (panting breath)

Sit in bhadrasana, keeping the big toes in contact with each other. Place the hands on the knees and close the eyes.

Relax the whole body for a few minutes, especially the abdomen.

Straighten the arms and lean forward slightly.

Keep the head erect.

Open the mouth wide and extend the tongue outside.

Breathe in a panting manner through the mouth, with the tongue extended.

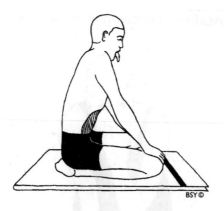

Contract and expand the abdomen rapidly.

While contracting the abdomen, breathe out and while expanding the abdomen, breathe in.

The breathing should be passive, only occurring because the movement of the abdomen is being accentuated. It should resemble the panting of a dog.

Keep the chest as still as possible. Do not strain.

Breathe in and out 10 to 20 times.

This is one round. Practise 3 rounds.

Relax and breathe normally between rounds.

Awareness: Physical – on synchronizing the breath rhythmically with the abdominal movement.

Spiritual – on manipura chakra.

Practice note: This kriya is an excellent practice to strengthen and develop control over the abdominal muscles and the diaphragm. It is also used as a preparatory practice for uddiyana bandha and nauli.

Note: *The words* agni *and* vahni *both mean 'fire'; sara means 'essence', and* kriya *means 'action'. The essence or nature of fire is attributed to the digestive process. If the abdominal organs are not working properly, the digestive fire smoulders and needs to be stoked or fanned to increase its power. Agnisara kriya does just that, as well as purifying the digestive system and its associated organs, and allowing the optimum assimilation of nutrients from food ingested.*

507

VAMAN DHAUTI

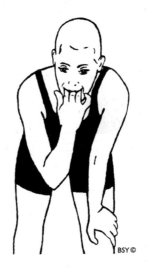

Vaman Dhauti (regurgitative cleansing)
Preparation: Wash the hands and make sure the nails are
   carefully trimmed.
   Prepare about 2 litres of lukewarm (body temperature)
   water per person, adding 1 teaspoonful of salt per litre
   according to taste.

Technique I: Kunjal Kriya (the practice of vomiting water)
   Stand near a sink or toilet, or if the weather is warm, in
   a suitable place outside in the garden or near an open
   drain.
   Drink at least 6 glasses of the prepared water, one after
   the other, as quickly as possible, until the stomach cannot
   hold any more. It is most important to drink fast and not
   just sip the water.
   When the stomach is full, the urge to vomit will occur
   automatically.
   Lean forward, keeping the trunk as horizontal as possible.
   Open the mouth and place the middle and index fingers
   of the right hand as far back on the tongue as possible.
   Gently rub and press the back of the tongue.

This should induce the water to gush out from the stomach.
If there is no expulsion of water, it means the tips of the fingers are not far enough down the throat or that the tongue is not being pressed.
The more the practitioner relaxes into the practice, the easier it will be.
During the expulsion of water the fingers may be removed from the mouth, although this is not necessary.
When the flow of water ceases, again place the fingers in the mouth and repeat the process.
Continue in this way until the stomach is empty.

Technique 2: Gaja Karma Kriya (elephant action)
Drink at least 6 glasses of the prepared, warm, salted water.
Fill the stomach with water until it will hold no more.
Stand with the feet a comfortable distance apart, bend forward and place the hands on the knees.
Relax the whole body.
Open the mouth and breathe in slowly, making a whispering 'ah' sound from the deeper part of the throat.
Simultaneously, contract the upper part of the abdomen just below the ribcage.
At the end of inhalation, retain the compression of the abdomen and exhale.
If this is performed correctly, the water should gush out of the mouth in a steady stream.
It is important that the body remains relaxed during expulsion so that the water is not impeded.

Additional practices: Both techniques of kunjal should be followed by jala neti.
Time of practice: Kunjal is best practised early in the morning before breakfast. However, if it is very cold, wait until the day has warmed up a little. It is essential that no food be taken before the practice.
Frequency: Kunjal may be performed once a week unless otherwise directed by a competent teacher.

Precaution: When the vomiting reflex ceases to bring up any water, stop the technique as it is a sure sign that the stomach is empty. These techniques remove some of the stomach lining, leaving it temporarily vulnerable. For this reason, it is advised to eat a light meal half an hour after completion of the practice.

Contra-indications: These practices should not be performed by people suffering from hernia, high blood pressure, raised intracranial pressure, heart disease, stroke, acute peptic ulcer or by diabetics with eye problems. They are not recommended during pregnancy.

Benefits: These techniques tone and stimulate all the abdominal organs by inducing strong muscular contractions in the stomach walls. Excess mucus is removed, helping respiratory functions.

These techniques help to release pent-up emotions and emotional blocks or feelings of heaviness in the heart caused by inner and external conflict and pressures.

Practice note: Plain water may be used on the advice of a competent teacher. Salt water, however, dissolves mucus and also inhibits the secretion of acid in the stomach, making it generally preferable, and a must for those suffering from excess mucus and hyperacidity.

The biggest obstacle to these techniques is the mental block which people have towards the idea of vomiting. Some people are unable to bring up the water at first. The water in the stomach will then simply pass through the system in the normal way.

The expelled water might be discoloured, especially on the first few attempts. This can be caused by fermented food particles, bile or mucus from the stomach. When the stomach is completely clean, the water will become clear. Gaja kriya is an advanced form of kunjal. In this practice, the water is expelled from the stomach by contracting the abdominal muscles. This action requires practice and good control over the muscles of the stomach.

Technique 3: Vyaghra Kriya (tiger practice)

While there is undigested or partially digested food in the stomach, drink at least 6 glasses of the prepared, warm, salted water.

Fill the stomach with water until it will hold no more.

Expel the water in the same way as for kunjal kriya.

All the food in the stomach will be removed.

Benefits: This practice prevents burdening the intestines when either excessive amounts of food or rotten food has been eaten.

Although the modern remedy is to take indigestion tablets, the most natural and least harmful way to relieve the stomach is to vomit.

Time of practice: Vyaghra kriya may be practised three hours after eating food, whenever the stomach feels uncomfortable. If the stomach has been severely overloaded or bad food has been taken, it may be performed earlier.

Frequency: Vyaghra kriya should be performed only when necessary.

Practice note: Vyaghra kriya is performed in the same way as kunjal kriya; however, it is done on a full or loaded stomach.

Note: Vyaghra *means 'tiger'. The tiger has the habit of gorging his stomach with his prey and then vomiting out the semi-digested food after three or four hours. This technique is a voluntary form of what the body does involuntarily if food is not digestible. The body will vomit as a last resort after trying unsuccessfully to digest the impure or excessive food that has been dumped into it. The easiest way to relieve heaviness, nausea and indigestion is to make the stomach expel the food through the mouth.*

VASTRA DHAUTI

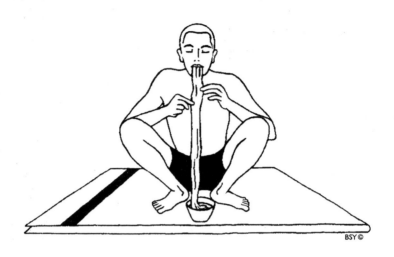

Vastra Dhauti (cloth cleansing)
Preparation: A cloth is required for this practice, which should be clean and new. Finely woven, unstarched, undyed cotton such as white muslin is best. Synthetic material should be avoided. The fabric should be about 2½ cm wide (no wider than the tongue or it will fold as it passes down the throat) and 3 metres long. After some months of practice, the width may be increased to 5 or 6 cm and the length to 6½ metres. Any frayed edges or loose threads should be removed.

The cloth should be thoroughly washed and boiled in water before using. It should then be placed in a mug or bowl of lukewarm water. Salt may be added to the water, but is not essential. The water keeps the cloth wet so that it slips smoothly down the oesophagus into the stomach. The cloth may be soaked in warm milk or even sweetened milk, if this makes it easier to swallow.

The same cloth may be used several times. After the practice, boil it thoroughly in hot water as it will be thick with mucus. Dry it well, preferably in direct sunlight, and store it in a clean place.

Ingestion: Squat comfortably, or sit on a low stool.

Place the bowl containing the cloth on the ground between the feet.

Relax the whole body.

Take hold of one end of the cloth, leaving the other end immersed in the water.

Fold the two corners of the end of the cloth so that it is slightly pointed; this will allow it to pass down the throat more easily.

Place the pointed end as far back on the tongue as possible. Hold the remaining cloth outside the mouth with the index fingers and thumbs as shown in the diagram.

Begin to swallow the cloth.

If it catches in the throat, take a sip or two of warm water, but just a little, as the stomach is to be filled with the cloth and not with water.

The jaws should move as though gently chewing the cloth, but do not actually chew it. This will induce copious secretions of saliva and enable the cloth to slip down with ease.

The cloth may stick in the lowest part of the throat, causing a vomiting sensation to be experienced. Stop for a few moments until this passes and then continue swallowing. Once the cloth passes through the junction of the windpipe and the oesophagus, the problem will end and the cloth will slide smoothly into the stomach.

Gradually feed more and more of the cloth into the mouth as the end slips down the oesophagus, but do not feed it too quickly or it will bunch up in the mouth and make the practice difficult.

Do not swallow the whole cloth; allow at least 30 cm to protrude from the mouth.

Churning: Stand up.

Practise dakshina (right) and vaman (left) nauli first, then perform rotations.

Finally perform madhyama (middle) nauli.

3 to 5 minutes of nauli is sufficient for cleaning the stomach. Beginners should only practise for one minute.

As an alternative to nauli, agnisara kriya may be practised. The cloth may be left in the stomach for 5 to 20 minutes, but no longer or it may start to enter the intestinal tract.

Removing the cloth: The cloth must be slowly removed from the stomach.

Sit back in the squatting position once more.

Take hold of the cloth and pull it gently but firmly.

Do not pull too hard or it may damage the delicate walls of the stomach and oesophagus.

There may be some resistance to the withdrawal of the cloth at first, but this will pass after a few seconds and the cloth will come out easily.

Remove the whole cloth and let it fall into the mug or bowl.

Sequence: It is necessary to become proficient in nauli before practising vastra dhauti.

Time of practice: This practice should be performed in the morning before any food or drink are taken. The stomach must be completely empty before commencing.

Precautions: Do not talk while practising. Do not attempt this practice without the guidance of a competent teacher.

Contra-indications: This practice should not be performed by people suffering from hypertension, heart disease, stroke, peptic ulcer, acute gastritis, during a time of general illness or when the body is in a weakened state.

It should not be practised until 6 months after any surgery, particularly abdominal surgery, or during pregnancy.

Benefits: The mucus from the chest is loosened and expelled, while the muscles of the bronchial tubes are relaxed, improving respiratory functions.

Vastra dhauti induces strong reflexes in the throat and chest region. The practitioner has to wilfully control the urge to vomit which, as a result, tones the autonomic nervous system. One gains self confidence, willpower and a feeling of detachment from the body.

Practice note: It may take some practice before being able to swallow the cloth. Remain relaxed, do not strain and the process will become easier. Do not hurry; just swallow the cloth gently. Once the mind accepts the idea, the technique will soon be mastered.

After swallowing the cloth, the stomach should be massaged by the churning process of nauli, so that the cloth rubs and cleans the stomach walls.

NAULI

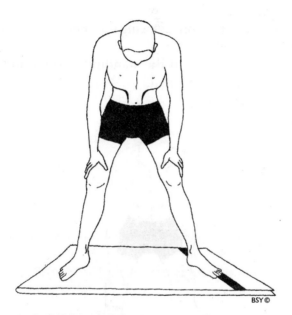

BSY©

Nauli (abdominal massaging)
Stage I: Madhyama Nauli (central abdominal contraction)

Stand with the feet about a metre apart.

Take a deep breath in through the nose and then exhale through the mouth, emptying the lungs as much as possible. Bend the knees slightly and lean forward, placing the palms of the hands on the thighs just above the knees. The fingers may point either inward or outward. The weight of the upper body should rest comfortably on this area above the knees. The arms should remain straight.

Perform jalandhara bandha while maintaining bahir kumbhaka, external breath retention.

Keep the eyes open and watch the abdomen.

Suck in the lower abdomen

Contract the rectus abdominii muscles, so that they form a central arch, running vertically in front of the abdomen. Contract the muscles as much as possible, without straining. Hold the contraction for as long as it is comfortable to hold the breath.

Release the contraction, raise the head and return to the upright position.

Inhale slowly and deeply, allowing the abdomen to expand. This is one round.

Relax the whole body in the standing position until the heartbeat returns to normal.

Repeat the practice.

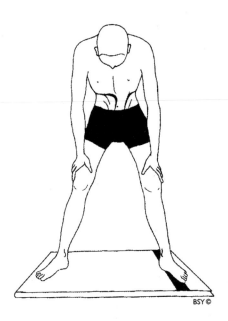

Stage 2: Vama Nauli (left isolation)

Follow the instructions for madhyama nauli as described above to the point where the lower abdomen is contracted and the rectus abdominii muscles form a central, vertical arch down the abdomen.

Isolate the rectus abdominii muscles at the left side.

Contract the muscles to the left side as strongly as possible, without straining.

Return to madhyama nauli.

Release the abdominal contraction, raise the head and return to the upright position.

Inhale slowly and deeply, allowing the abdomen to expand. This is one round.

Relax while standing until the heartbeat returns to normal.

Proceed to stage 3.

Stage 3: Dakshina Nauli (right isolation)

After completing vama nauli, practise the same way but on the right side.

After completing one round, relax in the upright position until the heartbeat returns to normal.

Stage 4: Abdominal rotation or churning

This practice should not be attempted until the previous three stages have been mastered.

Practise vama nauli on the left side, then rotate the muscles to the right, practising dakshina nauli, and back to the left, vama nauli.

Continue rotating the muscles from side to side. This process is known as churning.

Start by practising 3 consecutive rotations, then release the abdominal contraction.

Next start with dakshina nauli first, this time rotating the muscles from right to left, then left to right, 3 times consecutively.

Finally, perform madhyama nauli, isolating the muscles at the centre.

Raise the head and return to the upright position.

Inhale slowly and deeply, allowing the abdomen to expand. This is one round.

Relax in the upright position until the heartbeat returns to normal.

Time of practice: Nauli should be practised only when the stomach is completely empty, at least 5 to 6 hours after meals. The best time to practise is early in the morning before any food or drink is taken.

Duration: Start with 5 rounds of madhyama nauli and work up to 10. Vama and dakshina nauli should be performed together: 5 to 10 rounds each.

Start abdominal churning with 5 to 10 rotations and slowly increase to 25 rotations over a period of months as more control is gained over the muscles. Do not strain.

Precautions: Nauli should only be practised under the guidance of a competent teacher. If any pain is felt in the abdomen during nauli, stop the practice immediately. Try again the following day with more awareness and less force.

Contra-indications: Nauli should not be attempted by people suffering from heart disease, hypertension, hernia, high blood pressure, abdominal pain, gallstones, acute peptic ulcer, constipation, or those who are recovering from surgery, especially abdominal surgery.

Pregnant women should not practise nauli. However, six months after normal childbirth the practice can help strengthen the abdominal and pelvic muscles.

Benefits: Nauli massages and tones the entire abdominal area, including the muscles, nerves, intestines, reproductive, urinary and excretory organs. It generates heat in the body and stimulates appetite, digestion, assimilation, absorption and excretion. It helps to balance the adrenal component of the endocrine system.

Nauli stimulates and purifies manipura chakra, the storehouse of prana. It helps to increase mental clarity and power by harmonizing the energy flows in the body.

Practice note: Madhyama nauli should be perfected before proceeding to vama or dakshina nauli.

Before attempting, nauli the practices of agnisara kriya and uddiyana bandha should be mastered.

When nauli has been perfected in the standing position, it may be practised in siddha/siddha yoni asana.

Note: *The word* nauli *comes from the root* nala *or* nali, *which means a 'reed' or 'hollow stalk' and refers to a tubular vessel, vein or nerve of the body. The word* nala *is the Sanskrit term for the rectus abdominii muscles.* Nauli *is also known as* lauliki karma. *The*

518

word lauliki *is derived from the root* lola, *meaning 'to move hither and thither' or 'rolling and agitation' which is exactly what this technique does. It rolls, rotates and agitates the entire abdomen and the associated muscles and nerves.*

BASTI

Basti (yogic enema)
Technique I: Jala Basti (yogic enema with water)
Stand in pure water up to the navel. A flowing river used to be an ideal place.
Lean forward and place the hands on the knees.
Expand the anal sphincter muscles and simultaneously perform uddiyana bandha and nauli in such a way that water is drawn up into the bowels.
Hold the water in the bowels for some time and then expel it through the anus.
Benefits: The colon is cleaned and purified. Old stool is removed and gas expelled. Advanced practitioners of pranayama use basti to cool down the abdominal heat produced by their practices.
Practice note: This technique should be learned under the guidance of a competent teacher. A short tube may be inserted into the anus by beginners to make the practice easier.
Variation: Benefits of basti may also be obtained by sitting in cool, fresh water up to the navel and performing ashwini mudra.

Note: *The word* basti, *also widely written as* vasti *or* wasti, *is a general term pertaining to the lower abdomen, belly, pelvis and bladder. The technique is also known as basti karma,* karma *meaning 'process' or 'technique'.*

519

Technique 2: Sthal Basti (dry yogic enema)

Sit with both legs outstretched in front and perform paschimottanasana.

Hold the position and perform ashwini mudra 25 times, sucking air into the bowels.

Retain the air for some time and then expel it through the anus.

Benefits: Cleans the colon and removes gas and wind.

Technique 3: Moola Shodhana (anal cleansing)

Insert the soft root of a raw tumeric (haldi) plant gently into the anus.

Alternatively, the index or middle finger may be utilized.

Rotate the root or the finger around the inner surface of the anal sphincter 10 times clockwise and then 10 times counter-clockwise.

Remove the root or the finger and wash the anus with cold water.

Benefits: This practice purifies the anal region.

Practice note: A tumeric root is recommended for this practice because it has a high medicinal value as an antiseptic, blood purifier and general cleanser of physical impurities.

Note: *The word* moola *literally means 'root' or 'base'. The word* shodhana *means 'purification'. This technique is also known as* moola dhauti, *and* Ganesha kriya *or 'the obstacle removing action'.*

Kapalbhati (frontal brain cleansing)
Technique 1: Vatkrama Kapalbhati (air cleansing)

This practice is the same as kapalbhati pranayama, technique 1.

Technique 2: Vyutkrama Kapalbhati (sinus cleansing)

Fill a bowl with pure warm water and add salt to the ratio of one teaspoon per half litre, ensuring the salt is well dissolved.

Stand comfortably and bend over the bowl of water.

Relax the whole body as much as possible in this position.

Scoop the water up in the palm of the hand and sniff it in through the nostrils.

Let the water flow down to the mouth and then expel it.

Practise in this way several times.

Dry the nostrils properly as described for jala neti.

This completes the practice.

Technique 3: Sheetkrama Kapalbhati (mucus cleansing)

Prepare the water as above.

Stand comfortably and bend over the bowl of water.

Take a mouthful of the warm saline water. Instead of swallowing it, however, push it up and expel it through the nose.

Practise in this way several times.

Dry the nostrils as described for jala neti.

This completes the practice.

Time of practice: The best time is early in the morning. However, vyutkrama and sheetkrama kapalbhati may be performed at any time of the day except after meals.

Duration: Vyutkrama and sheetkrama kapalbhati should take only a few minutes each and may be performed as a weekly routine.

Contra-indications: People who experience frequent nasal bleeding should not perform these practices.

Benefits: Vyutkrama and sheetkrama kapalbhati remove mucus from the sinuses and help to relax the facial muscles and nerves. Other effects, both physical and spiritual, are the same as for jala neti, but intensified.

Practice note: Before attempting vyutkrama and sheetkrama kapalbhati, the practitioner should be proficient in the practice of jala neti.

Note: *The word* kapal *means 'cranium', 'forehead' or 'frontal lobe of the brain'.* Bhati *means 'light' or 'splendour' and also 'perception' or 'knowledge'.*

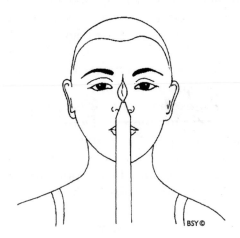

Trataka (concentrated gazing)

Light a candle and place it on a small table so that the flame is exactly at eye level when sitting. Trim the wick and protect the flame from draughts so that it remains steady.

Sit in any comfortable meditation asana with the head and spine erect.

Adjust the position so that the candle is an arm's length away from the body.

Close the eyes and relax the whole body, especially the eyes.

Be aware of body steadiness for a few minutes. Keep the body absolutely still throughout the practice.

Open the eyes and gaze steadily at the flame.

Try not to blink or move the eyeballs in any way.

Do not strain as this will cause tension and the eyes will flicker.

The awareness should be so completely centred on the flame that body awareness is lost.

If the mind begins to wander, gently bring it back to the practice.

After a minute or two, when the eyes become tired or begin to water, close them gently.

Gaze at the after-image of the flame in the space in front of the closed eyes. If the image moves up or down, or from side to side, observe it and try to stabilize it.

When the image of the flame begins to fade, try to bring it back.

When the image can no longer be retained, gently open the eyes an 1 gaze at the flame once more.

Repeat the procedure for external gazing.

Close the eyes once more and gaze at the inner image.

Continue in this way 3 or 4 times.

'After completing the final round, practise the technique of palming 2 or 3 times, before opening the eyes.

This completes the practice.

Time of practice: Trataka may be performed at any time, but the best time is at dawn or dusk when the stomach is empty.

Duration: Beginners should gaze for 1 or 2 minutes only, and then close the eyes. For general purposes 5 to 10 minutes is sufficient. For spiritual purposes, trataka may be performed for extended periods of time under the guidance of a competent teacher. Those who suffer from insomnia and mental tension should perform this practice for 10 to 15 minutes before sleeping at night.

Sequence: Trataka should be performed after asanas, pranayamas, mudras and bandhas to steady the body and mind.

Precautions: In the case of eye ailments, such as eyestrain, astigmatism and even the early symptoms of cataract, see the alternative practices on the following page.

People with myopia (short-sightedness) severe enough to warrant glasses should retain their glasses while practising trataka on a flame.

Contra-indications: People suffering from glaucoma should not practise trataka.

Epileptics should not practise trataka on a candle flame (see the alternative practice on the following page).

Avoid practising trataka on the sun, as the delicate membranes of the eyes may be damaged.

Benefits: This practice makes the eyes clear and bright. It balances the nervous system, relieving nervous tension.

It improves the memory and helps to develop good concentration and strong willpower. It activates ajna chakra and is an excellent preparation for meditation.

Practice note: When trataka is practised on a steady flame, there should be no draught in the vicinity. The practitioner should always avoid undue strain. The ability to keep the eyes open without blinking should be developed gradually with consistent practice.

Trataka is an excellent method for clearing accumulated complexes, problems and suppressed thoughts from the mind, enabling the practitioner to witness what is surfacing. It is also possible, however, for these problems to manifest too rapidly, which may be mentally disturbing. If this occurs, stop the practice and seek advice from a competent teacher.

Trataka focuses the mind and curbs oscillating tendencies, making it one-pointed and awakening inner vision. All the attention and power of the mind is channelled into one continuous stream. Once this has been achieved, the latent potential within the mind is able to arise spontaneously.

Alternative practices: In the case of eye ailments, such as eyestrain, astigmatism and even the early symptoms of cataract, a black dot should be used, instead of gazing at a candle flame. Practise in daylight or with steady background lighting.

Epileptics should not practise trataka on a candle flame, but should choose a black dot or some other completely steady object to gaze at, with steady background light.

Note: *The word* trataka *means 'to look' or 'to gaze'. Trataka is the last of the shatkarmas. It acts as a stepping-stone between physically oriented practices and mental practices which lead to higher states of awareness. It forms a bridge between hatha yoga and raja yoga. Traditionally, it is a part of hatha yoga, but it may also be considered a part of raja yoga.*

Psychic Physiology of Yoga

In this book, together with each practice, a particular point is recommended for concentration. If the aim is to relax and gain optimum physical benefit from yoga practices, it is necessary to concentrate on something. By directing the mind to a specific region of the body or to the breath, the effect of a particular practice is increased. Sometimes one of the chakras or psychic centres is also used as a point for spiritual concentration.

On a physical level, chakras are associated with the major nerve plexuses and endocrine glands in the body. Many asanas have a particularly powerful and beneficial effect on one or more of these glands or plexuses. For example, sarvangasana exerts a strong pressure on the thyroid gland in the throat region, which is associated with vishuddhi chakra. The thyroid is given a good massage and its functioning is greatly improved. However, if the concentration is directed to this chakra while performing the asana, the beneficial effects will be increased.

Definition of chakra

The word *chakra* literally means 'wheel' or 'circle', but in the yogic context a better translation is 'vortex' or 'whirlpool'. The chakras are vortices of pranic energy at specific areas in the body which control the circulation of prana permeating the entire human structure. Each chakra is a switch which turns on or opens up patterns of behaviour, thought or emotional reactions which may have been unconscious in our everyday life. They relate to specific areas of the brain, and in most people

526

these psychic centres lie dormant and inactive. Concentration on the chakras while performing yogic practices stimulates the flow of energy through the chakras and helps to activate them. This in turn awakens the dormant areas in the brain and the corresponding faculties in the psychic and mental bodies, allowing one to experience planes of consciousness which are normally inaccessible.

The major chakras are seven in number and are located along the pathway of *sushumna*, an energy channel which flows through the centre of the spinal cord. Sushumna originates at the perineum and terminates at the top of the head. The chakras are connected to a network of psychic channels called *nadis*, which correspond to the nerves, but are more subtle in nature. The chakras are depicted symbolically as lotus flowers, each having a particular number of petals and a characteristic colour. The lotus symbolizes the three stages the aspirant must pass through in spiritual life: ignorance, aspiration and illumination. It represents spiritual growth from the lowest state of awareness to the highest state of consciousness.

The petals of the lotus, inscribed with the *bija mantras* or seed sounds of the Sanskrit alphabet, represent the different manifestations of psychic energy connected with the chakras, and the nadis or psychic channels leading into and out of them. Within each chakra is a *yantra,* comprised of the geometrical symbol of its associated element and its bija mantra. Within the yantra there is also a presiding deity, which represents particular aspects of consciousness, along with the corresponding *vahana* or vehicle which is an animal form, representing the centre's other psychic aspects.

Description of the seven chakras

Mooladhara chakra: The lowest of the chakras is situated at the perineum in the male body and at the cervix in the female body. The word *mool* means 'root' and *adhara* means 'place'. Therefore, it is known as the root centre. Mooladhara chakra is associated with the sense of smell and the anus. It is symbolized by a deep red lotus with four petals. In the centre is a yellow square, the yantra of *prithvi tattwa*, the earth element,

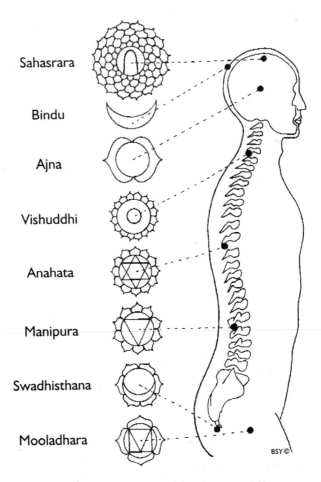

Location of the Chakras

Sahasrara	
Bindu	
Ajna	
Vishuddhi	
Anahata	
Manipura	
Swadhisthana	
Mooladhara	

and the bija mantra *lam*. In the centre of the square is a red triangle, the symbol of *shakti* or creative energy, with its apex pointing downward. Within the triangle is the smoky coloured *swayambhu linga*, symbolizing the astral body. A red serpent, representing the dormant *kundalini*, is coiled three and a half times around the linga. The red triangle is supported by an elephant with seven trunks, which symbolizes the stability and solidarity of the earth.

Mooladhara chakra is the seat or dwelling place of primal energy, *kundalini shakti*. Kundalini is the serpent coiled in deep slumber around swayambhu linga. It is the source of all energy in humankind and the universe, whether sexual, emotional, mental, psychic or spiritual. While this energy is one, it takes on various qualities and attributes, depending on the psychic centre through which it manifests. The aim of yoga is to awaken the dormant kundalini through self-purification and concentration of mind and to lead it up through the chakras to sahasrara where, as pure energy or Shakti, it unites with pure consciousness, Shiva.

For concentration on mooladhara chakra, visualize the red inverted triangle or the yellow square, symbols of energy and solidity, to enhance inner stability and balance.

Swadhisthana chakra: Approximately two fingers' width above mooladhara chakra, in the spine, is the concentration point for swadhisthana chakra. The literal meaning of the word *swadhisthana* is 'one's own abode'. The Sanskrit word *swa* means 'self' and *sthan* means 'dwelling place'. This chakra is symbolized by a crimson lotus with six petals. In the centre is a white crescent moon, the yantra of *apas tattwa*, the water element, and the bija mantra *vam*. The crescent moon yantra and the bija mantra are riding on a crocodile, symbolizing the underlying movement of the karmas.

Swadhisthana chakra is associated with seeking pleasure and security. It is associated with the tongue and genital organs. In swadhisthana the emphasis is on overcoming fear, and on enjoyment, on pleasurable sensations and sexual interaction. When swadhisthana becomes active, it may manifest as overwhelming desires or cravings.

On a deeper level, swadhisthana is the seat of the individual and collective unconscious; it is the storehouse of all *samskaras*, past mental impressions stored in the form of archetypes. It is the centre of humankind's most primitive and deep-rooted instincts. By purifying this centre, the animal nature is transcended. For concentration on this centre, visualize a vast, deep ocean with dark waves beneath a night sky. The tides of the ocean represent the ebb and flow of awareness.

529

Manipura chakra: Situated in the spine behind the navel is manipura chakra. The word *mani* means 'gem' and *pura* means 'city'. Therefore, *manipura* means 'city of jewels'. It is so called because, being the fire centre, it is lustrous like a jewel and radiant with vitality and energy. This chakra is depicted as a bright yellow lotus with ten petals. Within the lotus is a fiery red triangle, the yantra of *agni tattwa*, the fire element, and the bija mantra *ram*. The animal which serves as the vehicle for manipura is the ram, the symbol of assertiveness and energy.

Manipura is the centre of self-assertion, dynamism and dominance. It is associated with vision and the feet, with ambition and the will and ability to rule. On the negative side, this may be expressed in despotism and in seeing things and people merely as a means to gain personal power or to satisfy personal needs.

The solar plexus is the centre chiefly concerned with the vital process of digestion and food metabolism. It governs the functioning of the gastric glands, the pancreas, gall bladder and so on, which produce and secrete enzymes, acids and juices necessary for the digestion and absorption of nutrients. Manipura chakra is the psychic centre which controls these activities and the instinctive drive to find food and nurture oneself.

The adrenal glands located above the kidneys are also related with manipura. They secrete adrenaline into the blood during an emergency situation. This has the effect of speeding up all the physiological processes, making the mind sharp and alert, the heart beat faster, the respiration rate more rapid and so on. The body is then prepared for a more intense level of activity than normal in what is commonly called the 'fight or flight' reaction. Those people who suffer from sluggishness and depression or malfunctions of the digestive system, such as diabetes and indigestion, should concentrate on manipura chakra and try to feel energy radiating from this region.

For concentration on this centre, visualize the blazing sun or a ball of fire. Experience energy in the form of light radiating from this region and permeating the whole body.

Anahata chakra: Situated in the spine, behind the sternum, level with the heart, is anahata chakra. The word *anahata* literally means 'unstruck'. All sound in the manifested universe is produced by the striking together of two objects, which sets up vibrations or sound waves. However, the primordial sound, which issues from beyond this material world, is the source of all sound and is known as *anahad nada*, the unstruck sound. The heart centre is where this sound manifests. It may be perceived by the yogi as an internal, unborn and undying vibration, the pulse of the universe.

This chakra is symbolized by a blue lotus with twelve petals. In the centre of the lotus is a hexagon, formed by two interlacing triangles. This is the yantra of *vayu tattwa*, the air element. The bija mantra is *yam* and the vehicle is a swift black antelope, the symbol of alertness. Anahata chakra is the centre associated with the sense of touch (feeling), the hands (giving and taking), and emotions, ranging from the narrow attachments of jealousy to unconditional love. As this level is purified, the feelings of universal fellowship and tolerance begin to develop and all beings are accepted and loved for what they are.

On the physical level, anahata is associated with the heart and lungs, and the circulatory and respiratory systems. For meditation on anahata chakra, visualize a blue lotus or a blue hexagon, formed by two interlacing triangles, with a tiny, bright flame burning at the centre. Imagine it to be steady and unflickering like a flame in a windless place. This is the symbol of the *jivatma*, the individual soul, the indwelling spirit of all beings which is undisturbed by the winds of the world.

Vishuddhi chakra: Situated at the back of the neck, behind the throat pit, is vishuddhi chakra, the centre of purification. The word *shuddhi* means 'purification' and the prefix *vi* enhances this quality. It is symbolized by a violet lotus with sixteen petals. In the centre of the lotus is a white circle, the yantra of *akasha tattwa*, the ether element, and the beeja mantra is *ham*. The animal related to vishuddhi chakra is a white elephant. Right understanding and discrimination develop at vishuddhi chakra. Here the dualities of life are accepted, allowing one to flow with life and let things happen as they will.

531

Vishuddhi chakra governs the ears and the vocal cords, the region of the larynx, and the thyroid and parathyroid glands. It is the centre related with communication. The throat centre is the place where the divine nectar called *amrita*, the mystical elixir of immortality, is tasted. This nectar is a kind of sweet secretion which is produced at bindu chakra and then falls down to vishuddhi where it is purified and processed for further use throughout the body.

For concentration on this centre, visualize a large white drop of nectar. Try to experience icy cold drops of sweet nectar falling down to vishuddhi, giving a feeling of blissful intoxication.

Ajna chakra: Situated in the midbrain, behind the eyebrow centre, at the top of the spine, is ajna chakra. This centre is also known by various names such as: the third eye; *jnana chakshu*, the eye of wisdom; *triveni*, the confluence of three rivers; guru chakra and the eye of Shiva. The word *ajna* means 'command'. In deeper states of meditation the disciple receives commands and guidance from the guru, and from the divine or higher self, through this chakra.

Ajna chakra is depicted as a silver lotus with two petals, which represent the sun and the moon, or *pingala*, the positive force, and *ida*, the negative force. These two pranic flows, which are responsible for the experience of duality, converge at this centre with *sushumna*, the spiritual force. In the centre of the lotus is the sacred bija mantra *Aum*. The element of this chakra is the mind. This is the centre where wisdom and intuition develop. When ajna is awakened, the mind becomes steady and strong, and full control over prana is gained.

Ajna corresponds to the pineal gland, which has almost atrophied in the adult human being. On the psychic plane, this point is the bridge between the mental and psychic dimensions. Therefore, ajna chakra is responsible for supramental faculties such as clairvoyance, clairaudience and telepathy.

Thought is also a very subtle form of energy. When ajna chakra is awakened, it is possible to send and receive thought transmission through this centre. It is like a psychic doorway opening into deeper and higher realms of awareness. Stimu-

532

lating ajna chakra develops all the faculties of the mind, such as intelligence, memory and concentration.

For concentration on ajna chakra, the point of *bhrumadhya* at the eyebrow centre is used. Visualize a tiny point of light or an *Aum* symbol at this centre and let the thoughts dwell on the inner guru.

Bindu: At the top of the back of the head, where Hindu brahmins grow a small tuft of hair, is a point known as bindu. The word *bindu* means 'point' or 'drop'. Bindu is symbolized by a tiny crescent moon on a dark night. Bindu is the centre of *nada*, psychic sound. This centre is used for concentration on the psychic sounds that may manifest there in practices such as bhramari pranayama and shanmukhi mudra, which are used to develop the awareness of nada.

Sahasrara: Situated at the crown of the head is sahasrara. It is the abode of highest consciousness. The word *sahasrara* means 'one thousand'. Sahasrara is visualized as a shining lotus of a thousand petals, containing the fifty letters of the Sanskrit alphabet twenty times over. In the centre of the lotus is a shining *jyotirlinga*, lingam of light, symbol of pure consciousness. In sahasrara the mystical union of Shiva and Shakti takes place, the fusion of consciousness with matter and energy, the individual soul with the supreme soul. When kundalini awakens, it ascends through the chakras to sahasrara and merges into the source from whence it originated. Matter and energy merge into pure consciousness in a state of intoxicating bliss. Having attained this, the yogi gains supreme knowledge and passes beyond birth and death.

Nadis

The word *nadi* literally means 'flow' or 'current'. The ancient texts say that there are 72,000 nadis in the psychic body. These are visible as currents of light to a person who has developed psychic vision. In recent times the word nadi has been translated as 'nerve', but actually nadis are blueprints for physical manifestation. Like the chakras, they are not part of the physical body, although they correspond with the nerves. Nadis are the subtle channels through which the pranic forces flow. Out of the large number of nadis in the psychic body, ten are major. Of these, three are most significant: ida, pingala and sushumna. The most important of these three is sushumna. All the nadis in the psychic body are subordinate to sushumna.

Ida, pingala and sushumna

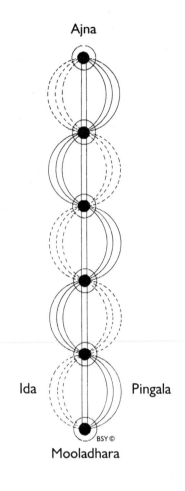

Sushumna nadi is the spiritual channel, and to concentrate on it, awareness is taken to the centre of the spinal cord. Sushumna originates from mooladhara chakra and terminates at sahasrara. Ida nadi flows from the left side of mooladhara in spirals, passing through each chakra in turn, forming a criss-cross pathway which terminates at the left side of ajna chakra. Pingala nadi flows from the right side of mooladhara, mirroring ida, terminating at the right side of ajna. Ida and pingala represent the two opposites forces flowing within us. Ida is passive, introvert and feminine; it is also known as the *chandra* or moon nadi. Pingala, on the other hand, is active, extrovert and masculine, and is called the *surya* or sun nadi.

Pranic currents and the breath

These pranic currents, ida, pingala and sushumna, operate alternately. The current that is flowing at any particular time may be gauged by noting the flow of the breath in the nostrils. When the left nostril has a greater flow of air, then ida nadi is predominant. When the flow is greater in the right nostril, then pingala is predominant. If the flow is equal, then sushumna is predominant. When the right nostril (pingala) flows, there is more vital energy for physical work, digestion of food and so on. The mind is extroverted and the body generates more heat. When the left nostril (ida) is flowing, mental energy is dominant. The mind is introverted and any kind of mental work may be undertaken. During sleep, ida nadi flows predominantly. If pingala flows at night, sleep will be restlessness and disturbed. Likewise, if ida flows while taking food, the digestive process may be slow, causing indigestion.

Altering the flow of nadis and breath

All activities are influenced by the flow of these nadis, which alternate approximately every sixty to ninety minutes. It is possible to alter the flow voluntarily by using yogic techniques such as asana and pranayama. For example, if ida nadi is flowing and there is physical work to be done, it is possible to redirect the flow of the breath to pingala nadi to obtain the necessary energy. On the other hand, one may adjust the activities to the energy flow.

Purpose of hatha yoga

The main aim of hatha yoga is to bring about a balanced flow of prana in ida and pingala nadis. The word hatha is comprised of two bija mantras: *ham,* representing the sun or solar force, and *tham,* representing the moon or lunar force. To bring about a balance between these two forces, the body must first be purified by the shatkarmas, asanas, pranayamas, mudras and bandhas. The aim of hatha yoga is to balance these two flows.

When ida and pingala nadis are purified and balanced, and the mind is controlled, then sushumna, the most important nadi, begins to flow. Sushumna must be flowing for success in meditation. If pingala flows, the body will be restless; if ida flows, the mind will be overactive. When sushumna flows, kundalini awakens and rises through the chakras.

Nadis and the nervous system

At the physical level, ida and pingala correspond to the two aspects of the autonomic nervous system. Pingala coincides with the sympathetic nervous system and ida with the parasympathetic nervous system. The sympathetic nervous system is responsible for the stimulation and acceleration of activities concerned with the external environment and the deceleration of the organs which tend to utilize a lot of energy internally. The sympathetic nerves speed up the heart, dilate the blood vessels, increase the respiration rate and intensify the efficiency of the eyes, ears and other sense organs. The parasympathetic nerves directly oppose the sympathetic nerves because they reduce the heartbeat, constrict the blood vessels and slow the respiration. This results in introversion. The flow of prana in ida and pingala is completely involuntary and unconscious until controlled by yogic practices.

Sensitivity and awareness

The primary requirements for locating the chakras and nadis and visualizing their symbols and pathways on the psychic plane are sensitivity and awareness. The practices presented in this text all relate to specific chakras and nadis. The actual purpose of these practices is to purify and balance the chakras and nadis so that the kundalini can awaken and uplift human consciousness. As the chakras and nadis become regulated, the awareness of these subtle dimensions is automatically stimulated and the spiritual vision opens. This has been the experience of yogis from time immemorial. In order to attain this experience for oneself, regularity in practice is essential.

Index of Practices